BEHAVIORAL EPIDEMIOLOGY
PRINCIPLES AND APPLICATIONS

RAY M. MERRILL, PHD, MPH, MS, FACE, FAAHB
BRIGHAM YOUNG UNIVERSITY
DEPARTMENT OF HEALTH SCIENCE
PROVO, UT

CARA L. FRANKENFELD, PHD
GEORGE MASON UNIVERSITY
DEPARTMENT OF GLOBAL AND
  COMMUNITY HEALTH
FAIRFAX, VA

NANCY FREEBORNE, DRPH, MPH, PA-C
GEORGE MASON UNIVERSITY
DEPARTMENT OF GLOBAL AND
  COMMUNITY HEALTH
FAIRFAX, VA

MICHAEL MINK, PHD, MPA
SOUTHERN CONNECTICUT STATE
  UNIVERSITY
DEPARTMENT OF PUBLIC HEALTH
NEW HAVEN, CT

D0557409

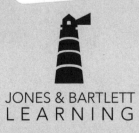

JONES & BARTLETT
LEARNING

World Headquarters
Jones & Bartlett Learning
5 Wall Street
Burlington, MA 01803
978-443-5000
info@jblearning.com
www.jblearning.com

Production Credits

VP, Executive Publisher: David D. Cella
Publisher: Michael Brown
Associate Editor: Lindsey Mawhiney
Associate Editor: Nicholas Alakel
Production Manager: Tracey McCrea
Senior Marketing Manager: Sophie Fleck Teague
Manufacturing and Inventory Control
   Supervisor: Amy Bacus
Composition: Cenveo® Publisher Services
Cover Design: Michael O'Donnell
Rights and Media Research Coordinator: Mary Flatley
Media Development Assistant: Shannon Sheehan
Cover Image: © Dmytro Hurnytskiy/ShutterStock, Inc.
Printing and Binding: Edwards Brothers Malloy
Cover Printing: Edwards Brothers Malloy

Library of Congress Cataloging-in-Publication Data
Merrill, Ray M., author.
  Behaviorial epidemiology : principles and applications / Ray M. Merrill, Cara L. Frankenfeld, Nancy Freeborne, Michael Mink.
    p. ; cm.
  Includes bibliographical references and index.
  ISBN 978-1-4496-4827-5 (pbk.)
  I. Frankenfeld, Cara L., author.   II. Freeborne, Nancy, author.   III. Mink, Michael, author.   IV. Title.
  [DNLM: 1. Health Behavior.   2. Epidemiologic Methods.   3. Public Health.   W 85]
  R726.5
  614.401'9—dc23
                                    2015014286
6048

Printed in the United States of America
19 18 17 16 15   10 9 8 7 6 5 4 3 2 1

Contents

Preface

The primary aim of this text is to advance the field of public health by providing epidemiologic tools to behavioral scientists and behavioral context to epidemiologists. This text focuses on how the principles of human behavior, as understood in a variety of disciplines such as sociology and psychology, can be applied to public health. Using epidemiology to then assess these behaviors and their outcomes allows researchers to obtain quantifiable data. These data are essential to justifying or developing any program or intervention.

Behavioral science and epidemiology are two core areas of public health, along with environmental health, biostatistics, and health services, policy, and management. There are excellent textbooks about the methods to study specific topics of behavior, such as nutrition and physical activity, but there is little that addresses behavioral epidemiology as an overall discipline. This text is designed to be of utility to advanced behavioral science students and researchers who seek to expand their work to epidemiologic study and practice and to epidemiologists who want to focus their research on behavior.

Sometimes, different behaviors can be studied by the same method—for example, frequency questionnaires for both food intake and physical activity. Other times, different behaviors require different research methods, for instance, nonrandom sampling is needed to reach stigmatized populations. This text reviews health-related behavior and puts behavior into the context of how we study behavior and disease, the complexities of such study, ways to minimize these complexities, and how to use this knowledge to develop interventions to prevent and control health problems in human populations. The purpose of combining sometimes seemingly disparate research foci, such as physical activity and sexual behaviors, is to provide a foundation for students and researchers in the methods used to study behavior and to teach when these research foci need to be approached differently, when these research foci can draw upon mutually successful methods, and what to do when these research foci overlap or interact.

Health conditions are often associated with human behavior. An interesting aspect of behavior-related conditions is that some conditions are the result of behavior, some conditions influence behaviors, and some are both a result of and can influence behaviors; for many conditions, this last category is common. For example, in some cases of depression, the illness results in individuals engaging in behaviors that could negatively impact their health, such as not eating well or not being physically active, and these behaviors, in turn, can influence the severity of depression or frequency of depressive episodes. While it is not possible to address all behavior-associated health conditions in one text, several will be highlighted, including injuries, cardiovascular diseases, cancer, diabetes, obesity, sexually transmitted infections, addictions, and depression. A goal of this text is to provide a foundation of methods that readers can bring to their research on these and other behaviors and health conditions.

This text is primarily designed for students studying behavior, epidemiology, or public health, but it may be useful to research scientists and clinicians in peripheral fields for a better understanding of the literature or in conducting research about disease risk associated with behavior in human populations. The text is designed to be an extension of introductory courses. However, as is necessary to make the text accessible to both behavioral scientists and epidemiologists, and to thereby enhance both disciplines, there will be some review of foundational behavioral science and epidemiologic principles.

The text is organized to guide readers through the background of behavioral epidemiology research, methods of behavioral epidemiology research, and implications of research results. In the applications section at the end of the text, the reader is provided with topical case studies. Each case study is designed to guide the reader through the study of disease risk in relation to a health behavior or in the application of public health practice to the alteration of health behavior to the benefit of population health. At the conclusion of this text, the reader should feel comfortable describing the distribution of behavioral risk factors in the population and the overall role of behavior in public health, communicating the history of behavioral research and what factors determine selected behavior, calculating measurements of behavior-related diseases, identifying and conducting appropriate study designs and analyses for behavioral epidemiology and interpretation of research results, interpreting the nature of how a behavior and disease are related, applying logistics of data collection and management to behavioral epidemiology studies, and describing factors that influence the choice of behavioral intervention targets and the expected impact of effective interventions. Readers will also be introduced to interdisciplinary study designs and how they can be applied to behavioral epidemiology.

We hope that our work in this collaborative discipline will be of benefit to your teaching, research, or practice.

Acknowledgments

This text is the combined work of individuals with many years of cumulative research and teaching experience in behavioral sciences or epidemiology. We appreciate our mentors and colleagues who helped us get to where we are today (e.g., Eric [Rocky] Feuer, Lap-Ming Wun, and Lawrence Mayer) and individuals who reviewed and provided valuable feedback on the text (i.e., Cerissa Hayhurst, Brittanie Steele, Lauren Christoffersen, and Chella Palmer). We would also like to express appreciation to our students, who have contributed to our learning over the years. Finally, we could not have devoted the time and effort to writing this book had it not been for the extraordinary support and patience of our families.

© Dmytro Hurnytskiy/ShutterStock, Inc.

Introduction

Epidemiology is the study of the distribution and determinants of health-related states or events, and the prevention and control of health problems in human populations (Last, Abramson, & International Epidemiological Association, 1995). Its roots are in the study of infectious diseases, but it has expanded to include anything that threatens health on the population level. Epidemiology focuses on the collection of individuals who share one or more observable characteristics from which data may be collected and evaluated. The purpose of this chapter is to describe public health, the role of epidemiology in public health, and the specific subfield of epidemiology that we refer to as *behavioral epidemiology*.

Public Health and Epidemiology

Public health is the field of medicine concerned with safeguarding and improving the health of a community as a whole (Dorland's Medical Dictionary, 2007). It is a social institution, a service, and a practice that promotes, protects, and restores the people's health (Stedman's

Medical Dictionary, 2005). Public health is concerned with threats to health in communities or populations. Population refers to a collection of people that share one or more observable personal or observational characteristics. Social, economic, family, work and labor force, and geographic factors can characterize populations. Efforts to protect and improve the public's health include the following (U.S. Department of Health and Human Services, 1998):

- Assessment: Monitoring health status and environmental hazards
- Policy development: Informing and educating people about health issues; mobilizing community partnerships and taking action to identify and solve health problems; and developing policies and plans to support health efforts
- Assurance: Ensuring that laws and regulations protect health and safety; preparing competent public and personal healthcare workers; linking people with health services; evaluating effectiveness, accessibility, and quality of personal and population-based health services; and researching for new insights and innovative solutions to health problems

The primary disciplines upon which public health is built are epidemiology, biostatistics, and health services. Epidemiology provides an approach to assess and monitor the health of populations at risk and to identify health problems and priorities, identify risk factors (items that increase the probability that an adverse health outcome will occur), identify effective health interventions, and provide a basis for predicting the effects of certain exposures. In turn, epidemiologic information is useful in policy development, individual decision making, and initiating new research for protecting and promoting the public's health.

Health-related states or events include disease (an interruption, cessation, or disorder of body functions, systems, or organs), events (e.g., injuries, accidents, drug overdoses, and suicides), behaviors (e.g., physical activity, diet, and safety precautions), and conditions that already exist (e.g., an unhealthy state, a state of fitness, something that is essential to the occurrence of something else). Modern epidemiology has expanded its scope of investigation to each of these health-related states or events, with the primary aim to apply study findings to prevent and control health problems.

Public health is impacted by physical, chemical, biological, and social environments, behaviors, and genetic factors. Physical, chemical, and biological environments related to health include work site risks/exposures, environmental hazards, vehicular hazards, household hazards, medical care risks, radiation exposures, infectious pathogens, and engineering/design hazards; the social environment that influences health includes culture, income, education, work skills, family, sociodemographic status, and so on; behaviors shown to influence health include smoking or tobacco use, alcohol use/abuse, nutrition/diet, lack of exercise/fitness, high blood pressure, cholesterol levels, overweight/obesity, stress, drug use/abuse, lack of seat belt use, general lack of safety precautions, and more; and genetic factors related to health include chromosome/genetic defects, congenital anomalies, and developmental defects. A growing understanding of how these various factors influence health is attributed to epidemiologic research. As epidemiologic research has identified important risk factors for disease, disability, and death, attempts have been made to effectively modify these factors to prevent disease and promote better health.

Behavioral Sciences

Although many of the risk factors for health-related states or events are not modifiable, many are, especially the behavior-related risk factors. Behavior is defined as any response emitted by or elicited from an organism; any mental or motor act or activity; or parts of a total response pattern (Stedman's Medical Dictionary, 2005).The word *behavioral* refers to overt actions, underlying psychological processes (e.g., cognition, emotion, temperament, and motivation), and behavioral interactions with psychosocial and biological processes. In medicine, there are several extensions to these words, such as behavioral sciences, behavioral epidemic, behavioral pathogen, behavioral psychology, behavior disorder, behavior modification, and behavior therapy. *Behavioral sciences* refer to those disciplines or branches of science (e.g., psychology, sociology, and anthropology) that derive their theories and methods from the study of the behavior of living organisms. *Behavioral epidemic* is an epidemic that originates from behavior patterns (e.g., disease related to increased obesity). *Behavioral pathogens* are personal habits and lifestyle behaviors of an individual that places him or her at increased risk of physical illness and dysfunction. *Behavioral psychology* is the formulation of the laws and principles that underlie the behavior of humans and animals, based on observation and experiment. *Behavior disorder* is a general term that refers to a mental illness. *Behavior modification* is a systematic treatment technique that tries to change a person's behavior by creating rewards or developing skills to promote a desired response or to stop an undesirable behavior or attitude. *Behavior therapy involves* procedures and techniques associated with conditioning and learning for a variety of psychological problems (Stedman's Medical Dictionary, 2005).

Behavioral science has shown that human behavior is the product of several interrelated factors. The influences on behavior can be broadly characterized as genetics, individual thoughts and feelings, the physical environment, social interaction (with other individuals), social identity (interaction within and between groups), and the macrosocial environment (e.g., state of the economy) (United Kingdom Parliamentary Archives, 2011). Behavioral psychology attempts to understand the underlying reasons for behavior and behavioral disorders, while behavioral pathogens, the consequences of epidemics related to behavior, and interventions designed to modify behavior with assessments for efficiency and effectiveness are understood through epidemiology.

Several behavior change theories have tried to make sense of the complex behavioral process, such as learning theories, social cognitive theory, theories of reasoned action and planned behavior, the transtheoretical model, and the health action process approach. Research has also examined specific elements of these theories, such as self-efficacy, which is common to several of the theories. Methods commonly employed in the social sciences for studying human behavior include controlled experiments and observational studies (e.g., case reports, case series, and cross-sectional surveys).

Behavior change models are based on the idea that health education is an important component, but it is often not sufficient to motivate behavior change. The Health Belief Model is a widely used conceptual framework for understanding health behavior (Prochaska & DiClemente, 1992). In this model, behavior change involves a rational decision-making process that considers perceived susceptibility to illness, perceived consequences or seriousness of the illness, belief that recommended action is appropriate or efficacious to reduce risk, and belief that the benefits of action outweigh the costs (Janz & Becker, 1984; Rosenstock, 1966, 1974). Two extensions of these concepts in more recent years include cues to action and self-efficacy (Glanz, Lewis, & Rimer, 1997). Epidemiologic information can influence the different stages of the Health Belief Model by identifying population risk levels and personalized risk based on a person's characteristics or behaviors; by describing the natural history or course of disease; by identifying prevention and treatment benefits through clinical trials; and by recommending programs designed to reduce barriers to health, promote awareness, provide training, and give guidance to motivate readiness to change and action.

Behavioral Epidemiology

Epidemiologists identify health problems in the population through surveillance, evaluating disease in relation to potential risk factors, and using surveillance to monitor the effects of policy and behavioral interventions at the population level. When a public health concern is identified, such as increased disease frequency or severity, information gathered by epidemiologists can be used, along with social science theory and collaboration with public health and policy professionals, to identify suspect behavioral factors that might explain increased disease frequency or severity. Working together, epidemiologists, behavioral scientists, and core public health professionals develop testable hypotheses. Although there are often overlapping roles, epidemiologists collect, analyze, and interpret research data, often in collaboration with behavioral scientists and other health professionals, to generate results that can be used to develop additional research or create programs or policies that target modifiable risk factors.

The definition of epidemiology given in the introduction of this chapter involves careful examination of a phenomenon with the use of sound methods of scientific inquiry. A description of the distribution (frequency and pattern) of a health-related state or event according to person, place, and time factors is central to epidemiologic research. The definition also emphasizes the importance of identifying determinants or factors that produce an effect, result, or consequence on another factor in human populations. Epidemiology is built on the premise that human health problems do not occur at random and that there are identifiable and often preventable risk factors. If ways do not exist to improve health through disease prevention or treatment efforts, there would be no need to identify causes of disease.

Human health can be influenced by a broad array of factors, such as physical stresses (excessive heat, cold, noise, radiation, climate change, ozone depletion, housing, etc.), chemicals (drugs, acids, alkali, heavy metals, poisons, and some enzymes), biological agents (pathogens), and psychosocial milieu (families and households, socioeconomic status, social networks and social support, neighborhoods and communities, access to health care, formal institutions, and public policy).

We see that the study of how behaviors influence health falls within the definition of epidemiology. Therefore, behavioral epidemiology involves the study of personal behaviors (the manner of conducting oneself), how these behaviors influence health-related states or events in human populations, and how behaviors can be modified to prevent and control health problems.

Behavioral epidemiology combines behavioral theory and methods to relate overt actions with health-related outcomes to understand ways to modify behaviors in order to prevent and control health problems. In epidemiology, the study of behavior should involve describing it according to person, place, and time factors and determining the link between certain behaviors and health. It should also consist of identifying factors that influence health-related behaviors, evaluating interventions designed to modify these behaviors, and translating study results into practice (Sallis, Owen, & Fotheringham, 2000).

The importance of behavioral epidemiology is emphasized by the fact that many health outcomes have been linked to modifiable behaviors. For example, cancer is largely lifestyle related. Doll and Peto (1981) estimated that smoking explains about 30% of all cancer deaths, diet explains about 35%, and the remainder is due to viruses, bacteria, radiation, industrial carcinogens, family predisposition, and so on. Cancer is generally not an inherited illness, with only 5–10% of all cancer cases attributed to genetic defects, and the remaining 90–95% associated with environmental and behavioral factors (Anand, Kunnumakara, Sundaram, Harikumar, Tharakan, et al., 2008). This is similarly true for many other chronic diseases. Hence, it is essential to understand how selected behaviors are associated with health; characterize these behaviors according to person, place, and time factors; identify ways to influence these behaviors; and evaluate interventions designed to modify these behaviors.

After epidemiologic research has established a link between selected behaviors and health problems, behavioral therapy and modification can be implemented to promote better health. Health promotion is the process of enabling people to increase control over and, thereby, improve their health (World Health Organization, 2014). It includes the endorsement of ideas and concepts that motivate healthy behaviors and actions directed at changing social, economic, and environmental conditions that can more positively influence public health. Health promotion efforts may target a great number of factors at the personal, social, and environmental levels, but the ultimate goal is to create conditions that generate improved health behaviors.

Descriptive Epidemiology of Health Behaviors

Descriptive epidemiology provides a description of health-related states or events in human populations. It is used to monitor the health of a community or population and to identify health problems and priorities according to person, place, and time factors. Describing data by person allows identification of the frequency of disease and who is at greatest risk. High-risk populations can be identified by investigating inherent characteristics of people (age, gender, race, ethnicity), acquired characteristics through behavior choices (immunity, marital status, education), behavioral activities (exercise, leisure, medication use), and conditions (access to health care, environmental state). Describing data by place (residence, birthplace, place of employment, country, state, county, census tract, etc.) allows the epidemiologist to understand the geographic extent of disease, where the causal agent of disease resides and multiplies, and how the disease is transmitted and spread. Describing data by time can reveal the extent of the public health problem according to when and whether the health problem is predictable. Assessing whether interactions exist among persons, places, and time may also provide insights into the health outcome. In general, the core public health function involving assessment is completed by descriptive epidemiology wherein we identify who is at greatest risk for experiencing the public health problem, where the public health problem is greatest, and when the public health problem is greatest so we can monitor potential exposures and intervention-related health outcomes over time.

Some descriptive epidemiologic studies have shown that the frequency of health-related states or events differs considerably in different settings, situations, or conditions. For example, if a certain behavior such as a high-fat, low-fiber diet is more common where the frequency of colon cancer is greater, this may implicate diet as a possible causal factor. If an increasing trend in smoking, for example, is associated with an increasing trend in coronary heart disease, this can implicate smoking as a possible causal factor. If a greater level of an activity, such as repetitive motion on an assembly line, for example, is associated with an increase in carpal tunnel syndrome, then the activity is implicated as a possible causal factor. In essence, if health-related states or events that differ in various settings, situations, or conditions have a similar trend with some factor, or vary in direct relation to the strength of some factor, then researchers gain important clues as to what is causing the health problems.

Natural History of Disease

When allowed to run their course without medical intervention, every disease has a natural history of progression. There are four common stages for most diseases: stage of susceptibility; stage of presymptomatic disease; stage of clinical disease; and stage of recovery, disability, or death. Epidemiologic methods are useful for identifying who is susceptible to the disease; identifying the types of exposures capable of causing the disease, describing the pathologic changes that occur and the stage of subclinical disease, and identifying the expected length of this subclinical phase of the disease; identifying the types of symptoms that characterize the disease; and identifying probable outcomes (recovery, disability, or death) associated with different levels of the disease. The stage of susceptibility precedes the disease and involves the likelihood a host has of developing the health problem from a physical, chemical, biological or social environment, behavior, or genetic factor.

Primary prevention strategies seek to avoid the biological onset of disease and, therefore, tend to target the general population. Primary prevention occurs during the stage of susceptibility prior to disease occurrence. Fundamental public health measures and activities basic to primary prevention include sanitation; infection control; immunizations; protection of food, milk, and water supplies; environmental protection; and protection against occupational hazards and accidents. Basic personal hygiene and public health measures have had a major impact on halting communicable disease epidemics (Centers for Disease Control and Prevention [CDC], 1999). Secondary prevention may occur during the stage of presymptomatic disease or the stage of clinical disease. Secondary prevention strategies seek to minimize adverse health outcomes through screening and early detection, when some risk factors are present but typically before symptoms occur. Tertiary prevention may occur during the stage of clinical disease or in the final stage. Tertiary prevention seeks to reduce further damage, disability, and risk of death in known disease cases. Medical treatment is a common form of tertiary prevention, as are improvements in diet, exercise, and stress management in response to many chronic disease diagnoses. For example, after suffering a heart attack, a person might start taking daily medication and reduce saturated fat and cholesterol intake. Many intervention strategies can be used at any of these levels of prevention. The defining factor is the degree to which the target group has been exposed to risk. For example, increasing moderate physical activity to 30 minutes per day would be a primary prevention strategy for a young healthy person, a secondary prevention strategy for an obese person, and tertiary prevention strategy for a person who has been diagnosed with hypertension.

Health behaviors cross the different levels of prevention. For example, the development and availability of most vaccinations are conducted for the population, but whether someone chooses to be vaccinated or have his or her child vaccinated is an individual-level behavior. Similarly, requirements for means to reduce microbial contamination and fortification of foods with micronutrients have made safer food available. Increased food distribution has made healthier foods, such as seasonal fruits and vegetables, available year round, but food selection is an individual-level behavior. Secondary prevention (screening) is an important way to improve the prognosis in somebody who has a disease. Effective screening programs presuppose an understanding of the natural history of disease, which improves our ability to target high-risk groups and time the screening program.

Health policy related to screening must consider several questions: Who should be screened? What diseases should we screen? What is the appropriate age when screening should occur? How should risk status influence screening? Screening may be conducted on the total population level (mass screening), or it may be applied to high-risk groups (selective screening). Selective screening is more likely than mass screening to result in a greater yield of true cases and be the most economical.

The World Health Organization published a set of guidelines that epidemiologists should consider when planning and implementing a screening program (Wilson & Jungner, 1968):

1. Acceptable treatment should be available for individuals with diseases discovered in the screening process.
2. Access to healthcare facilities and services for follow-up diagnosis and treatment for the discovered disease should be available.
3. The disease should have a recognizable course, with identifiable early and latent stages.
4. A suitable and effective test or examination for the disease should be available.
5. The test and the testing process should be acceptable to the general population.
6. The natural history of the disease or condition should be adequately understood, including the regular phases and course of the disease, with an early period identifiable through testing.
7. Policies, procedures, and threshold levels on tests should be determined in advance to establish who should be referred for further testing, diagnostics, and possible treatment.
8. The process should be simple enough to encourage large groups of persons to participate.

These guidelines are each meant to maximize the public's health and to minimize any adverse effects of the screening process.

Although tertiary prevention often takes the form of medical treatment, it is a critical component of the public health approach to reducing the impact of any illness. Tertiary prevention in public health takes three common forms: closing the gap in clinical care; maximizing quality of life after diagnosis; and reducing the spread of illness to others. Millions of Americans lack health insurance coverage and forgo essential medical care because of prohibitive cost. Public health departments in every state provide low-cost or free medical treatment to people who would otherwise not receive it. These medical treatments can often cure disease or ameliorate their negative impact. Public health programs also provide patient-centered health education on how to live with, and even reduce, the negative impact of chronic medical conditions on a patient's ability to function and enjoy life. People living with chronic conditions such as heart disease, diabetes, and HIV can now expect to live for many years, even decades, but they must learn how to manage their illness to maximize their quality of life. Public health programs also educate patients on how to reduce their exposure to medical complications and prevent infecting or hurting others. In this way, tertiary prevention for a person diagnosed with an illness can function as primary prevention for the healthy individuals who may come into contact with him or her.

It may seem obvious that the ideal approach to maximize public health and minimize suffering would be to employ primary prevention for every possible health problem. In theory, that is correct, but in reality, it is not feasible. Limited resources will always force public health professionals to make difficult choices between what potential threats will receive primary prevention efforts and which ones will only receive tertiary prevention efforts.

It is important to understand where your population lies overall in the pathway of disease and injury. For example, imagine a population in one geographic area in which all the residents already have diagnosed coronary heart disease. In this case, primary prevention strategies will be ineffective at reducing disease burden, and screening will be unnecessary. Tertiary prevention is the most appropriate because everyone in the population has been diagnosed with the illness. However, rarely are all individuals in the target population at the same point in the pathway. As noted previously, the responsible incident or series of incidents that lead to the onset of a biological disease is often unknown. This becomes important when evaluating the effectiveness of an intervention. For example, in Population A, of 1,000 people without cancer, there are 200 people who already have experienced an irreversible mutation that will result in cancer. In Population B, of 1,000 people without cancer, there are 400 people who have also experienced the same irreversible mutation. Imagine that two health promotion strategies to improve people's diets (Strategy Y used in Population A and Strategy Z used in Population B) are 100% effective at preventing this mutation. Strategy Y will appear to be more effective than Strategy Z, even though the actual effectiveness for primary prevention is the same. This example illustrates one way that an epidemiologist can add to the discussion of interpreting program effectiveness. Therefore, any population-based intervention will have to (1) identify subgroups based on risk level and (2) devise different strategies that target each subgroup. The overall mechanics of how to develop programs and evaluate their effectiveness is addressed in other sources, and interested readers are encouraged to consult relevant health promotion, program planning, and program evaluation sources.

Behavior and the Epidemiologic Transition

The *epidemiologic transition* describes changing patterns in age distribution, fertility, life expectancy, disease, and death. McKeown (2009) classified the transition as changes in the population composition and growth trajectories, particularly movement toward an older age distribution, and changes in patterns of mortality, related life expectancy, and causes of death. The epidemiologic transition is a way of looking at and understanding the relationship among population dynamics, disease, and death.

Improvements in life expectancy over the past few centuries, throughout many places in the world, have been attributed to cultural adaptations (Caspari & Lee, 2006; Jones, Martin, & Pilbeam, 1994), ecobiologic and socioeconomic factors (Omran, 1971) and, more recently, advances in public health (e.g., hygiene and nutrition, housing conditions, sanitation, water supply, antibiotics, and immunization programs) (CDC, 1999). Consequently, the causes of death have shifted from primarily infectious diseases (e.g., pneumonia, tuberculosis, and diarrhea) and conditions (e.g., maternal mortality) to chronic diseases such as heart disease and cancer. Degenerative diseases that are often associated with the aging process (e.g., arteriosclerosis, gout, and mental decline) have also increased. Children and young women showed the greatest improvement in survival, possibly because of their relatively high susceptibility to infectious diseases, pestilence, and famine (Omran, 1971).

In 1950, the world's population consisted of about 2.6 billion people. In 2014, it was about 7.2 billion, and it is projected to reach almost 9.4 billion by 2050 (U.S. Census Bureau, 2013). Increasing population growth has paralleled an older age distribution (longer life expectancy) and downward trends in mortality. For example, in 1900–1902, life expectancy in the United States was 49.2 years (Arias, 2010) and was one of the highest life expectancies worldwide. In 2014, life expectancy in the United States was 78.75 years (Canty, Frischling, & Frischling, 2014). In 2014, the estimated life expectancy in 228 countries was greater than 50 years, and life expectancy exceeded 80 years in 36 countries (Canty, Frischling, & Frischling, 2014).

As changing patterns have occurred in the population age distribution, mortality, fertility, life expectancy, and causes of death, the scope of epidemiology has broadened. By the end of the 19th century, several vitamin-related and nutritional diseases were identified, germ theory had been developed, the importance of personal hygiene and sanitation was known for reducing the spread of disease, and the multifactorial etiology for many diseases was known. By the mid-20th century, public health shifted focus to chronic disease prevention and control. There began to be an emphasis on behavior- and lifestyle-related risk factors and interventions and an interest in understanding how the broader contextual and environmental factors influenced health. Advances in study designs and epidemiologic methods have kept pace with the expanding role of the discipline.

Epidemiologic studies have now shown that many chronic diseases and conditions can be prevented and controlled by behaviors such as maintaining a healthy weight; eating no more than two or three servings of red meat per week; taking a multivitamin with folate every day; drinking less than one alcoholic drink per day; eating five or more servings of fruit and vegetables per day; eating more high-fiber foods, such as whole grains, wheat cereals, bread, pasta, and cruciferous vegetables (such as broccoli and cabbage); not smoking; getting adequate sleep; protecting oneself from the sun; avoiding certain workplace exposures; protecting oneself and partner(s) from sexually transmitted infections; and exercising regularly. A primary way in which health-related behaviors are monitored in the United States is by the Behavioral Risk Factor Surveillance System (CDC, 2014), an ongoing national cross-sectional survey that monitors selected health behaviors. The information obtained from this survey can be particularly useful for planning, initiating, supporting, and evaluating disease prevention programs.

Summary

1. Public health is the field of medicine concerned with safeguarding and improving the health of a community as a whole. It has a population focus. Efforts to protect and improve the public's health include assessment, policy development, and assurance. The primary foundation disciplines of public health are epidemiology, biostatistics, and health services.

2. Epidemiology is the study of the distribution and determinants of health-related states or events and the prevention and control of health problems in human populations. It provides an approach to assess and monitor the health of populations at risk and to identify health problems and priorities, identify risk, identify effective health interventions, and provide a basis for predicting the effects of certain exposures. It provides information that is useful in policy development, individual decision making, and for initiating new research.

3. An important aspect of public health and epidemiology is behavior. Behavior is any response emitted by, or elicited from, an organism; any mental or motor act or activity; or parts of a total response pattern.

4. Behavioral sciences refer to those disciplines or branches of science (e.g., psychology, sociology, and anthropology) that derive their theories and methods from the study of the behavior of living organisms. The influences on behavior can be broadly characterized as genetics, individual thoughts and feelings, the physical environment, social interaction (with other individuals), social identity (interaction within and between groups), and the macrosocial environment (e.g., state of the economy).

5. Working together, epidemiologists, behavioral scientists, and core public health professionals develop testable hypotheses. Although there are often overlapping roles, epidemiologists collect, analyze, and interpret research data, often in collaboration with behavioral scientists and other health professionals, to generate results that can be used to develop additional research or create programs or policies that target modifiable risk factors.

6. Behavioral epidemiology involves the study of personal behaviors (the manner of conducting oneself), how these behaviors influence health-related states or events in human populations, and how behaviors can be modified to prevent and control health problems.

7. The study of behavior in epidemiology should involve describing behavior according to person, place, and time factors; determining the link between certain behaviors and health; identifying factors that influence behaviors; and applying and evaluating interventions designed to modify health-related behaviors.

8. Population-based risk factors can be identified by investigating inherent characteristics of people (age, gender, race, ethnicity); acquired characteristics through behavior choices (immunity, marital status, education); behavioral activities (exercise, leisure, medication use); and conditions (access to health care, environmental state).

9. In epidemiology, behavioral variables are treated as risk factors for disease. They are also sometimes treated as outcome variables in which we investigate factors that influence these behaviors.

10. Epidemiologic methods are useful for providing an understanding of the natural history of disease: who is susceptible to the disease; the types of exposures capable of causing the disease; the pathologic changes that occur during the subclinical phase of disease; the signs and symptoms that characterize the disease; and the probable outcomes associated with different stages of the disease.

11. Health behaviors can reflect primary, secondary, and tertiary prevention.

12. As changing patterns have occurred in population age distribution, mortality, fertility, life expectancy, and causes of death, the scope of epidemiology has accordingly broadened.

References

Anand, P., Kunnumakara, A. B., Sundaram, C., Harikumar, K. B., Tharakan, S. T., Lai, O. S.,…, Aggarwal, B. B. (2008). Cancer is a preventable disease that requires major lifestyle changes. *Pharmaceutical Research*, 25(9), 2097-2116.

Arias, E. (2010). United States life tables, 2006. *National Vital Statistics Reports*, 58(21). Hyattsville, MD: National Center for Health Statistics.

United Kingdom Parliamentary Archives. (2011). Chapter 3: Understanding what influences behaviour. Retrieved from http://www.publications.parliament.uk/pa/ld201012/ldselect/ldsctech/179/17906.htm

Canty, J. L., Frischling, B., & Frischling, D. (2014). The world: Life expectancy (2014)—top 100+. Retrieved from http://www.geoba.se/population.php?pc=world&type=015&year=2014&st =rank&asde=&page=1

Caspari, R., & Lee, S-H. (2006). Is human longevity a consequence of cultural change or modern biology? *American Journal of Physical Anthropology*, 129(4), 512–517.

Centers for Disease Control and Prevention. (1999). Ten great public health achievements—United States, 1900–1999. *Morbidity and Mortality Weekly Report*, 48(12), 241–243. Retrieved from http://cdc.gov/mmwr/preview°/mmwrhtml/00056796.htm

Centers for Disease Control and Prevention. (2014). Behavioral Risk Factor Surveillance System. Retrieved from http://www.cdc.gov/brfss/

Doll, R., & Peto, R. (1981). Quantitative estimates of avoidable risk of cancer in the United States today. *Journal of the National Cancer Institute, 66,* 1191–1308.

Dorland's Medical Dictionary for Health Consumers. (2007). Philadelphia, PA: Saunders.

Glanz, K., Lewis, F. M., & Rimer, B. K. (1997). *Theory at a glance: A guide for health promotion practice.* Bethesda, MD: National Institutes of Health.

Janz, N. K., & Becker, M. H. (1984). The health belief model: A decade later. *Health Education Quarterly, 11,* 1–47.

Jones, S., Martin, R., & Pilbeam, D. (Eds.). (1994). *The Cambridge encyclopedia of human evolution.* Cambridge, MA: Cambridge University Press.

Last, J. M., Abramson, J. H., & International Epidemiological Association. (1995). *A dictionary of epidemiology.* New York, NY: Oxford University Press.

McKeown, R. E. (2009). The epidemiologic transition: Changing patterns of mortality and population dynamics. *American Journal of Lifestyle Medicine, 3*(Suppl. 1), 19S–26S.

Omran, A. R. (1971). The epidemiologic transition. *Milbank Memorial Fund Quarterly, 49,* 509–538.

Prochaska, J. O., & DiClemente, C. C. (1992). Stages of change in the modification of problem behaviors. *Progress in Behavior Modification, 28,* 184–218.

Rosenstock, I. M. (1966). Why people use health services. *Milbank Memorial Fund Quarterly, 44,* 94–127.

Rosenstock, I. M. (1974). Historical origins of the health belief model. *Health Education Quarterly, 2,* 328–335.

Sallis, J. F., Owen, N., & Fotheringham, M. J. (2000). Behavioral epidemiology: A systematic framework to classify phases of research on health promotion and disease prevention. *Annals of Behavioral Medicine, 22*(4), 294–298.

Stedman's Medical Dictionary for the Health Professions and Nursing (Illustrated 5th ed.). (2005). New York, NY: Lippincott Williams & Wilkins.

U.S. Census Bureau. (2013). International data base. Retrieved from http://www.census.gov/population/international/data/idb/worldpoptotal.php

U.S. Department of Health and Human Services. (1998). The public health workforce: An agenda for the 21st century. Retrieved from http://www.health.gov/phfunctions/pubhlth.pdf

Wilson, J. M. G., & Jungner, F. (1968). *Principles and practice of screening for disease* [Paper No. 34]. Geneva, Switzerland: World Health Organization.

World Health Organization. (2014). Health promotion. Retrieved from http://www.who.int/topics/health_promotion/en/

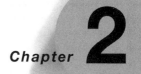

Behavioral Sciences Research

The definition of behavioral and social sciences research involving health was developed in 1996 by the National Institutes of Health (NIH) based on consultation with behavioral and social scientists and science organizations. The definition divided behavioral and social sciences research into two areas: (1) core areas of research (basic or fundamental research, and applied research); and (2) adjunct areas of research (many types of neurological research and some pharmacological interventions) (NIH, 2010). The NIH recognized that behavioral and social factors play an important role in explaining health and illness, and they often interact with each other and with other factors (e.g., biological environments) to impact health. Health-related behavioral and social factors also provide useful targets for prevention and treatment efforts.

The behavioral sciences represent many disciplines. However, all derive their theories and methods from the study of behavior among living organisms. Behavioral research is the study of those factors that impact our actions or reactions. The purpose of this chapter is to present the core area of behavioral research, which consists of basic research and applied research, with basic research often providing the foundation of applied research. These areas of behavioral research are related to health, whereas health may be thought of as complete physical, mental, and social well-being, not just the absence of disease, as defined by the World Health Organization.

Basic Research in the Behavioral Sciences

Basic research in the behavioral sciences does not address disease outcomes per se, but it is designed to provide knowledge about underlying mechanisms and patterns, which helps us better explain, predict, prevent, and manage illness, as well as promote better health and well-being. Basic research involves the study of behavioral processes, interactions of biological and social factors with behavioral variables, and methodology and measurement.

RESEARCH ON BEHAVIORAL PROCESSES

Research on behavioral processes involves the study of human functioning. This study may be conducted on various levels: individual, group, organization/institution, or larger societies. On an individual level, research involves the study of behavioral factors like cognition, memory, perception, personality, emotion, motivation, and others. Study may also focus on small groups such as couples, families, and work groups; or on organizations/institutions and communities; or on larger economic, political, cultural, and demographic systems. Research on behavioral processes also includes the study of interactions within and between these various levels of aggregation (e.g., the influence of cultural factors on emotional responses) and with environmental factors (e.g., climate, noise, environmental hazards, and residential or other built environments) (NIH, 2010).

BIOPSYCHOSOCIAL RESEARCH

Biopsychosocial research posits that biological, psychological, and social factors each influence human functioning in the context of health. It involves the study of the interactions of biological factors with behavioral or social variables and how they affect each other. For example, behavioral genetics research has shown that inherent factors can influence addictions, heart disease, cancer risk, diabetes, and oral health. This research model was theorized by George Engel in the mid-1970s (Engel, 1977).

METHODOLOGY AND MEASUREMENT

Research on methodology and measurement involves developing new types of research design, data collection, measurement, and data analysis. New behavioral research methodology and measurement can involve ways to assess complex dynamic systems; ways to collect and measure data; statistical modeling techniques; innovative research designs such as multi-informant designs; methods to reduce sampling, survey, and nonresponse bias; behavioral observation procedures; and new measurement procedures for behavioral phenomena (NIH, 2010).

Applied Research in the Behavioral Sciences

Although basic research in the behavioral sciences helps us understand mechanisms and patterns of behavioral functioning that are relevant to health, the aim of applied research is to predict or influence behavior-related health risks, protective health factors, and health outcomes. It is also concerned with identifying the impact of illness or risk for illness on behavioral functioning. The NIH presented applied research in five categories (NIH, 2010). We have modified these categories to specifically address applied behavior research:

1. Identification and understanding of behavioral factors associated with the onset and course of illness and with health conditions:

    ❑ How do specific behavioral factors influence mental and physical health outcomes? What mechanisms explain these associations? What behavioral factors damage health (i.e., are risk factors), and which promote health (i.e., are protective factors)?

    ❑ Examples of research in this area include the study of risk and protective factors such as tobacco smoking, alcohol drinking, substance abuse, dietary practices, physical inactivity, stress, social support, culture, and socioeconomic status.

2. The effects of illness or physical condition on behavioral functioning:

    ❑ This area of research addresses topics like psychological and social behaviors that can result from genetic testing; behavioral effects of head injury across developmental stages; emotional behaviors resulting from being diagnosed with a disease (e.g., HIV infection or cancer); coping behaviors linked to chronic pain; effects of illness on employment and economic status; and coping responses to disability (impairment, activity limitation, and/or participation restriction).

3. Treatment outcomes research:

    ❑ This area of research involves designing and evaluating behavioral interventions that treat mental and physical illnesses. It also consists of interventions designed to minimize the effects of disease on behavioral functioning.

❑ Examples of research topics in this area are behavioral interventions for dealing with anxiety disorders and depression; interventions for restoring behavioral and brain functioning following a traumatic head injury; lifestyle choices (dietary change, exercise, stress reduction) to reverse coronary atherosclerosis; measures to improve adherence to medical interventions.

4. The study of health promotion and disease prevention:

❑ This area of research consists of designing, implementing, and evaluating behavioral interventions to prevent health problems. Health promotion research also involves evaluating approaches that assist in optimal health functioning.

❑ Examples of research topics include designing, implementing, and evaluating interventions aimed at discouraging tobacco use, increasing physical activity, altering dietary intake to promote better health, preventing injuries in children, providing health knowledge, and promoting approaches for preventing sexually transmitted diseases.

5. The study of institutional and organizational influences on health:

❑ This area of research includes health services research—how access and effectiveness of health care are related to cost, and social and cultural acceptability. It also involves research on how behaviors related to consumption and choice of health care is influenced by the structure and functioning of families, community and neighborhood organizations, and the economy.

❑ Examples of research in this area include studying the impact of providing patients who smoke with information and brief counseling from healthcare workers; the accessibility of vaccinations to immigrants; rural dental health care for migrant workers; the cost-effectiveness of work site wellness programs; the use of churches as sites for the delivery of mental health services; the effects of restricting healthcare utilization; the effects of race/ethnicity, gender, and age on referral for mental health services; and identifying the association between physician counseling behavior and patient adherence to medical treatments.

Behavioral Psychology

Returning to the area of basic research in the behavioral sciences, behavioral psychology has greatly advanced our understanding of behavioral processes and interactions of biological and social factors with behavioral variables. The branch of psychology that formulates the theories underlying behavior through observation and experimentation is *behaviorism*. The term refers to the belief that behaviors can be measured, trained, and modified. Behaviorism was introduced by John B. Watson in his classic article, "Psychology as the Behaviorist Views It," which was published in 1913 (Watson, 1913). He proposed that all of our responses are simply patterns of stimulus and response. He believed that people behave differently because of different experiences of learning.

Along with Watson, B. F. Skinner was a pioneer of modern behaviorism. He proposed that behaviors were reflexes. His hypothesis-based research was conducted through laboratory experiments and elucidates a mechanism for describing and measuring behavior (Hilgard, 1988). Most of his trials involved rats or pigeons and observations of their behaviors when they were exposed to food. He investigated the animals' habits, extinctions, operant behaviors, and respondent behaviors (Hilgard, 1988). Extinctions occur when an organism tries an activity and does not get a response; eventually the organism will stop doing the activity, producing extinction of the behavior (Lattal, St. Peter, & Escobar, 2013). Skinner's explanation of operant behavior or conditioning is that which occurs when a behavior changes after the organism experiences consequences of a behavior (O'Donohue & Ferguson, 2001; Skinner, 1966). Respondent behavior is that which happens when a stimulus is provoked, such as saliva production in an animal after the animal knows that pressing a lever will eventually cause food to be provided (Skinner, 1963). Skinner endorsed the idea that all of psychology relates to behavior, and that many relationships between behavior and the environment are predictable. His work helped other investigators determine research strategies such as *behavioral analysis*, whereby behaviors are carefully monitored and observed as in other scientific experiments—an approach that remains popular today (Toates, 1986).

The theoretical goal of behaviorist is to predict and control behavior based on objective events. Behaviorism has contributed to our understanding of behavioral learning, including contiguity, classical conditioning, and operant conditioning theories:

1. Contiguity theory:

   ❑   This theory is based on the work of E. R. Guthrie (1938), which concludes that a stimulus and response linked in time and/or space will be associated.

❏ An example of this theory is a person who is vaccinated and does not get sick, so they make the association between the vaccination and not getting sick.

2. Classical conditioning theory:

❏ This is the first (classical) type of learning theory among behaviorists.

❏ *Classical conditioning* involves learning a new behavior by the process of association; it is a type of learning by which a stimulus has the capacity to evoke a response that was originally a response to another stimulus.

❏ Russian scientist Ivan Pavlov introduced this theory as he observed that dogs deprived of food began to salivate when an assistant would walk into the room. His investigation of this phenomenon resulted in the laws of classical conditioning. Pavlov hypothesized that the central nervous system is responsible for stimuli-activated responses suggesting that certain pathways in the brain work to evoke the conditioned response (Morgulis, 1914).

❏ An example of this is a health coach saying that a certain exercise is easy just before you experience considerable discomfort through the exercise process. The next time you hear that something is easy, you cringe in skepticism. Another example is if you get food poisoning at a church picnic. The next time you hear that your church is having a picnic, you become nauseous.

3. Operant conditioning theory:

❏ *Operant conditioning* is the study of the impact of consequences from a voluntary behavior—a reinforcing or punishing stimulus results after a behavior. The consequences that follow a behavior determine whether the behavior will be repeated. Those behaviors that are followed by punishment tend not to be repeated. The theory was developed by B. F. Skinner (Skinner, 1938).

❏ Unlike classical conditioning, in which the response is drawn out of the organism, in operant conditioning a voluntary behavior occurs as a way of achieving an outcome.

❏ Four types of operant conditioning are positive reinforcement (consequences of the behavior are positive), negative reinforcement (a negative stimulus is removed from the environment because of a given behavior), punishment (the behavior results in a negative consequence, thereby reducing the chance of the behavior in the future), and extinction (the behavior discontinues because of the absence of reinforcement). Positive and negative reinforcement result in an increase in the behavior, whereas negative consequences or no reinforcement result in a decrease and elimination of the behavior.

❏ For example, a health coach can use reinforcement to positively impact motivation and human behavior according to the principles of operant conditioning. A positive reinforcement, through praise, can inform an individual about his or her performance with respect to some behavior change and enhance a feeling of self-worth and competence. Praise can be a positive reinforcement if it is accurate and timely, tailored to the individual, ability and achievement is connected with effort, and the process is made as positive as possible (e.g., build a social support team to make the activities fun). An example of negative reinforcement is that when you use sunscreen, you remove the chance of sunburn. The punishment of severe sunburn in the absence of sunscreen will cause you to consider using sunscreen in the future.

❏ Extinction occurs in both operant conditioning and classical conditioning. When operant behavior that had been reinforced no longer receives reinforcement, the behavior gradually stops occurring (Miltenberger, 2012).

❏ For example, an individual takes extreme risks such as longboarding at high speeds, which is reinforced by the attention of friends. However, when the friends grow up and move on, the attention-seeking behavior declines and eventually stops. Of course, there could be a resurgence in the behavior if the individual makes new delinquent friends and the behavior reappears. In classical conditioning, extinction occurs when a conditioned stimulus is no longer paired with an unconditioned stimulus. For example, hearing that there will be a church dinner (unconditioned stimulus) had been paired with being nauseous (conditioned stimulus). If the unconditioned stimulus is no longer paired with the conditioned stimulus, the conditioned response (nausea) will disappear. Perhaps your next church dinner or two did not result in food poisoning.

Another type of behavioral learning theory is cognitive dissonance. *Cognitive dissonance* is a motivational state that exists when a person experiences incongruous beliefs and attitudes simultaneously. For example, a person may have a fondness for donuts but learns that they are harmful to their health. New information can lead to a conflict in one's beliefs or assumptions. Psychologist Leon Festinger introduced the concept of cognitive dissonance in the late 1950s (Festinger, 1957, 1962). Festinger and later researchers showed that in light of challenging new information, people tend to preserve their current understanding of the world by rejecting or refuting the information, seeking support from others who share their beliefs, convincing themselves that no conflict really exists, attempting to persuade others, or avoiding the new information altogether (Harmon-Jones, 2002). Nevertheless, cognitive dissonance does provide an explanation for attitude change.

Group Influences on Behavior

Many behaviors are influenced by group dynamics. For example, a married individual may have a better diet, have more consistent sleep patterns, and engage in less risky behaviors; one's family environment can influence diet, stress, physical activity, hygiene, and many other behaviors; and a group of friends may reinforce certain behaviors (e.g., not driving while intoxicated, regular exercise, and church activity). Further, the presence of people can cause us to act differently, depending on who those people are. Most of us are concerned to some degree about our social image or what other people think of us. Various theories have been put forward about our behaviors in group settings, including social facilitation, groupthink, and group polarization. Each of these has application in public health.

Research has shown an increase in awareness of our surroundings when others are present (Zajonc, 1965). *Social facilitation* is the tendency for people who are being watched or observed to perform better than they would alone on simple tasks or activities they are familiar with and are good at performing (Guerin, 1993). On the other hand, if the task is not simple or familiar, the theory indicates there is a larger margin of error because of nervousness. For example, in a work site setting, monitoring employees doing simple tasks may improve production, whereas if a task is not simple or familiar, the presence of other people may lead to mistakes and possible injuries. Injuries may also occur if the presence of others causes individuals to attempt to do more than they are physically capable of.

A group decision-making process typically has one of two outcomes: groupthink or group polarization. Social psychologist Irving L. Janis introduced the term *groupthink* in 1972. It refers to the unrealistic thought processes and decision making that results within a group in which group harmony is a primary objective. If the group has a tendency to agree on most issues and the group members are happy with that agreement, there is an inclination to stifle dissent or opposing argument (Janis, 1972). Groupthink can have the advantage of allowing large groups to make decisions, complete tasks, and finish projects efficiently. However, this tendency can lead to impulsive decisions and a failure to consider side arguments or alternatives. Groupthink is more common when group members are homogeneous or if the group has a powerful, persuasive leader.

Groupthink is an issue that should be considered when conducting focus groups. To avoid a dominant figure hijacking group thoughts and feelings, allow each member of the group to express his or her opinions and/or divide the group into smaller independent groups. Groupthink can also be an issue in public health decision making. Similar strategies should be employed, along with epidemiologic information.

Group polarization refers to the enhancement of a group's prevailing tendencies through discussion that tends to accentuate the group's differences from other groups (Moscovici & Zavalloni, 1969). The decisions and opinions of group members become more extreme than their actual privately held beliefs. This phenomenon has shown that after participating in a group discussion, the participants advocate more extreme positions such as a riskier course of action (Isenberg, 1986). Although a group may recommend a riskier course of action, a group of conservative individuals may recommend a more conservative course of action. Group polarization may occur because when somebody takes a stand in a group setting, there is more pressure to maintain that stand to avoid appearing unsure or indecisive; because affirmation by other group members can give individuals greater confidence to express preferences and opinions; because moderate opinions expressed in a group become more real with group expectations of commitment; and because in a group of like-minded individuals, one person's arguments can be combined with others to strengthen group polarization. The theory of group polarization suggests that health behavior change efforts would work better by bringing together groups of individuals who have a similar desire to improve their health. Strategies and commitment can be developed and encouraged at the group level, with better health behaviors achieved by members of the group than had the individuals acted alone.

Health Behavior in the Workplace

Behavior change theory, expert opinion, and best practice standards indicate that work site policies and environments supporting a culture of safety and health are an important aspect for helping individuals adopt and maintain healthy behaviors (Aldana et al., 2012). Studies have shown that the work site has the potential to promote healthy lifestyle choices through organizational and environmental policies and supports that encourage the adoption and maintenance of healthy behaviors (Berry, Mirabito, & Baun, 2010; Schult, Galway, Awosika, Schmunk, & Hodgson, 2013). For example, work site administrative actions can promote safe behaviors and surround employees with much of what is needed to avoid injury (Purdue, 2007). A culture of safety has been associated with fewer injuries (Kowalski-Trakofler & Barrett, 2007; Zacharatos, Barling, & Iverson, 2005), more accurate reporting of accidents (Probst & Estrada, 2010), safer driving (Wills, Watson, & Biggs, 2006), and other safety-related conditions and behaviors (Lu & Tsai, 2010).

Work site health promotion efforts that help employees adopt and maintain healthy behaviors include experiences that *"enhance awareness, increase motivation, and build skills* and, most importantly, *that create supportive policies and environments* that make positive health practices the easiest choice" (O'Donnell, 2009, iv).

Creating supportive policies and environments is an important aspect of health promotion and is fundamental to behavior change theory (Bandura, 1988; Prochaska & Velicer, 1997). Behavior change is an important aspect of work site wellness programs. For change to occur, the following seven benchmarks have been suggested: capturing CEO support, creating cohesive wellness teams, collecting data to drive health efforts, carefully crafting an operating plan for health and wellness within the organization, choosing appropriate interventions, creating a supportive environment, and carefully assessing outcomes (Wellness Council of America, 2007).

A quarter of a century ago some of the first information and rationales for the need to create a work site culture of health was reported (Allen, Allen, Certner, & Kraft, 1987; Allen & Allen, 1987). Researchers adopted an existing generic work site culture change framework, which posits that the behavioral choices made by employees are influenced by five organizational dimensions (Allen, 2007; Golaszewski, Hoebbel, Crossley, Foley, & Dorn, 2008). *Norms* are the social boundaries that define the expected and accepted ways of behaving with respect to health issues. *Shared values* reflect the collective beliefs about what health-related issues are important. *Touch points* are the system-wide provision of informal and formal structures, services, policies, and procedures that influence the organizational culture in matters of health. *Work climate* includes a set of temporary employee attitudes, feelings, and perceptions that is influenced by workplace social and structural characteristics and serves as a catalyst to individual health behavior change. The last component in the framework is *peer support.*

Health Behavior Affected by Larger Systems

Health behaviors are also influenced by larger political, economic, cultural, and demographic systems. In this section, we will discuss selected ways health behaviors are affected by these larger systems.

POLITICAL INFLUENCES ON HEALTH BEHAVIOR

In the United States, tobacco control laws and government policies help prevent people, particularly children, from starting to use tobacco; help people quit using tobacco; and protect people from the harmful effects of tobacco use. A comprehensive approach is taken that includes education and clinical, regulatory, economic, and social strategies. Federal laws aimed at modifying tobacco use are passed by Congress and signed by the president. The laws are then enforced through an agency of the executive branch, like the Food and Drug Administration (FDA). Laws may also be made on the state and local levels to make tobacco products less accessible, attractive, or affordable. Research has shown that as cigarette prices increase, cigarette use decreases, fewer young people start smoking, and smokers have a greater incentive to quit (Centers for Disease Control and Prevention [CDC], 1998; Chaloupka, 1999; Chaloupka, Tauras, & Grossman, 1997; Gallus, Schiaffino, La Vecchia, Townsend, & Fernandez, 2006; Harris & Chan, 1998; Oredein & Foulds, 2011; Ringel, Wasserman, & Andreyeva, 2005; Tauras, 2004; Tauras, O'Malley, & Johnston, 2001; U.S. Department of Health and Human Services [USDHHS], 2000).

The executive branch of the federal government, under the authorization of Congress, can enact federal regulations. Regulations can also be introduced by states. For example, the Tobacco Control Act allows the FDA to issue tobacco-related regulations. Some key tobacco product regulations by the FDA include banning flavored cigarettes (September 2009), restricting youth access to tobacco products (March 2010), banning misleading advertising to avoid the perception that tobacco products are safe (June 2010), establishing new smokeless tobacco warnings (June 2010), establishing a list of harmful constituents (March 2012), issuing draft guidance on submitting a modified risk tobacco product application (March 2012), announcing the first decision to authorize and deny marketing of new tobacco products (June 2013), releasing a preliminary scientific evaluation about menthol (July 2013), awarding $53 million to establish 14 tobacco centers of regulatory science (September 2013), and launching the first public campaign to help prevent youth tobacco use (February 2014) (USDHHS, 2014).

There are several highlights of tobacco control efforts in the United States and elsewhere. Some of these efforts occurring in the United States are described in **Table 2-1**.

ECONOMIC INFLUENCES ON HEALTH BEHAVIOR

The Food Research and Action Center (FRAC) prepared a report on why low-income and food-insecure people are vulnerable to

Table 2-1

Highlights of Tobacco Control Efforts in the United States

Year	Title	Description
1964	First Report of the Surgeon General's Advisory Committee on Smoking and Health	• Identifies smoking as a cause of increased mortality
1965	Federal Cigarette Labeling and Advertising Act	• Requires a health warning on cigarette packages • Requires the Federal Trade Commission to submit an annual report to Congress on tobacco industry advertising and labeling practices • Requires the Department of Health, Education, and Welfare to submit an annual report to Congress on the health consequences of smoking
1970	Public Health Cigarette Smoking Act	• Requires a health warning on cigarette packages • Prohibits cigarette advertising on television and radio
1984	Comprehensive Smoking Education Act	• Institutes the use of four rotating health warning labels, all listed as Surgeon General's Warnings, on cigarette packages and advertisements
1986	Comprehensive Smokeless Tobacco Health Education Act	• Institutes the use of three rotating health warning labels on smokeless tobacco packages and advertisements • Prohibits smokeless tobacco advertising on television and radio • Requires the U.S. Department of Health and Human Services to submit a report every 2 years to Congress on smokeless tobacco • Requires the Federal Trade Commission to report annually to Congress on smokeless tobacco sales, advertising, and marketing • Requires the smokeless tobacco industry to submit a confidential list of additives and nicotine content in smokeless tobacco products
1988	Amendment to Federal Aviation Act	• Makes domestic flights of 2 hours or less smoke free
1992	Synar Amendment to the Alcohol, Drug Abuse, and Mental Health Administration Reorganization Act	• Enacts laws prohibiting the sale and distribution of tobacco products to minors • Enforces these laws in a way that can reasonably be expected to reduce the availability of tobacco products to youth younger than age 18 years • Conducts random, unannounced inspections of tobacco outlets • Reports annual findings to the secretary of the U.S. Department of Health and Human Services
1996	Regulations restricting the sale and distribution of cigarettes and smokeless tobacco to protect children and adolescents	• Asserts jurisdiction over tobacco products, issuing this final rule restricting the sale and distribution of cigarettes and smokeless tobacco to protect youth; in 2000, the U.S. Supreme Court ruled that FDA did not have the authority to regulate tobacco and that such regulation required authorization by Congress
2000	Wendell H. Ford Aviation Investment and Reform Act	• Prohibits smoking on all flights between the United States and foreign destinations

Table 2-1 (Continued)		
Highlights of Tobacco Control Efforts in the United States		
Year	**Title**	**Description**
2009	Family Smoking Prevention and Tobacco Control Act (Tobacco Control Act); some parts of this law, and FDA regulations authorized by it, are currently subject to litigation, making the implementation of these provisions uncertain	• Grants the FDA authority to regulate the manufacture, distribution, and marketing of tobacco products • Requires prominent graphic warning labels for cigarettes and larger text warnings for smokeless tobacco products • Prohibits the advertising or labeling of tobacco products with the descriptors "light," "low," "mild," or similar terms without an FDA order • Requires tobacco companies to submit research on health, toxicological, behavioral, or physiologic effects of tobacco use • Allows the FDA to conduct compliance check inspections of tobacco retailers; penalties for violations include fines, and, for repeated violations, a potential no-tobacco sale order prohibiting the sale of tobacco products • Prohibits the sale of cigarettes containing certain characterizing flavors (such as strawberry, grape, orange, and others) • Requires tobacco manufacturers to get an order or exemption from the FDA before they may introduce new tobacco products
2010	Prevent All Cigarette Trafficking (PACT) Act; some parts of this law are currently subject to litigation	• Prohibits the mailing of cigarettes (including roll-your-own tobacco) and smokeless tobacco through the U.S. Postal Service • Requires Internet and mail-order sales retailers to comply with age verification requirements • Among other things, requires Internet and other mail-order retailers to pay appropriate federal, state, local, and tribal taxes for cigarettes (including roll-your-own tobacco) and smokeless tobacco

Reproduced U.S. Department of Health and Human Services (HHS). (2014). Laws/Policies. Retrieved from http://betobaccofree.hhs.gov/laws/.

becoming overweight and obese. Some of the findings from the report are presented here because they relate to dietary behaviors (FRAC, 2010). The study found that low-income neighborhoods and people are often limited to affordable foods. They may not have access to full-service grocery stores and farmers' markets, which offer a large selection of fruit and vegetables, whole grains, and low-fat dairy products (Beaulac, Kristjansson, & Cummins, 2009; Larson, Story, & Nelson, 2009). Their access to reliable transportation may also be limited, restricting them to shop at small neighborhood stores, which may have a limited supply of these items. A comprehensive review of studies conducted in the United States found that neighborhood residents with better access to supermarkets generally had healthier diets and lower risk for obesity (Larson et al., 2009).

When healthy food is available, it tends to be more expensive. On the other hand, refined grains, sugars, and fats tend to be inexpensive and readily available in lower-income neighborhoods (Drewnowski, 2010; Drewnowski, Monsivais, Maillot, & Darmon, 2007; Drewnowski & Specter, 2004; Monsivais & Drewnowski, 2007, 2009). Low-income households often buy cheap, energy-dense foods that maximize calories per dollar (Basiotis & Lino, 2002; DiSantis et al., 2013; Drewnowski, 2009; Drewnowski & Specter, 2004). Although they are cheaper, these foods generally have lower nutritional value and, because they result in high calorie intake, contribute to obesity (Hartline-Grafton, Rose, Johnson, Rice, & Webber, 2009; Howarth, Murphy, Wilkens, Hankin, & Kolonel, 2006; Kant & Graubard, 2005).

When healthy food is available in low-income neighborhoods, it is often of poor quality, which is unappealing to buyers (Andreyeva, Blumenthal, Schwartz, Long, & Brownell, 2008; Zenk et al., 2006). Fast-food restaurants are often more common in low-income neighborhoods (Fleischhacker, Evenson, Rodriguez, & Ammerman, 2011; Larson et al., 2009; Simon, Kwan, Angelescu, Shih, & Fielding, 2008). The types of food consumed at fast-food restaurants tend to be high in calories and low in nutrients, and these foods contribute to weight gain (Bowman & Vinyard, 2004; Pereira et al., 2005).

The FRAC report also identified fewer opportunities for physical activity in low-income neighborhoods. This is because there are often fewer parks, green spaces, bike paths, and recreational facilities, which makes a physically active lifestyle more difficult (Cohen, McKenzie, Sehgal, Williamson, Golinelli et al., 2007). Estabrooks, Lee, & Gyurcsik, 2003; Powell, Slater, & Chaloupka, 2004). However, when they are available, the quality of these physical activity resources may be less attractive, with fewer natural features such as grass and trees, and they have more signs of disrepair and city noise (Neckerman et al., 2009). Crime, traffic, and unsafe equipment are other potential barriers (Duke, Huhman, & Heitzler, 2003; Gordon-Larsen et al., 2004; Neckerman et al., 2009; Suecoff, Avner, Chou, & Crain, 1999). Consequently, children may be more likely to stay indoors and watch television or play video games. They are less likely to be involved in organized sports (Duke et al., 2003), they spend less time being physically active during physical education classes, and they are less likely to have recess (Barros, Silver, & Stein, 2009; UCLA Center to Eliminate Health Disparities & Samuels and Associates, 2007).

The FRAC report associates high levels of stress with financial and emotional pressures and food insecurity. In addition to stress being associated with food insecurity, it may also stem from low-wage work, lack of access to health care, inadequate and long-distance transportation, poor housing, neighborhood violence, and other factors. Stress, in turn, can lead to unhealthful eating behaviors (Adam & Epel, 2007; Torres & Nowson, 2007), and it can trigger anxiety and depression (Anderson, Cohen, Naumova, Jacques, & Must, 2007; Simon et al., 2006).

CULTURAL INFLUENCES ON HEALTH BEHAVIOR

Social and cultural influences can influence many aspects of health behavior. In this section we will consider how these influences can impact contraception and reproductive health behaviors. Although contraception practices are very similar between western Europe and the United States, there is a noticeable difference in the rates of sterilization. Sterilization is not as popular in Europe as it is in the United States (Merrill, 2010).

There is enormous social and cultural pressure on women in India to bear many children. It is particularly important that women conceive in the first year of marriage, produce a son, and continue to have children throughout their fertile years (Wilson-Williams, Stephenson, Juvekar, & Andes, 2008). Most women do not get to choose when or how frequently to conceive because of India's male society, where a husband is allowed to beat his wife if she covertly uses a form of contraception or refuses to have sex (Wilson-Williams et al., 2008). He is often afraid of how he will be perceived if his wife is not conceiving, and this fear leads him to overcompensate, which leads to frequent pregnancies (Wilson-Williams et al., 2008).

Contraceptive practices in China are unique because of the policy of one child per family. Family planning in the Pacific Island culture is evolving from primitive notions that there is no place for contraception to the gradual acceptance that some form of birth control may be appropriate in certain circumstances. There is still room for improvement, but trends indicate that family planning is progressing in the Pacific Islands. Traditionally, men in island cultures have had control over when to have children and how many to have, although this has changed in recent years (Brewis, McGarvey, & Tu'u'au-Potoi, 1998). The islands still need to address the issue of family planning in a way that makes it culturally acceptable and widely available. Several of the cultural values inherent in island culture inhibit family planning. Many prevalent religious groups on the islands strongly discourage contraceptive use, and some clinics run by religious institutions refuse to dispense contraceptives, even if the person is not of the same faith (Kenyon & Power, 2003).

Multiple factors affect the methods of contraception used by Latinos, including tradition, religion, and wealth. Latino cultures, in general, are male dominated (the Argentine Civil Code of 1868 even sanctioned women's legal inferiority), and women have little control over the method of contraception used or whether contraception is used at all (Barrancos, 2006; Martin, 2004).

Induced abortions have traditionally been used as a form of birth control in Latin America. Abortion may be induced by ingesting highly toxic plants, and the procedure is overseen by healers, herbalists, and sorcerers (Conway & Slocumb, 1979). Today these procedures are gradually being replaced by natural family planning methods (including the rhythm method); however, abortion-related complications remain the leading cause of maternal death in many Latin American countries (Barrancos, 2006). Religion has heavily influenced the acceptance of contraception in Latin America. The majority of those living in Latin America are connected to the Catholic Church in some way; this group discourages its members from using all forms of contraception. As a result, natural family planning remains the predominant form of birth control practiced by Latin American women.

Economic factors also limit an individual's access to contraception. Women in upper and middle classes have greater access and more available options; poorer women are more likely to continue the use of dangerous traditional or herbal methods (Barrancos, 2006). As previously mentioned, women of lower socioeconomic status are more likely to participate in traditional induced abortions.

Africa is plagued by many of the same problems mentioned earlier in association with other regions. Several factors are associated with a woman's utilization of contraception. These factors include a lack of family planning services, lack of knowledge, cultural traditions, and socioeconomic status (Orji & Onwudiegwu, 2002). Religious affiliation and education were not found to have a significant impact on contraceptive use (Orji & Onwudiegwu, 2002).

Ethnicity has been found to be a contributing factor to contraceptive use (Addai, 1999). Abortion is a common form of contraception in Africa. This procedure is used especially by adolescents, who cite fear of future infertility as the overriding factor in their decisions to rely on induced abortion rather than contraception. A majority of these procedures are not performed by trained medical professionals in a proper clinical setting and can lead to serious complications (Fathella, 1994).

Female circumcision refers to a process in which female external reproductive tissues are altered (mutilated) for nonmedical purposes. The World Health Organization estimates the prevalence of this practice to be as high as 140 million girls and women (World Health Organization, 2014a). In Africa, more than 90 million females older than 9 years are living with the consequences of genital mutilation, and an estimated 3 million girls in Africa are at risk for the procedure each year (World Health Organization, 2014a). The reasons for female genital cutting stem from a mix of social, cultural, and religious roots. These societies assume that women are highly sexual, promiscuous beings. The clitoris and labia are considered unclean sexual body parts. Their removal symbolizes the emergence of a clean and chaste woman. Hence, female circumcision is used to achieve a society's ideal of beauty, femininity, and modesty. Removal of the unclean genitalia is also seen as a way to reduce a woman's libido and to ensure her virginity and fidelity to her husband (Morris, 1999). Therefore, some cultures view the procedure as a female's initiation into womanhood, a way to prepare her for marriage, and a method to maintain marital fidelity (World Health Organization, 2014b).

DEMOGRAPHIC INFLUENCES ON HEALTH BEHAVIOR

Demographic refers to characteristics of a population. A demographic is a section of the population sharing a common characteristic (e.g., age, sex, and income). Demographic analyses may involve people in a group, organization/institution, or larger society. Demographic trends describe changes in demographics in a population. The population (or age) pyramid is a graphical technique used by demographers to track and compare changes in the population age distributions over time. The number of persons in selected age groups for given populations are affected by behaviors (e.g., reproduction, migration, civil unrest, marriage, and immunization) and environmental conditions (famines, droughts, sanitation, clean water supply, and healthcare access). **Figure 2-1** shows the population pyramid for Russia in 2014. This is an example of a constrictive pyramid showing a lower number or percentage of younger people. Economic and other factors have contributed to a lower birth rate in Russia in the past 25 years.

Decreasing trends in marriage rates are seen throughout many places in the world (**Table 2-2**). In all but 4 of the 27 countries shown, marriage rates are declining. A Pew Research Center nationwide survey, in association with TIME and complemented by demographic and economic data from the U.S. Census Bureau, has brought insight into the declining marriage rates (Pew Research, 2010). The study found a class-based decline in marriage. In 1960, 72% of adults in this country were married, as opposed to 52% in 2008. The decline occurred by class. In the earlier year, 76% of college graduates were married, compared with 72% of those with a high school diploma or less. In the later year, the corresponding percentages were 64% and 48%, respectively. The report goes on to say that there are strong group differences in how changes in marriage and family life are perceived. Specifically, the young versus the old, the secular versus the religious, and the liberals versus the conservatives are more accepting of the emerging arrangements. Cohabitation has almost doubled since 1990,

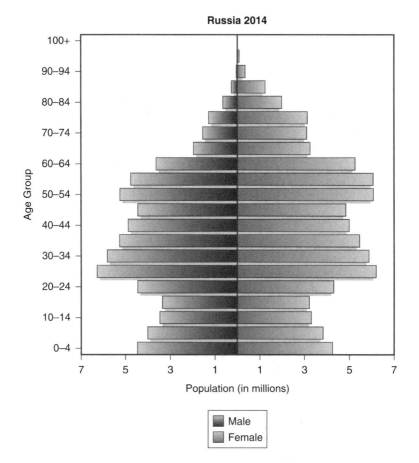

Figure 2-1 Population pyramid for the population of Russia, 2014
Data from the U.S. Census Bureau (2014).

with 44% of all adults, and more than 50% of adults ages 30 to 49 years, cohabitating at some time in their lives (2010).

Several suggestions have explained the change in marriage rates: the recession, which caused depressed wages and increased unemployment for many young adults; a growing income gap, with fewer financially stable partners in lower-income communities; shifting public attitudes, which may be partially due to a decline in religious orientation; a rise in contraception use; and an increase of women in the workforce, which has brought greater social and political freedoms (Sterbenz, 2014).

In the United States, research has shown that women, on average, are more health conscious in the sense that they are less likely to use illicit drugs, binge drink, or smoke cigarettes (USDHHS, 2009). They are also more likely than men to have health insurance and to

	1990	1999	2006	% change 1990 to 2006
Table 2-2				
Trends in Crude Marriage Rates per 1,000 People for Selected Countries				
Australia	6.9	6	5.4	−22%
Austria	5.8	4.8	4.5	−22%
Belgium	6.6	4.3	4.3	−35%
Bulgaria	6.7	4.2	4.3	−36%
Czech Republic	8.4	5.2	5.1	−39%
Denmark	6.1	6.6	6.7	10%
Finland	4.8	4.7	5.4	13%
France	5.1	—	4.4	−14%
Germany	6.5	5.2	4.5	−31%
Greece	5.8	6.4	5.2	−10%
Hungary	6.4	4.5	4.4	−31%
Ireland	5	4.9	4.1	−18%
Israel	7	5.9	5.9	−16%
Italy	5.4	—	4.1	−24%
Japan	5.8	6.3	5.8	0%
Luxembourg	6.2	4.9	4.1	−34%
Netherlands	6.4	5.6	4.4	−31%
New Zealand	7	5.3	5.1	−27%
Norway	5.2	5.3	4.7	−10%
Poland	6.7	5.7	5.9	−12%
Portugal	7.3	6.8	4.5	−38%
Romania	8.3	6.5	6.8	−18%
Russia	8.9	5.8	7.8	−12%
Sweden	4.7	4	5	6%
Switzerland	6.9	4.9	5.3	−23%
United Kingdom	6.8	5.1	5.1	−25%
United States	9.8	8.3	7.2	−27%

Data from United Nations, 2001; United Nations Statistics Division, 2009.

have access to regular and consistent medical care and better nutrition (CDC, 2011; USDHHS, 2009). Studies have consistently shown that women have a greater tendency to participate in work site wellness programs (Merrill, Anderson, & Thygerson, 2011a; Merrill, Hyatt, Aldana, & Kinnersley, 2011b; Polacsek, O'Brien, Lagasse, & Hammar, 2006; Robroek, van Lenthe, van Empelen, & Burdorf, 2009). Participation in these programs for women appears to be less driven by financial incentives than it is for men (Merrill & Merrill, 2014).

Linking Health Behaviors with Health Outcomes

The goal of applied research is to predict or influence behavior-related health risks, protective health factors, and health outcomes. Epidemiology provides the methods for identifying risk factors and for monitoring and predicting patterns of risk factors and health outcomes. The connection between certain behaviors and health goes back thousands of years. Hippocrates (460–377 BCE) believed that physicians should observe peoples' behavior, such as eating, drinking, and other activities; Thomas Sydenham (1624–1689) proposed that exercise, fresh air, and an appropriate diet were behaviors that could prevent and treat disease; Ignaz Semmelweis (1818–1865) discovered that puerperal fever could be drastically cut by the use of hand-washing standards in obstetrical clinics; Bernardino Ramazzini (1633–1714) observed that violent and irregular motions and unnatural postures imposed on the body were linked to various diseases and conditions; the Framingham study, which began in 1948 with 5,209 adults from Framingham, Massachusetts, identified poor diet and lack of physical activity as increasing the risk of heart disease; and many epidemiologic studies have identified poor diet, sedentary lifestyle, obesity, tobacco smoking and alcohol drinking, unprotected sexual relations, and certain occupational exposures as risk factors for disease (Agency for Toxic Substances & Disease Registry, 2002; Cumston, 1926; Dawber, Kannel, & Lyell, 1963; Dorland's Illustrated Medical Dictionary, 1974; Garrison, 1926; Hippocrates, 1988).

In the FRAC report discussed earlier, applied research studies were cited indicating that the risk of obesity was greater in lower-income neighborhoods where there was poorer access to supermarkets and farmer's markets; fewer opportunities for physical activity; higher levels of crime; higher levels of stress; and disproportionately higher exposure to marketing and advertising for obesity-promoting products that encourage consumption of unhealthy foods and discourage physical activity (FRAC, 2010).

Epidemiology also provides methods for assessing the impact of certain health outcomes on behavioral functioning. For example, research on the effects of severe traumatic brain injury (TBI) have shown that children and adult survivors of TBI were more susceptible to global impairments, including poor school performance, greater employment difficulties, poor quality of life, and increased mental health problems (Di Battista, Soo, Catroppa, & Anderson, 2012; Stancin et al., 2002). Research has also shown that children and adults with attention-deficit hyperactivity disorder are more likely to be engaged in risky behaviors that result in more frequent and severe injuries (Merrill, Lyon, Baker, & Gren, 2009).

Adjunct Areas of Research

In the outset of this chapter we presented the NIH definition of behavioral and social sciences research as consisting of two areas: (1) core areas of research (basic or fundamental research, and applied research); and (2) adjunct areas of research (many types of neurological research and some pharmacological interventions) (NIH, 2010). Thus far in this chapter we have addressed the core areas of research. This final section will briefly address some of the adjunct areas of research in the behavioral and social sciences.

Neurology is the branch of medical science concerned with the various nervous systems (central, peripheral, autonomic, and neuromuscular junction and muscular) and its disorders (Stedman's Medical Dictionary, 2005). This area of study has investigated diseases and conditions that can affect the nervous system, as well as how brain chemistry is related to disorders such as schizophrenia and depression or conditions like epilepsy.

Neuroscience is any or all of the sciences concerned with the development, structure, function, chemistry, pharmacology, clinical assessments, and pathology of the nervous system and brain (Stedman's Medical Dictionary, 2005). A growing area of research is behavioral neuroscience, which investigates how the brain and nervous system work in the expression of behavior. Behavioral neuroscience generally examines basic biological processes, brain circuitry, and molecular biology of nerves and nervous tissue that underlie both normal and abnormal behavior. In the mid-1950s, neuroscience researchers began to investigate the roles of dopamine and the neurotransmitter norepinephrine in the brain reward centers (Wise, 2008). Similarly, recent neuroscience studies (Sesack, 2009) indicate that dopamine factors can regulate many behaviors. In particular, researchers have connected dopamine stimulation to enhanced reward and reinforcement of behaviors (Wise, 2008).

Neuroscience and psychology together have influenced a newer approach to behavioral research, that of cognitive psychology. Cognitive psychology allows for conscious thought to contribute to behaviors rather than just stimuli affecting a response (Bargh & Ferguson, 2000). Recent psychological research shows a role for cognitive-behavioral therapy. In this therapeutic approach, psychologists or therapists work with persons to help extinguish troublesome thoughts or behaviors such as obsessive-compulsive thoughts (Freeman et al., 2009), and they help with protective behaviors for anxiety and phobias (Silverman, Ortiz, Viswesvaran, Burns, Kolko et al., 2008).

Pharmacological interventions frequently target modifying behavior. For example, disruptive behavioral disorder (DBD) describes a group of similar psychiatric disorders in childhood and adolescence (e.g., aggression, defiance, and tantrums). Several temperamental, biological, and environmental factors have been associated with an increased risk of DBDs. Temperamental risk factors include a short attention span and callous-unemotional traits; biological risk factors include lower salivary cortisol levels, greater increase in heart rate in response to frustration, and low birth weight; and environmental risk factors include maternal smoking, substance use, illness, stress, anxiety, and depression (Latimer, Wilson, Kemp, Thompson, Sim et al., 2012; Loeber, Green, Lahey, Frick, & McBurnett, 2000; McKinney & Morse, 2012; Van Goozen, Matthys, Cohen-Kettenis, Gispen-de, Wiegant et al., 1998). Children experiencing abuse, neglect, and early separation from their parents are also at increased risk of DBDs (Latimer et al., 2012). Psychotherapy and/or psychotropic medication management is the most common intervention for DBDs (Agency for Healthcare Research and Quality, 2014).

Summary

1. Basic research in the behavioral sciences is designed to provide knowledge about underlying mechanisms and patterns that can help us explain, predict, prevent, and manage illness, as well as promote better health and well-being. Basic research involves the study of behavioral processes, interactions of biological and social factors with behavioral variables, and methodology and measurement.

2. The goal of applied research in the behavioral sciences is to predict or influence behavior-related health risks, protective health factors, and health outcomes. It is also concerned with identifying the impact of illness or risk for illness on behavioral functioning.

3. Five categories of behavioral applied research are as follows: identification and understanding of behavioral factors associated with the onset and course of illness and with health conditions; the effects of illness or physical condition on behavioral functioning; treatment outcomes research; the study of health promotion and disease prevention; and the study of institutional and organizational influences on health.

4. The theoretical goal of behaviorists is to predict and control behavior based on objective events. Behaviorism has contributed to our understanding of behavioral learning (contiguity, classical conditioning, and operant conditioning).

5. Cognitive dissonance is a motivational state that exists when a person experiences incongruous beliefs and attitudes simultaneously.

6. Many behaviors are influenced by group dynamics. Theories have been developed on our behaviors in group settings, including social facilitation, groupthink, and group polarization. Creating supportive policies and environments is an important aspect of health promotion and is fundamental to behavior

change theory. We developed these ideas in a work site setting. We also identified selected ways that health behaviors are influenced by larger political, economic, cultural, and demographic systems.

7. Neurology has involved studies investigating diseases and conditions that can affect the nervous system, as well as how brain chemistry is related to disorders such as schizophrenia and depression or conditions like epilepsy. Neuroscience is any or all of the sciences concerned with the development, structure, function, chemistry, pharmacology, clinical assessments, and pathology of the nervous system and brain. Behavioral neuroscience investigates how the brain and nervous system work in the expression of behavior.

References

Adam, T. C., & Epel, E. S. (2007). Stress, eating and the reward system. *Physiology and Behavior, 91*(4), 449–458.

Addai, I. (1999). Ethnicity and contraceptive use in sub-Saharan Africa: The case of Ghana. *Journal of Biosocial Science, 31*(01), 105–120.

Agency for Healthcare Research and Quality. (2014). Psychosocial and pharmacologic interventions for disruptive behavior disorder. Retrieved from http:// effectivehealthcare.ahrq.gov/ehc/products/555/1932/disruptive-behavior -disorder-protocol-140701.pdf

Agency for Toxic Substances & Disease Registry. (2002). Cancer fact sheet. Retrieved from http://www.atsdr.cdc.gov/com/cancer-fs.html

Aldana, S. G., Anderson, D. R., Adams, T. B., Whitmer, R. W., Merrill, R. M., George, V., & Noyce, J. (2012). A review of the knowledge base on healthy worksite culture. *Journal of Occupational and Environmental Medicine, 54*(4), 414–419.

Allen, J. (2007). *Not alone: Healthy habits, helpful friends.* Burlington, VT: Healthyculture.

Allen, R., Allen, J., Certner, B., & Kraft, C. (1987). *The organizational unconscious: How to create the corporate culture you want and need* (2nd ed.). Burlington, VT: Human Resources Institute.

Allen, R. F., & Allen, J. (1987). A sense of community, a shared vision and a positive culture: Core enabling factors in successful culture based health promotion. *American Journal of Health Promotion, 1*(3), 40–47.

Anderson, S. E., Cohen, P., Naumova, E. N., Jacques, P. F., & Must, A. (2007). Adolescent obesity and risk for subsequent major depressive disorder and anxiety disorder: Prospective evidence. *Psychosomatic Medicine, 69*(8), 740–747.

Andreyeva, T., Blumenthal, D. M., Schwartz, M. B., Long, M. W., & Brownell, K. D. (2008). Availability and prices of foods across stores and neighborhoods: The case of New Haven, Connecticut. *Health Affairs, 27*(5), 1381–1388.

Bandura, A. (1988). Organizational application of social cognitive theory. *Australian Journal of Management, 13*(2), 275–302.

Bargh, J. A., & Ferguson, M. J. (2000). Beyond behaviorism: On the automaticity of higher mental processes. *Psychological Bulletin, 126*(6), 925–945.

Barrancos, D. (2006). Problematic modernity: Gender, sexuality, and reproduction in twentieth-century Argentina. *Journal of Women's History, 18*(2), 123–150.

Barros, R. M., Silver, E. J., & Stein, R. E. (2009). School recess and group classroom behavior. *Pediatrics, 123*(2), 431–436.

Basiotis, P. P., & Lino, M. (2002). Food insufficiency and prevalence of overweight among adult women. *Nutrition Insight*, 26. Alexandria, VA: U.S. Department of Agriculture, Center for Nutrition Policy and Promotion.

Beaulac, J., Kristjansson, E., & Cummins, S. (2009). A systematic review of food deserts, 1966–2007. *Preventing Chronic Disease*, 6(3), A105.

Berry, L. L., Mirabito, A. M., & Baun, W. B. (2010). What's the hard return on employee wellness programs? *Harvard Business Review*, 88(12), 104–112, 142.

Bowman, S. A., & Vinyard, B. T. (2004). Fast food consumption of U.S. adults: Impact on energy and nutrient intakes and overweight status. *Journal of the American College of Nutrition*, 23(2), 163–168.

Brewis, A., McGarvey, S., & Tu'u'au-Potoi, N. (1998). Structure of family planning. *Australian and New Zealand Journal of Public Health*, 22(4), 424–427.

Centers for Disease Control and Prevention. (1998). Responses to cigarette prices by race/ethnicity, income, and age groups—United States 1976–1993. *Morbidity and Mortality Weekly Report*, 47(29), 605–609.

Centers for Disease Control and Prevention. (2011). Prevalence and trends data: Nationwide (States and DC). Retrieved from http://apps.nccd.cdc.gov/brfss/

Chaloupka, F. J. (1999). Macro-social influences: The effects of prices and tobacco control policies on the demand for tobacco products. *Nicotine and Tobacco Research*, 1(Suppl. 1), S105–S109.

Chaloupka, F. J., Tauras, J., & Grossman, M. (1997). Public policy and youth smokeless tobacco use. *Southern Economic Journal*, 64(2), 503.

Cohen, D. A., McKenzie, T. L., Sehgal, A., Williamson, S., Golinelli, D., & Lurie, N. (2007). Contribution of public parks to physical activity. *American Journal of Public Health*, 97(3), 509–514.

Conway, G., & Slocumb, J. (1979). Plants used as abortifacients and emmenagogues by Spanish New Mexicans. *Journal of Ethnopharmacology*, 1(3), 241–261.

Cumston, C. G. (1926). *An introduction to the history of medicine.* New York, NY: Alfred A. Knopf.

Dawber, T. R., Kannel, W. B., & Lyell, L. P. (1963). An approach to longitudinal studies in a community: The Framingham study. *Annals of the New York Academy of Sciences*, 107, 539–556.

Di Battista, A., Soo, C., Catroppa, C., & Anderson, V. (2012). Quality of life in children and adolescents post-TBI: A systematic review and meta-analysis. *Journal of Neurotrauma*, 29(9), 1717–1727.

DiSantis, K. I., Grier, S. A., Odoms-Young, A., Baskin, M. L., Carter-Edwards, L., Young, D. R., ... Kumanyika, S. K. (2013). What "price" means when buying food: Insights from a multisite qualitative study with black Americans. *American Journal of Public Health*, 103(3), 516–522.

Dorland's Illustrated Medical Dictionary (25th ed.). (1974). Philadelphia, PA: Saunders.

Drewnowski, A. (2009). Obesity, diets, and social inequalities. *Nutrition Reviews*, 67(S1), S36–S39.

Drewnowski, A. (2010). The cost of US foods as related to their nutritive value. *American Journal of Clinical Nutrition*, 92(5), 1181–1188.

Drewnowski, A., Monsivais, P., Maillot, M., & Darmon, N. (2007). Low-energy-density diets are associated with higher diet quality and higher diet costs in French adults. *Journal of the American Dietetic Association*, 107, 1028–1032.

Drewnowski, A., & Specter, S. E. (2004). Poverty and obesity: The role of energy density and energy costs. *American Journal of Clinical Nutrition, 79,* 6–16.

Duke, J., Huhman, M., & Heitzler, C. (2003). Physical activity levels among children aged 9–13 years—United States, 2002. *Morbidity and Mortality Weekly Report, 52*(33), 785–788.

Engel, G. L. (1977). The need for a new medical model: A challenge for biomedicine. *Science, 196,* 129–136.

Estabrooks, P. A., Lee, R. E., & Gyurcsik, N. C. (2003). Resources for physical activity participation: Does availability and accessibility differ by neighborhood socio-economic status? *Annals of Behavioral Medicine, 25*(2), 100–104.

Fathella, M. (1994). Women's health: An overview. *International Journal of Gynecology & Obstetrics, 46,* 105–118.

Festinger, L. (1957). *A theory of cognitive dissonance.* Stanford, CA: Stanford University Press.

Festinger, L. (1962). Cognitive dissonance. *Scientific American, 207*(4), 93–107.

Fleischhacker, S. E., Evenson, K. R., Rodriguez, D. A., & Ammerman, A. S. (2011). A systematic review of fast food access studies. *Obesity Reviews, 12*(5), e460–e471.

Food Research and Action Center. (2010). Why low-income and food insecure people are vulnerable to overweight and obesity. Retrieved from http://frac.org /initiatives/hunger-and-obesity/why-are-low-income-and-food-insecure -people-vulnerable-to-obesity/

Freeman, J. B., Choate-Summers, M. L., Garcia, A. M., Moore, P. S., Sapyta, J. J., Khanna, M. S., … Franklin, M. E. (2009). The pediatric obsessive-compulsive disorder treatment study II: Rationale, design and methods. *Child and Adolescent Psychiatry and Mental Health, 3*(1), 4.

Gallus, S., Schiaffino, A., La Vecchia, C., Townsend, J., & Fernandez, E. (2006). Price and cigarette consumption in Europe. *Tobacco Control, 15*(2), 114–119.

Garrison, F. H. (1926). *History of medicine.* Philadelphia, PA: Saunders.

Golaszewski, T., Hoebbel, C., Crossley, J., Foley, G., & Dorn, J. (2008). The reliability and validity of an organizational health culture audit. *American Journal of Health Studies, 23*(3), 116–123.

Gordon-Larsen, P., Griffiths, P., Bentley, M. E., Ward, D. S., Kelsey, K., Shields, K., & Ammerman, A. (2004). Barriers to physical activity: Qualitative data on caregiver–daughter perceptions and practices. *American Journal of Preventive Medicine, 27*(3), 218–223.

Guerin, B. (1993). *Social facilitation.* New York, NY: Press Syndicate of the University of Cambridge.

Guthrie, E. R. (1938). *The psychology of human conflict.* New York, NY: Harper.

Harmon-Jones, E. (2002). A cognitive dissonance theory perspective on persuasion. In J. P. Dillard & M. Pfau (Eds.), *The persuasion handbook: Developments in theory and practice* (p. 101). Thousand Oaks, CA: Sage.

Harris, J., & Chan, S. (1998). The continuum-of-addiction: Cigarette smoking in relation to price among Americans aged 15–29. *Health Economics Letters, 2*(2), 3–12. Retrieved from http://www.mit.edu/people/jeffrey/HarrisChanHEL98.pdf

Hartline-Grafton, H. L., Rose, D., Johnson, C. C., Rice, J. C., & Webber, L. S. (2009). Energy density of foods, but not beverages, is positively associated with body mass index in adult women. *European Journal of Clinical Nutrition, 63*(12), 1411–1418.

Hilgard, E. R. (1988). Review of B. F. Skinner's *The Behavior of Organisms. Journal of the Experimental Analysis of Behavior*, 50(2), 283–286.

Hippocrates. (1988). Airs, waters, places. In C. Buck, A. Llopis, E. Najera, M. Terris (Eds.), *The challenge of epidemiology: Issues and selected readings* (pp. 18–19). Washington, DC: World Health Organization.

Howarth, N. C., Murphy, S. P., Wilkens, L. R., Hankin, J. H., & Kolonel, L. N. (2006). Dietary energy density is associated with overweight status among 5 ethnic groups in the multiethnic cohort study. *Journal of Nutrition*, 136, 2243–2248.

Isenberg, D. J. (1986). Group polarization: A critical review and meta-analysis. *Journal of Personality and Social Psychology*, 50(6), 1141–1151.

Janis, I. L. (1972). *Victims of groupthink: A psychological study of foreign-policy decisions and fiascoes*. Boston, MA: Houghton Mifflin.

Kant, A. K., & Graubard, B. I. (2005). Energy density of diets reported by American adults: Association with food group intake, nutrient intake, and body weight. *International Journal of Obesity*, 29, 950–956.

Kenyon, M., & Power, J. (2003). *Family planning in the Pacific Region: Getting the basics right*. Paper presented at Population Change in Asia and the Pacific: Implications for Development Policy, Australian National University, Canberra, Australia.

Kowalski-Trakofler, K., & Barrett, E. (2007). Reducing non-contact electric arc injuries: An investigation of behavioral and organizational issues. *Journal of Safety Research*, 38(5), 597–608.

Larson, N. I., Story, M. T., & Nelson, M. C. (2009). Neighborhood environments: Disparities in access to healthy foods in the U.S. *American Journal of Preventive Medicine*, 36(1), 74–81.

Latimer, K., Wilson, P., Kemp, J., Thompson, L., Sim, F., ..., Minnis, H. (2012). Disruptive behaviour disorders: A systematic review of environmental antenatal and early years risk factors. *Child: Care, Health and Development*, 38(5), 611–628.

Lattal, K. A., St. Peter, C., & Escobar, R. (2013). Operant extinction: Elimination and generation of behavior. *APA Handbook of Behavior Analysis*, 2, 77–107.

Loeber, R., Green, S. M., Lahey, B. B., Frick, P. J., & McBurnett, L. (2000). Findings on disruptive behavior disorders from the first decade of the Developmental Trends Study. *Clinical Child and Family Psychology Review*, 3(1), 37–60.

Lu, C. S., & Tsai, C. L. (2010). Relating safety, productivity and company type for motor-manual logging. The effect of safety climate on seafarers' safety behaviors in container shipping. *Accident Analysis & Prevention*, 42(6), 1999–2006.

Martin, A. (2004). Emergency contraception in Latin America and the Caribbean (Trans.). *Revista Panamericana de Salud Pública*, 16(6), 424–431.

McKinney, C., & Morse, M. (2012). Assessment of disruptive behavior disorders: Tools and recommendations. *Professional Psychology-Research and Practice*, 43(6), 641–649.

Merrill, R. M. (2010). *Reproductive epidemiology: Principles and methods*. Sudbury, MA: Jones and Bartlett Publishers, LLC.

Merrill, R. M., Anderson, A. E., & Thygerson, S. M. (2011a). Effectiveness of a worksite wellness program on health behaviors and personal health. *Journal of Occupational and Environmental Medicine*, 53(9), 1008–1012.

Merrill, R. M., Hyatt, B., Aldana, S. G., & Kinnersley, D. (2011b). Lowering employee health care costs through the Healthy Lifestyle Incentive Program. *Journal of Public Health Management and Practice*, 17(3), 225–232.

Merrill, R. M., Lyon, J. L., Baker, R. K., & Gren, L. H. (2009). Attention deficit hyperactivity disorder and increased risk of injury. *Advances in Medical Sciences*, 54(1), 20–26.

Merrill, R. M., & Merrill, J. G. (2014). Improving health through an accountability-based worksite telephonic health coaching program. *International Journal of Workplace Health Management*, 7(2), 74–88.

Miltenberger, R. (2012). *Behavior modification, principles and procedures* (5th ed.). Belmont, CA: Wadsworth Cengage Learning.

Monsivais, P., & Drewnowski, A. (2007). The rising cost of low-energy-density foods. *Journal of the American Dietetic Association*, 107, 2071–2076.

Monsivais, P., & Drewnowski, A. (2009). Lower-energy-density diets are associated with higher monetary costs per kilocalorie and are consumed by women of higher socioeconomic status. *Journal of the American Dietetic Association*, 109, 814–822.

Morgulis, S. (1914). Pawlow's theory of the function of the central nervous system and a digest of some of the more recent contributions to this subject from Pawlow's laboratory. *Journal of Animal Behavior*, 4(5), 362–379.

Morris, R. I. (1999). Female genital mutilation: Perspectives, risks, and complications. *Urologic Nursing*, 19(1), 13–19.

Moscovici, S., & Zavalloni, M. (1969). The group as a polarizer of attitudes. *Journal of Personality and Social Psychology*, 12(2), 125–135.

National Institutes of Health. (2010). Behavioral and social sciences (BSSR) definition. Retrieved from http://obssr.od.nih.gov/about_obssr/BSSR_CC/BSSR_definition /definition.aspx

Neckerman, K. M., Lovasi, G. S., Davies, S., Purciel, M., Quinn, J., Feder, E., … Rundle, A. (2009). Disparities in urban neighborhood conditions: Evidence from GIS measures and field observation in New York City. *Journal of Public Health Policy*, 30(Suppl. 1), S264–S285.

O'Donnell, M. P. (2009). Definition of health promotion 2.0: Embracing passion, enhancing motivation, recognizing dynamic balance, and creating opportunities. *American Journal of Health Promotion*, 24(1), iv.

O'Donohue, W. T., & Ferguson, K. E. (2001). *The psychology of B. F. Skinner.* Thousand Oaks, CA: Sage.

Oredein, T., & Foulds, J. (2011). Causes of the decline in cigarette smoking among African American youths from the 1970s to the 1990s. *American Journal of Public Health*, 101(10), e1–e11. doi:10.2105/AJPH.2011.300289

Orji, E., & Onwudiegwu, U. (2002). Prevalence and determinants of contraceptive practice in a defined Nigerian population. *Journal of Obstetrics and Gynecology*, 22(5), 540–543.

Pereira, M. A., Kartashov, A. I., Ebbeling, C. B., Van Horn, L., Slattery, M. L., Jacobs, D. R., Jr., & Ludwig, D. S. (2005). Fast-food habits, weight gain, and insulin resistance (the CARDIA study): 15-year prospective analysis. *Lancet*, 365(9453), 36–42.

Pew Research. (2010). The decline of marriage and rise of new families. Retrieved from http://www.pewsocialtrends.org/2010/11/18/the-decline-of-marriage -and-rise-of-new-families/

Polacsek, M., O'Brien, L. M., Lagasse, W., & Hammar, N. (2006). Move and improve: A worksite wellness program in Maine. *Preventing Chronic Disease*, 3(3), A101.

Powell, L. M., Slater, S., & Chaloupka, F. J. (2004). The relationship between community physical activity settings and race, ethnicity, and socioeconomic status. *Evidence-Based Preventive Medicine*, 1(2), 135–144.

Probst, T. M., & Estrada, A. X. (2010). Accident under-reporting among employees: Testing the moderating influence of psychological safety climate and supervisor enforcement of safety practices. *Accident Analysis & Prevention*, 42(5), 1438–1444.

Prochaska, J. O., & Velicer, W. F. (1997). The transtheoretical model of health behavior change. *American Journal of Health Promotion*, 12(1), 38–48.

Purdue, R. (2007). Making safety a culture, not just an initiative. Retrieved from http://www.industryweek.com/safety-culture

Ringel, J. S., Wasserman, J., & Andreyeva, T. (2005). Effects of public policy on adolescents' cigar use: Evidence from the National Youth Tobacco Survey. *American Journal of Public Health*, 95, 995–998.

Robroek, S. J. W., van Lenthe, F. J., van Empelen, P., & Burdorf, A. (2009). Determinants of participation in worksite health promotion programmes: A systematic review. *International Journal of Behavioral Nutrition and Physical Activity*, 6, 26.

Schult, T. M., Galway, A. M., Awosika, E. R., Schmunk, S. K., & Hodgson, M. (2013). Management support, worksite culture, and local resources for healthier employees: The Veterans Affairs experience. *Journal of Occupational and Environmental Medicine*, 55(3), 310–317.

Sesack, S. R. (2009). Functional implications of dopamine D2 receptor localization in relation to glutamate neurons. In A. Bjorklund, S. Dunnett, L Iversen, S. Iversen (Eds.), *Dopamine handbook*, Oxford University Press; New York.

Silverman, W., Ortiz, C., Viswesvaran, C., Burns, B., Kolko, D., Putnam, F., & Amaya-Jackson, L. (2008). Evidence-based psychosocial treatments for children and adolescents exposed to traumatic events. *Journal of Clinical Child & Adolescent Psychology*, 37(1), 156–183.

Simon, P. A., Kwan, D., Angelescu, A., Shih, M., & Fielding, J. E. (2008). Proximity of fast food restaurants to schools: Do neighborhood income and type of school matter? *Preventive Medicine*, 47, 284–288.

Simon, G. E., Von Korff, M., Saunders, K., Miglioretti, D. L., Crane, P. K., van Belle, G., & Kessler, R. C. (2006). Association between obesity and psychiatric disorders in the U.S. adult population. *Archives of General Psychiatry*, 63(7), 824–830.

Skinner, B. F. (1938). *The behavior of organisms: An experimental analysis*. New York, NY: Appleton-Century-Crofts.

Skinner, B. F. (1963). Operant behavior. *American Psychologist*, 18(8), 503–515.

Skinner, B. F. (1966). What is the experimental analysis of behavior? *Journal of the Experimental Analysis of Behavior*, 9(3), 213–218.

Stancin, T., Drotar, D., Taylor, H. G., Yeates, K. O., Wade, S. L., & Minich, N. M. (2002). Health-related quality of life of children and adolescents after traumatic brain injury. *Pediatrics*, 109(2), E34.

Stedman's Medical Dictionary for the Health Professions and Nursing (Illustrated 5th ed.). (2005). New York, NY: Lippincott Williams & Wilkins.

Sterbenz, C. (2014). Marriage rates are near their lowest levels in history—here's why. Retrieved from http://www.businessinsider.com/causes-of-low-marriage-rates-2014-5

Suecoff, S. A., Avner, J. R., Chou, K. J., & Crain, E. F. (1999). A comparison of New York City playground hazards in high- and low-income areas. *Archives of Pediatrics and Adolescent Medicine, 153*(4), 363–366.

Tauras, J., O'Malley, P. M., & Johnston, L. D. (2001). Effects of price and access laws on teenage smoking initiation: A national longitudinal analysis. National Bureau of Economic Research Working Paper Series.

Tauras, J. (2004). Public policy and smoking cessation among young adults in the United States. *Health Policy, 6*, 321–332.

Toates, F. M. (1986). *Motivational systems.* Cambridge, UK: Cambridge University Press.

Torres, S. J., & Nowson, C. A. (2007). Relationship between stress, eating behavior, and obesity. *Nutrition, 23*(11–12), 887–894.

UCLA Center to Eliminate Health Disparities & Samuels and Associates. (2007). *Failing fitness: Physical activity and physical education in schools.* Retrieved from http://www.calendow.org/uploadedFiles/failing_fitness.pdf

United Nations. (2001). Monthly bulletin of statistics, April 2001. Retrieved from http://unstats.un.org/unsd/mbs/data_files/MBS_Apr_1991.pdf

United Nations Statistics Division. (2009). Demographic yearbook. Table 23. Retrieved from http://unstats.un.org/unsd/demographic/products/dyb/dyb2006.htm

U.S. Census Bureau. (2014). International data base. Retrieved from http://www.census.gov/population/international/data/idb/informationGateway.php

U.S. Department of Health and Human Services. (2000). *Reducing tobacco use: A report of the surgeon general.* Atlanta, GA: U.S. Department of Health and Human Services, Centers for Disease Control and Prevention, National Center for Chronic Disease Prevention and Health Promotion, Office on Smoking and Health. Retrieved from http://profiles.nlm.nih.gov/NN/B/B/L/Q/_/nnbblq.pdf

U.S. Department of Health and Human Services. (2009). *Healthy People 2010 women's and men's health: A comparison of select indicators.* Washington, DC: U.S. Government Printing Office.

U.S. Department of Health and Human Services. (2014). Laws/policies. Retrieved from http://betobaccofree.hhs.gov/laws/

Van Goozen, S. H., Matthys, W., Cohen-Kettenis, P. T., Gispen-de, W. C., Wiegant, V. M., & Van Engeland, H. (1998). Salivary cortisol and cardiovascular activity during stress in oppositional-defiant disorder boys and normal controls. *Biological Psychiatry, 43*(7), 531–539.

Watson, J. B. (1913). Psychology as the behaviorist views it. *Psychological Review, 20,* 158–177.

Wellness Council of America. (2007). WELCOA's well workplace initiative. *Absolute Advantage, 6*(1), 3–4.

Wills, A. R., Watson, B., & Biggs, H. C. (2006). Comparing safety climate factors as predictors of work-related driving behavior. *Journal of Safety Research, 37*(4), 375–383.

Wilson-Williams, L., Stephenson, R., Juvekar, S., & Andes, K. (2008). Domestic violence and contraceptive use in a rural Indian village. *Violence Against Women, 14*(10), 1181–1198.

Wise, R. A. (2008). Dopamine and reward: The anhedonia hypothesis 30 years on. *Neurotoxicity Research, 14*(2–3), 169–183.

World Health Organization. (2014a). Female genital mutilation and other harmful practices. Retrieved from http://www.who.int/reproductivehealth/topics/fgm/prevalence/en/

World Health Organization. (2014b). Fact sheet: Female genital mutilation. Retrieved from http://www.who.int/mediacentre/factsheets/fs241/en/index.html

Zacharatos, A., Barling, J., & Iverson, R. D. (2005). High-performance work systems and occupational safety. *Journal of Applied Psychology, 90*(1), 77–93.

Zajonc, R. B. (1965). Social facilitation. *Science, 149*, 269–274.

Zenk, S. N., Schulz, A. J., Israel, B. A., James, S. A., Bao, S., & Wilson, M. L. (2006). Fruit and vegetable access differs by community racial composition and socioeconomic position in Detroit, Michigan. *Ethnicity and Disease, 16*(1), 275–280.

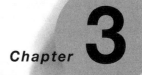

Chapter **3**

Health Behavior and Theory

$\mathbf{P}$ublic health is an effort, service, and practice organized by society to prevent disease, prolong life, and promote the people's health. In 1948, the World Health Organization proposed that "health is the state of complete physical, mental, and social well-being and not merely the absence of disease or infirmity" (1948, para. 2). This idea of treating health as more than just the absence of disease was novel at the time, but it was quickly accepted. More recently, three additional dimensions of health have been added to the definition: emotional, spiritual, and environmental (**Table 3-1**). Thus, public health is a societal effort to prevent disease, prolong life, and promote these six interactive dimensions of health in the community. Health behavior is an individual-level effort to achieve these same goals of disease prevention, prolonged life, and the promotion of the six dimensions of health.

On the community level, public health seeks to accomplish its task by incorporating interdisciplinary approaches of epidemiology, biostatistics, and health services. The three core functions of public health (assessment, policy development, and assurance) are enacted. On the individual level, disease prevention, extended life, and health

Table 3-1	
Six Dimensions of Health	
Dimension	**Definition**
Physical	Ability of the human body to function properly; includes physical fitness and activities of daily living
Social	Ability to have satisfying relationships; interaction with social institutions and societal mores
Mental	Ability to think clearly, reason objectively, and act properly
Emotional	Ability to cope, adjust, and adapt; self-efficacy and self-esteem
Spiritual	Feeling as if part of a greater spectrum of existence; personal beliefs and choices
Environmental	External factors (i.e., one's surroundings, such as habitat or occupation) and internal factors (i.e., one's internal structure, such as genetics)

promotion are achieved through specific behaviors. The purpose of this chapter is to address the role of health behavior in disease prevention, improved life expectancy, and health promotion.

Health Behavior and Disease Prevention

A focus of public health is disease prevention. Disease prevention occurs on both community and individual levels. On the community level, environmental hazards are monitored, people are informed about health issues, policies and plans to support health efforts are made, laws and regulations are put in place to protect health and safety, people are linked with health services, health services and programs are evaluated, and there is research for new insights and innovative solutions to health problems. These efforts can facilitate better health behaviors among individuals within the community.

Although primary prevention strategies seek to avoid the biological onset of disease and, therefore, tend to target the general population, prevention at this level has to be behaviorally directed and lifestyle oriented. Efforts at the primary prevention level have to focus on influencing individual behavior and protecting the environment. *Active primary prevention* requires behavior change on the part of the individual (e.g., begin exercising, stop smoking, reduce dietary fat intake), while *passive primary prevention* does not require behavior change on the part of the individual (e.g., drinking fluoridated water, eating vitamin-enriched foods, working in a setting that has made safety upgrades). *Secondary prevention* is aimed at the health screening and detection activities used to identify disease. The aim of this level of prevention is to block the progression of disease. Screening and detection behaviors are often influenced by health education, access, and resource allocation. *Tertiary prevention* consists of limiting any disability by providing rehabilitation where a disease, injury, or disorder has already occurred and caused damage. Several behavioral choices occur in tertiary prevention, including the decision to receive treatment and participate in rehabilitation. Health education can influence behavior at this level of prevention. The primary aim of tertiary prevention is to slow and check the progression of the disease, disorder, or injury.

Therefore, health behavior has an important presence at each level of disease prevention in public health. Several factors have facilitated healthier behaviors, as will be discussed more fully in the next section. In turn, there has been an unprecedented increase in life expectancy since the mid- to late 1800s.

Prolonged Life

One of society's greatest achievements in the past 150 years has been the global increase in life expectancy. The largest increase in life expectancy, referred to as the First Public Health Revolution, occurred between 1880 and 1920, before the advent of antibiotics and advanced surgical techniques (Novick, 2008; Rosen, 1993; Sigerist, 1956). From 1970 through 1998, life expectancy worldwide has increased on average by 4 months each year. This increase in life expectancy is most pronounced in low- and middle-income countries (World Bank, 2001). In the United States, the average number of remaining years of life from birth improved by 28.1 years for males and 30.2 years for females from 1900 through 2009 (**Figure 3-1**). From age 1 onward the improvement was 21.2 years for males and 24.2 years for females.

The majority of improvement in life expectancy since 1880 has been attributed to the control of infectious diseases, greater availability of food, safer food and water, better sanitary conditions, and other nonmedical social improvements (Bunker, Frazier, & Mosteller, 1994; Centers for Disease Control and Prevention [CDC], 1999c; CDC, 2011; McKeown, 1976; Riley, 2001). Improved sanitation in the form of public water treatment, sewage management, food inspection, and municipal garbage collection has nearly eliminated cholera, dysentery, and typhoid (Preston & Haines, 1991). Innovative methods of agricultural production, food transportation, and food preservation have improved the average diet, reducing or eliminating many nutritional deficiency-caused diseases and improving immune function against infectious diseases (Keusch, 2003). The second leading cause of death in the United States in 1900 was tuberculosis (Garrison, 1926). Improved housing, less crowded living conditions, and better

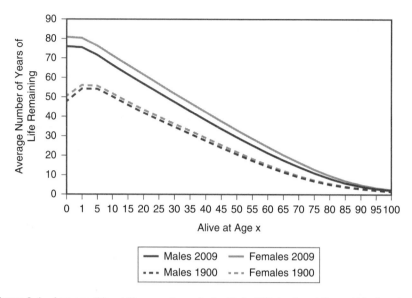

Figure 3-1 Age-conditional life expectancy in the United States for white and black males and females, 2009

Data from Arias, E (2014). United States life tables, 2009. United States life tables, 2009. *National vital statistics reports, 62*(7). Hyattsville, MD: National Center for Health Statistics.

nutrition greatly reduced this disease, many years before the first effective tuberculosis drug was developed in 1946 (CDC, 1999a). Death rates from occupational accidents were greatly reduced through regulations, education, and engineering changes (CDC, 1999b). Air quality has improved because of the elimination of coal-burning furnaces and leaded gasoline, as well as better industrial emissions regulations (Environmental Protection Agency, 2003). Higher education and literacy, child labor laws, and improved economic prosperity have also contributed to better life expectancy and health (Costa, 2003; McKinlay & McKinlay, 1997; Riley, 2001; Roggero, Mangiaterra, Bustero, & Rosuti, 2007).

Although many of the factors contributing to better life expectancy today are not directly related to behavior, many of them have made healthy behaviors more amenable. For example, in many places in the world today, one would have to go out of their way to find unsafe drinking water, to not eat vitamin-fortified foods, to avoid fluoridated water, or to not live in areas with sewage management and garbage disposal. Health education and public policy are also making health behaviors easier. For example, information about the health risks associated with cigarette smoking, and public policy related to tobacco products, resulted in a steady decrease in tobacco smoking in the United States from the mid-1960s through the 1990s, and it has leveled off thereafter. Roughly half of the decrease in the rate of death from coronary heart disease over the past 50 years was mostly because of a reduction in tobacco use (Goldman & Cook, 1984; Hunink et al., 1997).

The Health Impact Pyramid developed by Frieden (2010) is a five-tier pyramid that describes different types of public health interventions, with lower levels of the pyramid tending to have a broader reach on society (**Figure 3-2**). Public health action in interventions at the base of the pyramid generally requires less individual effort and has the greatest impact on the population. On the other hand, the top tiers focus more on helping individuals rather than the entire population. However, theoretically, they have a large population impact if universally accepted and effectively applied (Frieden, 2010). The different levels of the pyramid will be addressed in the remainder of this section.

At the base of the pyramid are interventions addressing socioeconomic factors (e.g., poverty reduction and education improvement). A graph showing the relation between life expectancy and gross domestic product illustrates the positive impact of income on health (**Figure 3-3**). However, when a certain level of income is reached, there does not appear to be much improvement in life expectancy beyond that point.

The second level of the pyramid is changing the context to make individuals' default decisions healthy (e.g., fluoridated water,

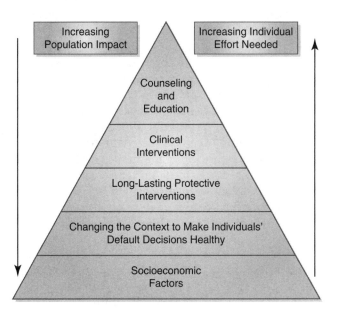

Figure 3-2 The Health Impact Pyramid

Data from Frieden, TR (2010). A framework for public health action: The health impact pyramid. *Am. J. Public Health, 100*(4), 590–595.

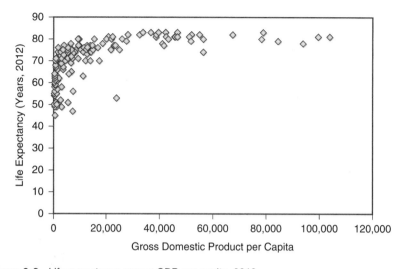

Figure 3-3 Life expectancy versus GDP per capita, 2012

Data from World Health Organization (1948). Constitution of the World Health Organization. Retrieved July 24, 2014, from http://apps.who.int/gb/bd/PDF/bd47/EN/constitution-en.pdf.

vitamin-fortified foods, clean water, elimination of lead and asbestos exposure, reducing sodium in packaged foods and restaurant meals, and iodization of salt). These changes involve passive primary prevention in which active behavior change is not required on the part of the individual, but community actions make the health behavior our default decision.

The third level of the pyramid is long-lasting protective interventions (e.g., immunization, colonoscopy, and smoking cessation programs). Interventions on this level involve active primary prevention where behavior change on the part of the individual is involved. The decision to receive a vaccination, undergo screening, or stop smoking is often influenced by health education and other factors.

The fourth level is clinical interventions (e.g., medication monitoring, blood pressure and cholesterol checks, updated electronic health records that can facilitate preventive and chronic care). Behavioral decisions are again involved, with utilization of clinical interventions often influenced by socioeconomic factors. There is also the decision of whether or not to comply with clinical recommendations and care.

The top level of the pyramid is health education and counseling (i.e., instructional activities and other strategies to change individual health behaviors). Health education and counseling aims to promote better health behaviors. Although health education is perceived by some as the essence of public health action, it is placed on the top of the pyramid because education alone is often considered the least effective of these interventions for promoting better health (Whitlock, Orleans, Pender, & Allan, 2002). Nevertheless, in many circumstances health education and counseling are the only interventions available.

Health Education and Promotion

The purpose of health education proposed by Griffiths was that it "attempts to close the gap between what is known about optimum health practice and that which is actually practiced" (1972, p. 13). Green, Kreuter, Partridge, and Deeds defined health education as "any combination of learning experiences designed to facilitate voluntary adaptations of behavior conducive to health." (1980, p. 7). Green and Kreuter referred to health education as "any combination of learning experiences designed to facilitate voluntary action conducive to health" (1999, p. 27). Key words in this definition are *combination, designed, facilitate, voluntary,* and *actions,* which the authors describe as follows:

- ▣ Combination "emphasizes the importance of matching the multiple determinants of behavior with multiple learning experiences or education interventions" (Green & Kreuter, 1999, p. 27)
- ▣ Designed "distinguishes health education from incidental learning experiences as a systematically planned activity" (p. 27).
- ▣ Facilitate "means predispose, enable, and reinforce" (p. 27).
- ▣ Voluntary "means without coercion and with full understanding and acceptance of the purposes of the action" (p. 27).
- ▣ Actions "means behavioral steps taken by an individual, group, or community to achieve an intended health effect or to build their capacity for health" (p. 27).

In 1960, Mayhew Derryberry, a leader in health education, noted that health education about certain behaviors requires thoughtful and thorough attention to what characterizes the public being considered, such as cultural traditions, social status, power structure, knowledge and attitudes, and so on (Derryberry, 1960). William Griffiths stressed that health education involves more than just individuals and their families, but also consideration of the institutions and social conditions that hinder or enable individuals reaching optimal health (1972). These comments are consistent with the predisposing, enabling, and reinforcing factors discussed by Green and Kreuter.

Green and Kreuter identify three general categories of factors that affect behavior: predispose, enable, and reinforce (Green & Kreuter, 2005). *Predisposing factors* are antecedents to behavioral change that provide the rationale or motivation for the behavior" (p. 147). *Enabling factors* "are antecedents to behavioral or environmental change that allow a motivation or environmental policy to be realized" (p. 147). *Reinforcing factors* "are factors following a behavior that provide the continuing reward or incentive for the persistence or repetition of the behavior" (p. 147).

Predisposing factors that are not modifiable include age, sex, race, and genetics. In cancer research, there are certain genetic factors that predispose a person to getting the disease. For example, families with Li-Fraumeni syndrome are predisposed to a higher risk of sarcomas, brain cancer, breast cancer, and leukemia. Predisposing factors may also protect a person from getting cancer. For example, Hispanics are at much lower risk of developing skin cancer. Similarly, there are many factors that predispose a person to certain health risk behaviors (**Table 3-2**). Suppose we are interested in identifying factors that predispose a person to binge drink. The behavior is likely to be influenced by the person's knowledge of the health risks associated with binge drinking, personal beliefs about whether binge drinking is good or bad, and values and attitudes about binge drinking shaped by their life experiences. The behavior is also likely to be influenced by their confidence and capacity to avoid or say no to binge drinking. Behavioral intentions about binge drinking may be influenced by prior planning and reasoning.

An enabling factor may cause a disease to spread (e.g., the absence of public health and medical care services) or help prevent and control the disease (e.g., access to public health and medical care services).

Table 3-2
Factors That Influence Behavior
Predisposing: Antecedents to behavior • Awareness, knowledge, and health literacy • Beliefs, values, attitudes • Self efficacy • Behavioral intention • Existing skills
Enabling: Antecedents to behavior • Availability, accessibility, and affordability of health resources • Community/government laws, priority, commitment to health • Health-related skills
Reinforcing: Subsequent to behavior • Social and physical benefits; tangible, imagined, or vicarious rewards • Family, peers, teachers, employers, healthcare providers, community leaders, decision makers

In the case of binge drinking behavior, enabling factors may include availability, accessibility, and affordability of the alcohol. These factors are influenced by laws and regulations. Perhaps the individual has developed some skills related to avoiding binge drinking, which may enable them when exposed to alcohol.

Reinforcing factors that help aggravate and perpetuate the health-related state or event are *negative reinforcing factors*. Negative reinforcing factors are repetitive patterns of behavior that occur and perpetuate and support the health-related state or event. *Positive reinforcing factors* are those that support, enhance, and improve the prevention or control of the health-related state or event. Binge drinking may be a recurring behavior because of perceived social rewards, or it may stop because of health information provided by a teacher.

Health education interventions may target one or a combination of these determinants of behavior. They are intended to motivate well thought out, planned, and voluntary actions. These actions, in turn, are intended to produce a specific health outcome or a greater capacity for health.

The term *health education* is often used interchangeably with health promotion, although health promotion is larger in scope. The term *health promotion* has a more recent origin than health education. Health promotion includes health education, but it also considers changes in social, economic, and environmental conditions that can positively influence public health. Green and Kreuter defined health promotion as "the combination of educational and environmental supports for actions and conditions of living conducive the health" (1991, p. 4). Glanz and Rimer note that behavior is both affected by and affects multiple levels of influence (1995). Five types of factors have been identified for influencing health-related behaviors: (1) intrapersonal or individual factors; (2) interpersonal factors; (3) institutional or organizational factors; (4) community factors; and (5) public policy factors (McLeroy, Bibeau, Steckler, & Glanz, 1988). In addition, it has been observed that behavior is influenced by the social environment, and the social environment influences behavior (Stokols, 1992).

The recent introduction of health promotion and education stems from the fact that little was known about the risk factors for certain diseases until the past century or so. The miasma theory was widely accepted from ancient times until the germ theory of disease took hold in the latter part of the 19th century. The theory held that diseases like cholera or the plague were caused by miasma, a noxious form of bad air, also called night air, resulting from rotting organic matter (Last, 2007). Not until the mid-1800s was hand washing identified as a way to reduce the risk of puerperal fever in obstetrical clinics; contaminated water was linked to cholera; and the cause of rabies and many other devastating diseases were identified (Merrill,

2013). Not until the late 1800s and into the past century did researchers connect several diseases with vitamin and nutritional deficiencies (Merrill, 2013).

At the heart of health education is information about risk behaviors, based on epidemiologic studies. For example, epidemiologic investigations have shown that deaths could be prevented if certain tenets were followed such as increasing physical activity and healthy food intake (fruits, vegetables, seafood with omega-3 fatty acids), decreasing smoking, and modifying alcohol consumption (Goodarz et al., 2009). One study emphasized that if individuals embraced just four health behaviors (not smoking; exercising; having moderate alcohol intake; and eating five servings of fruit and vegetables a day) they could add 14 years, on average, to their lives (Khaw et al., 2008). With such important information, health education is delivered in many different settings, including schools, hospitals, work sites, churches, and prisons. Health education is intended to motivate healthy behaviors by providing information, instruction, policy directives, economic assistance, mass media, and community-level programs.

Health Behavior Theories

Health behavior theories presuppose that many behaviors are modifiable and teachable. We have discussed several factors that can facilitate behavior. Health promotion and education programs designed to influence health behavior must consider the complexity of the factors and interaction of those factors involved. Health researchers can use the health behavior theories described in this section to formally test the relationship between factors that influence behaviors and the behaviors themselves. Health promotion and education specialists can use this research to support their health program activities and to positively influence behaviors.

This section will consist of individual-level theories, interpersonal-level theories, community-level theories, and planning models.

INDIVIDUAL-LEVEL THEORIES

Researchers have studied individual-level behaviors for more than a hundred years, while community-level models have been introduced and developed only in the past few decades (DiClemente, Crosby, & Kegler, 2003). Programs with specific goals and objectives for individual-level behaviors can be informed by theories founded in individualistic epistemology, whereas health communication campaigns can better be informed by macro-level theories such as the diffusion of innovations theory (Dutta-Bergman, 2005). Some individual-level theories include the Health Belief Model, the Theory of Reasoned Action or Planned Behavior, and the Stages of Change Model.

Health Belief Model

The Health Belief Model is one of the oldest theories of its kind. In trying to better understand why tuberculosis screenings were failing, social psychologists from the U.S. Public Health Service developed this theory in the 1950s (Rosenstock, 1974). This model is now widely used for a variety of purposes including better understanding behaviors regarding medical screenings and immunizations and behavioral responses to both acute and chronic illnesses.

The Health Belief Model is divided into six categories (**Table 3-3**). The first four (perceived seriousness, susceptibility, benefits, and barriers) focus on the reasons why an individual chooses to engage in or refrain from a particular behavior. The latter two, cues to action and self-efficacy, focus on sustaining a behavior change.

By targeting an individual's perceptions, beliefs surrounding a behavior can be changed, thus changing the individual's likeliness to engage in the behavior. Perceived seriousness refers to how the individual understands the intensity or possibility of a negative health outcome in regards to the behavior. Perceived susceptibility is how likely the individual thinks he or she is to be at risk. The perceived benefits

Table 3-3		
Health Belief Model		
Belief variable	**Definition**	**Application**
Perceived susceptibility	Belief of their risk for developing a certain condition	Define those at risk and their levels of risk; identify risk according to person, place, and time factors; heighten perceived susceptibility if too low
Perceived severity	Belief in the seriousness of the effects of a certain condition	Specify consequences of the risk and the condition
Perceived benefits	Belief in the positive results from adopting a certain behavior	Define action to take; how, where, when; clarify the positive effects to be expected
Perceived barriers	Belief about the negative consequences from adopting a certain behavior	Identify and reduce barriers through reassurance, incentives, assistance
Cues to action	Strategies to activate readiness	Provide how-to information, promote awareness, reminders
Self-efficacy	Confidence in one's ability to take action	Provide training, guidance in performing action

Data from Janz, NK, and Becker, MH (1984). The Health Belief Model: a decade later. Health Educ Q, 11(1), 1–47; Glanz, K, Marcus, LF, Rimer BK (1997). *Theory at a Glance: A Guide for Health Promotion Practice*. Bethesda, MD: National Cancer Institute.

are the positive outcomes an individual associates with performing or refraining from a behavior. Finally, perceived barriers are the inhibiting factors that an individual believes is prohibiting his or her engagement in a behavior.

To illustrate these perceptions, let us consider a screening for breast cancer. Perceived seriousness would reflect how serious a participant believes breast cancer to be. Perhaps the participant has had a close family member or friend die from breast cancer. This participant may view the seriousness of breast cancer to be more severe than a participant who has no connection to the disease. Next, the perceived susceptibility would be how likely the individual feels he or she is to develop breast cancer. If the participant's mother had breast cancer, she would likely believe herself to be at high risk for developing the disease. Participants who have no family history of breast cancer may believe themselves to be at low risk of developing breast cancer. The perceived benefits of this screening may vary according to how much the participant believes early detection can lead to better health outcomes. Lastly, barriers to the screening process may include cost, access, and the invasiveness of the screening. Participants who perceive many barriers will be less likely to seek out screening opportunities.

Interventions developed with this theory as its basis aim to adjust participants' perceptions to reflect reality. Continuing with the breast cancer example, this may mean developing an intervention in which participants walk away knowing how serious breast cancer is, how likely they are to develop it, the advantages and benefits of early detection, and the ease and availability of screening services in their area.

After these perceptions have been targeted, behavior change can be sustained. Cues to action remind participants to engage in their behavior change. A cue to action may be something such as a calendar reminder to make an appointment for a screening. Self-efficacy, a component found in multiple behavior change theories, is a measure of confidence a participant has in his or her ability to engage in a behavior. The goal of any behavior change intervention is to raise self-efficacy for the desired behavior.

Theory of Reasoned Action/Theory of Planned Behavior

The Theory of Reasoned Action was developed by Fishbein and Ajzen in 1975. It states that a person's behavior is determined by their intention to perform the behavior and that this intention is a function of their attitudes (i.e., sum of beliefs about a given behavior weighted by evaluations of these beliefs) and subjective norms (i.e., influence of people in a person's social environment on her behavioral intentions) toward the behavior (Fishbein & Ajzen, 1975). For example, you may believe that exercise is good for you and that it makes you look healthy, but that it takes time and is painful. Each of these beliefs may

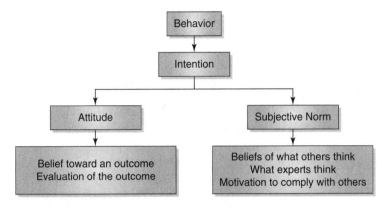

Figure 3-4 Flow model in the Theory of Reasoned Action

Modified from Ajzen, I, and Fishbein, M (1980). *Understanding attitudes and predicting social behavior.* Englewood Cliffs, NJ: Prentice-Hall.

be weighted to form an overall attitude about exercise. In addition, you may have friends who are sedentary, but your family members are avid exercisers. Weighing the importance of the behaviors of these individuals can influence your decision to exercise or not. Your attitudes and subjective norms about exercise, each with their respective weights, will influence your intention to exercise or not, which, in turn, will lead to the actual behavior. A flow model of the behavioral process in the Theory of Reasoned Action is shown in **Figure 3-4**.

The theory was subsequently expanded by Ajzen into the Theory of Planned Behavior (**Figure 3-5**). The extension adds another predictor to the model called *perceived behavioral control* to "account for times when people have the intention of carrying out a behavior, but the actual behavior is thwarted because they lack confidence or control over behavior" (Miller, 2005, p. 127).

Fishbein and Ajzen define beliefs as "a person's subjective probability judgments concerning some discriminable aspect of his world"

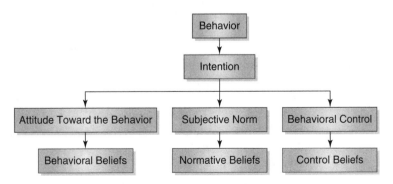

Figure 3-5 Flow model in the Theory of Planned Behavior

Modified from Ajzen, I (1991). The Theory of Planned Behavior. *Organizational Behavior and Human Decision Processes, 50*(2), 179–211.

(1975, p. 131). Beliefs can be formed by direct observation, inference, or an outside source. Belief development lies on a continuum with direct observation being more concrete and inference, on the other end of the continuum, being more abstract. Formation of beliefs via outside information leads to a more concrete belief, not too different from direct observation. Descriptive beliefs are ascertained by direct observation, while inferential beliefs are more likely to have been formed by past experience. Individual beliefs are the antecedent to individual attitudes. Some social psychologists maintain that beliefs do not differ much from attitude, but Fishbein posits that a belief concerns an individual's hypotheses about an object while attitudes are learned dispositions to an object (1967). Additionally, Fishbein suggests that beliefs are cognitive constructs, while attitudes are affective or related to motivation. For example, one would use likely/unlikely to measure a belief and harmful/beneficial to measure an attitude. Fishbein states that any belief about a certain object is a function of the individual's perception of the probability of the object existing or, in the case of relationships, the individual's perception of the probability of a relationship between an object and another object or concept. He further described "beliefs about the characteristics, qualities, or attributes of the object" (1967, p. 259).

While individual beliefs influence individual attitudes, *normative beliefs* influence the *subjective norm*. Normative beliefs refer to those beliefs of a collective group toward a behavior. These beliefs influence the subjective norm and can be viewed as pressures from a group or population to perform or not perform a behavior. In short, Fishbein and Ajzen describe beliefs as inferential or descriptive; cognitive rather than affective; and as an antecedent to attitude (1975). In the case of the Theory of Reasoned Action, beliefs are a combination of the belief regarding the outcome of a specific behavior and the individual's assessment of potential behavioral outcomes.

Fishbein and Ajzen (1974) did extensive evaluation of attitude formation and found more than 500 different measures for attitude. At the time they were developing the Theory of Reasoned Action, they reported that studies using more than one measure of attitude had different results about 70% of the time. They inferred that measures used at that time were unreliable. Fishbein (1967) reported on the history of the concept of attitude, stating that it first was studied in the mid-1800s. Many researchers describe the discipline of social psychology as the study of attitudes.

According to Fishbein and Ajzen (1974), the following characteristics are attributed to the attitude construct: (1) attitudes are typically stable—when attitude is measured, a person will give a similar response when presented with the same stimulus another time; (2) an attitude is a predisposition—a person is predisposed to have a favorable or unfavorable response toward a behavioral pattern; and (3) attitudes are learned or determined from past experience. However, Fishbein and Ajzen (1975) also assert that attitudes change over time as a person changes his or her belief system. According to the theorists, no more than five to nine beliefs contribute to an attitude, but this corollary appears to be conjecture and unmeasured.

Typically, theories are tested by individuals or researchers doing small-scale research before they are used in large-scale applications. The Centers for Disease Control and members of the Project Respect Study Group utilized the Theory of Reasoned Action for a large-scale intervention on HIV and other sexually transmitted diseases (Kamb et al., 1998). Participants in this trial (N = 5,758) who presented for sexually transmitted disease (STD) examinations were randomly assigned to four different arms. Participants in Arm 1 received enhanced counseling based on the Theory of Reasoned Action and the Social Cognitive Theory (E_1). The counseling sessions in this arm were aimed to change key constructs from the theories in individuals—self-efficacy, attitudes, and perceived norms. Participants in Arm 1 attended four sessions (session 1: 20 minutes; sessions 2–4: 60 minutes each) in which they were asked to devise their own personal risk-reduction plan and to work on behavior change. Participants assigned to Arm 2 (n = 1,447) also received theory-based counseling, but they attended only two, not four, sessions (E_2). In Arm 2, session 1 was identical to the Arm 1 enhanced session, and session 2 was 20 minutes of counseling and discussion of the HIV test. Participants in Arm 3 (n = 1,443) (E_3) and Arm 4 (n = 1,430) (E_4) received exclusively didactic messages.

The study outcomes were assessed when participants returned for follow-up visits every 3 months for 12 months. Outcomes were positive gonorrhea cultures, positive chlamydia tests, positive syphilis studies, and positive HIV tests. The key results are as follows: (1) 30% fewer participants at 6 months in both E_1 and E_2 counseling arms had STDs or HIV; and (2) 20% fewer participants at 12 months in both E_1 and E_2 had STDs or HIV. The results of this study support the Theory of Reasoned Action; both Arm 1/E_1 (enhanced counseling) and Arm 2/E_2 (brief counseling based on the theory constructs) showed improved outcomes.

A similar application was utilized among adolescents in Belize (Kinsler, Sneed, Morisky, & Ang, 2004). Researchers devised an intervention based on the Theory of Reasoned Action and the Social Cognitive Theory. Peer educators were selected to administer a theory-based intervention to half of the group. Seventy-five students from three schools received the intervention, while 75 students at three similar schools served as controls. The intervention consisted of a weekly 2-hour educational class over the course of 7 weeks. The classes were based on the Theory of Reasoned Action and the Social Cognitive

Theory. Sessions included discussion of attitudes toward condom use, normative beliefs of peers regarding sex and condom use, intention to use condoms, and self-efficacy. At the conclusion of the study, researchers determined that the intervention group was significantly more likely to have used condoms (4.84 versus 4.57 on a scale of 1–5); had significantly more positive attitudes toward condoms (2.33 versus 1.25 on a scale of 1–4); and was significantly more likely to express interest in using condoms in the future (3.83 versus 2.77 on a scale of 1–4). A serious limitation to the results regarding condom use and condom intention was that only respondents who had previously been sexually active (28 in the intervention group and 24 in the control group) were asked questions about condom use and condom use intention.

A summary of the factors and corresponding definitions that can influence behavior are presented in **Table 3-4**.

Stages of Change Model (Transtheoretical Model)
The Transtheoretical Model is based on a series of four core constructs that outline an individual's readiness and ability to change from not thinking about or considering the behavior to confidence in one's own ability to maintain a behavior (Prochaska & DiClemente, 2005). These core constructs are broken down into four areas: stages of change, processes of change, decisional balance, and self-efficacy.

The stages of change are broken down into five different stages: precontemplation, contemplation, preparation, action, and

Table 3-4	
Theory of Planned Behavior and Reasoned Action	
Belief variable	**Definition**
Subjective norm	An individual's perception of whether people will approve or disapprove of a certain behavior
Perceived behavioral control	An individual's perception of how difficult it will be to perform a certain behavior
Behavioral belief	An individual's perception about the outcomes of performing a certain behavior
Evaluation of behavioral outcome	Individuals evaluate the outcome of an action as either negative or positive, which influences the individuals' likelihood to perform that action
Normative beliefs	An individual's beliefs about whether people who are important to him or her will approve or disapprove of performing a certain behavior
Control beliefs	An individual's belief about his or her likelihood of confronting certain barriers and/or the facilitators for performing a certain behavior
Perceived power	An individual's belief about how difficult or easy each barrier or facilitating condition will make performing a certain behavior

Data from Ajzen, I, and Fishbein, M (1980). *Understanding attitudes and predicting social behavior.* Englewood Cliffs, NJ: Prentice-Hall; Ajzen, I (1985). From intentions to actions: A theory of planned behavior. In J. Kuhl & J. Beckmann (Eds.), *Action control: From cognition to behavior.* Berlin, Heidelberg, New York: Springer-Verlag; Ajzen, I (1991). The Theory of Planned Behavior. *Organizational Behavior and Human Decision Processes, 50*(2), 179-211.

maintenance. *Precontemplation* describes the first stage in which the individual is not yet ready or has not considered making a change in favor of a new or healthier behavior. In the *contemplation* stage, an individual is more aware of the benefits of changing their behavior, and they intend to make this change in the future, usually within 6 months. In the third stage, *preparation*, an individual is prepared to make a behavior change within 30 days and is getting ready for the change. This can include telling friends and family about the intention to change a behavior. In perhaps the most challenging stage, *action*, individuals must work to change their behavior. They must work to understand what triggers bad behavior and reward themselves for maintaining a positive behavior change. *Maintenance* is the final stage and is characterized by an individual who has committed to a behavior change for 6 months. During this stage it is important to not accidently fall back into old unhealthy behaviors.

The processes of change include 10 cognitive shifts that occur during the stages of change. These shifts facilitate behavior change. By better understanding the processes of change, enabling changes in a particular behavior can be better understood. The 10 processes of change are outlined in **Table 3-5**.

Table 3-5	
Ten Processes of Change	
Process of change	**Definition**
Consciousness raising	Seeking new information by increasing knowledge surrounding the behavior
Counterconditioning	Replacing the problem behavior with a new behavior
Dramatic relief	Communicating one's feelings toward the problem behavior and expressing a desire to change
Environmental reevaluation	Determining how the behavior affects both one's physical and social environment
Helping relationships	Gaining support and encouragement from peers
Reinforcement management	Using positive reinforcement/rewards to encourage good behavior
Self-liberation	Feeling as though one can and wants to change
Self-reevaluation	Cognitively reassessing one's views and understanding toward the behavior
Social liberation	An individual's acceptance of prosocial, positive behaviors
Stimulus control	Recognizing what aspects of one's social or physical environment trigger the problem behavior and determining ways to control or avoid these triggers

Data from Prochaska, JO, Velicer, WF, DiClemente, CC, Fava, J (1988). Measuring processes of change: applications to the cessation of smoking. *Journal of Consulting and Clinical Psychology, 56*(4), 520–528; Prochaska, JO and DiClemente, CC (1983). Stages and processes of self-change of smoking: toward an integrative model of change. *Journal of Consulting and Clinical Psychology, 51*(3), 390–395.

The decisional balance refers to the pros and cons to any behavior change that an individual must consider. Typically, the cons will outweigh the pros for an individual in the precontemplation stage. However, as an individual moves through the stages of change, the pros will outweigh the cons. This helps motivate and encourage behavior change. As seen in the Health Belief Model, it also employs a measure of self-efficacy. By measuring participants' self-efficacy both before and after an intervention, the effectiveness of the intervention can be assessed, and the likelihood that a behavior change will persist can be predicted.

INTERPERSONAL-LEVEL THEORIES

Social Cognitive Theory

Social Cognitive Theory outlines the idea that people tend to imitate what they see (Bandura, 2001). These social influences can be very direct, in the form of family and friends, or less direct, in the form of media influences. John Dollard and Neal E. Miller developed this theory in the 1940s. In the original theory, Miller and Dollard identified four factors in behavior: drives, cues, responses, and rewards. This theory was further expanded in the now well-known study conducted by Albert Bandura. In order to observe this concept, he had children observe then play with a Bobo doll. Children who observed gentle play tended to be gentler when given their chance to play. Those who observed violence toward the Bobo doll tended to act violently toward the doll (Bandura, Ross, & Ross, 1961).

Social Cognitive Theory develops the idea of interplay among the individual, the environment, and behavior. The individual refers to the person performing the behavior and their beliefs, cognitive abilities, and self-efficacy. The environment is the social and physical surroundings in which an individual makes observations. Behavior is then developed as interplay among these various factors. Interventions can thus be developed to target one of these three core elements.

COMMUNITY-LEVEL THEORIES

Diffusion of Innovation

The theory of diffusion of innovation seeks to explain the way a new idea spreads through a community or population. Everett Rodgers first developed this theory in 1962 with his book Diffusion of Innovation (Rogers, 1962). This concept points to four main factors that influence the rate and spread of an idea: innovation (the conception of a new idea), communication channels, time, and social system.

Communication channels and time are interrelated in that the diffusion of any new idea or innovation takes time to be communicated to the community. The process and timing of adoption is broken down into five steps. In the first step, *knowledge*, the individual is introduced to the idea but does not seek more information. During *persuasion*, the individual actively seeks information regarding the new idea. In the *decision* stage, the individual decides if he or she will ultimately accept or reject the innovation. Next, the individual engages in *implementation*, which eventually leads to *confirmation* in which the decision to adopt the new idea is finalized.

Social systems are any community or network of people through which an idea is transmitted. Adopters of a new idea are divided into six categories. *Innovators* are the first to adopt a new idea or innovation. They tend to be young, have financial resources, belong to the highest social class, and be willing to take risks. Next to adopt a new idea are *early adopters*. These people tend to share many of the same characteristics as the innovators. They also serve as opinion leaders in the community. *Opinion leaders* are community members who are influential in spreading positive or negative ideas regarding a new innovation. The *early majority* tends to be of average social status and have contact with early adopters. They adopt a new innovation slower than the innovators and early adopters. The *late majority* is very skeptical of any new innovation and has fewer financial resources than the preceding groups. The final group to adopt an innovation is the *laggards*. Laggards are often the oldest members of society and have a strong preference to tradition over change. These members of society generally have contact only with close friends and family.

Understanding how an innovation spreads through a community is important for those trying to market a new idea. Advertising can be targeted to whichever group is next in line to adopt an innovation. Skipping any one group and trying to target a group later in the chain of transmission proves to be unsuccessful. Health professionals can use this theory to better understand how health practices and behaviors are adopted on a community-wide level.

PLANNING MODELS

Precede–Proceed

The Precede–Proceed Model is highly favored in academia but is not often used in practice. Developed in 1974 by Dr. Lawrence W. Green, this model has two elements. The first element is the Precede portion. Considered the "education diagnosis" phase, Precede stands for predisposing, reinforcing, and enabling constructs in educational diagnosis and evaluation. Second is the "ecological diagnosis" or Proceed portion (Green & Kreuter, 2005, p. 9). Proceed stands for policy, regulatory, and organizational constructs in educational and environmental development (2005, p. 9). This model provides a framework through which programs and interventions can be analyzed and assessed on the basis of their costs and benefits.

The Precede portion of this model focuses on community diagnostics. By better understanding the predisposing, reinforcing, and enabling constructs present in the community, an intervention can be better developed. Predisposing factors are the beliefs, attitudes, and knowledge present in the community. Reinforcing factors are those that reward or punish a given behavior, and enabling factors are the presence or absence of factors that allow a behavior or action to be performed. For example, a person may know that exercising is essential in maintaining a healthy heart and weight. However, the individual may see little reward in weekly exercises and is not currently concerned about the health of his or her heart. Additionally, there are no sidewalks or nearby parks that enable exercise to be a part of everyday life. Assessing these constructs helps tailor an appropriate health intervention. For this individual and community, knowledge regarding exercise is not lacking. However, motivation and accessibility are lacking. The Proceed portion of the model involves the implementation and evaluation of the program.

Both the Precede and Proceed portion of this model are broken down into four phases. The phases of the Precede model are as follows: (1) social diagnosis; (2) epidemiologic, behavioral, and environmental diagnosis; (3) educational and ecologic diagnosis; and (4) administrative and policy diagnosis. Next, the phases of the Proceed model continue forward based on the conclusions of the Precede phases. These phases are as follows: (5) implementation; (6) process evaluation; (7) impact evaluation; and (8) outcome evaluation. Descriptions of theses phases can be found in **Table 3-6**.

Table 3-6			
Phases of the Precede–Proceed Model			
Precede		**Proceed**	
Phase 1: Social diagnosis	Program planners, community members, and other relevant stakeholders assess and discuss the social factors that impact the community's health and well-being.	Phase 5: Implementation	The program, developed from the information gathered in the previous four phases, is put into practice.
Phase 2: Epidemiologic, behavioral, and environmental diagnosis		Phase 6: Process evaluation	An analysis of the program is done to assess and confirm that the program is following protocol and meeting objectives.

Table 3-6 (Continued)

Phases of the Precede–Proceed Model

Precede	Proceed	
Phase 3: Educational and ecologic diagnosis	Phase 7: Impact evaluation	The effectiveness of the program is measured, and the changes in the predisposing, enabling, and enforcing constructs are assessed. This phase focuses on intermediate objects and the effectiveness of the educators.
Phase 4: Administrative and policy diagnosis	Phase 8: Outcome evaluation	The change in individual behavior and the overall impact on community health and well-being is measured.

Data from Green, LW, and Kreuter, MW. (2005). *Health Promotion Planning: an Educational and Ecological Approach.* 4th ed. Mountain View, CA: Mayfield Publishers.

Summary

1. The six dimensions of health are physical, mental, social, emotional, spiritual, and environmental.
2. Health behavior is an individual-level effort to achieve these same goals of disease prevention, prolonged life, and the promotion of the six dimensions of health.
3. Public health is a societal effort to prevent disease, prolong life, and promote the six interactive dimensions of health in the community.
4. The three core functions of public health are assessment, policy development, and assurance.
5. Primary prevention strategies seek to avoid the biological onset of disease and, therefore, tend to target the general population. Prevention at this basic level has to be behaviorally directed and lifestyle oriented. Efforts at the primary prevention level focus on influencing individual behavior and protecting the environment.
6. The Health Impact Pyramid is a five-tier pyramid that describes different types of public health interventions. The base of the pyramid consists of interventions addressing socioeconomic factors; the second level of the pyramid is changing the context to make individuals' default decisions healthy; the third level of the pyramid is long-lasting protective interventions; the fourth level is clinical interventions; and the top of the pyramid is health education and counseling.
7. Health education is a relatively new discipline, which was defined by Green and Kreuter as "any combination of learning experiences designed to facilitate voluntary action conducive to health" (1999, p. 27).
8. Health promotion has a more recent origin than health education. It includes health education and also social, economic, and environmental conditions that can positively influence public health. Green and Kreuter defined health promotion as "the combination of educational and environmental supports for actions and conditions of living conducive the health" (1991, p. 4).

9. Health behavior theories assume that several behaviors are modifiable and teachable. Several health behavior theories have been developed in the past 50 years or so to help explain individual-level, interpersonal-level, and community-level behaviors.

10. In the Precede–Proceed model, Precede stands for predisposing, reinforcing, and enabling constructs in educational diagnosis and evaluation. Proceed stands for policy, regulatory, and organizational constructs in educational and environmental development. The model provides a framework through which programs and interventions can be analyzed and assessed on the basis of their costs and benefits.

References

Ajzen, I. (1985). From intentions to actions: A theory of planned behavior. In J. Kuhl & J. Beckmann (Eds.), *Action control: From cognition to behavior.* New York: Springer-Verlag.

Ajzen, I. (1991). The theory of planned behavior. *Organizational Behavior and Human Decision Processes, 50*(2), 179–211.

Ajzen, I., & Fishbein, M. (1980). *Understanding attitudes and predicting social behavior.* Englewood Cliffs, NJ: Prentice-Hall.

Arias, E. (2014). United States life tables, 2009. *National Vital Statistics Reports, 62*(7). Hyattsville, MD: National Center for Health Statistics.

Bandura, A. (2001). Social cognitive theory: An agentic perspective. *Annual Review of Psychology, 52*(1), 1–26.

Bandura, A., Ross, D., & Ross, S. A. (1961). Transmission of aggression through the imitation of aggressive models. *Journal of Abnormal and Social Psychology, 63*(3), 575–582.

Bunker, J. P., Frazier, H. S., & Mosteller, F. (1994). Improving health: Measuring effects of medical care. *Milbank Quarterly, 72,* 225–258.

Centers for Disease Control and Prevention. (1999a). Ten great public health achievements—United States, 1900–1999. *Morbidity and Mortality Weekly Report, 48*(12), 241–243.

Centers for Disease Control and Prevention. (1999b). Achievements in public health, 1900–1999: Control of infectious disease. *Morbidity and Mortality Weekly Report, 48*(29), 621–629.

Centers for Disease Control and Prevention. (1999c). Improvements in workplace safety—United States, 1990–1999. *Morbidity and Mortality Weekly Report, 48*(22): 461–469.

Centers for Disease Control and Prevention. (2011). Ten great public health achievements—United States, 2001–2012. *Morbidity and Mortality Weekly Report, 60*(19), 619–623.

Costa, D. L. (2003). Causes of improving health and longevity at older ages: A review of the explanations. *Genus, LXI*(1), 21–38.

Derryberry, M. (1960). Health education: Its objectives and methods. *Health Education Monographs, 8,* 5–11.

DiClemente, R. J., Crosby, R. A., & Kegler, M. C. (2003). Emerging theories in health promotion practice and research: Strategies for improving public health. *Health Promotion Practice, 4,* 377–378.

Dutta-Bergman, M. (2005). Theory and practice in health communication campaigns: A critical interrogation. *Health Communication, 18*(2), 103–122.

Environmental Protection Agency. (2003). National air quality and emissions trends report: 2003 special studies edition. Retrieved from http://www.epa.gov/airtrends/aqtrnd03/pdfs/toc_figs_tables.pdf

Fishbein, M. (1967). *Readings in attitude theory and measurement.* New York, NY: Wiley.

Fishbein, M., & Ajzen, I. (1974). Attitudes towards objects as predictors of single and multiple behavioral criteria. *Psychological Review, 81*(1), 59–74.

Fishbein, M., & Ajzen, I. (1975). *Belief, attitude, intention, and behavior: An introduction to theory and research.* Reading, MA: Addison-Wesley.

Frieden, T. R. (2010). A framework for public health action: The health impact pyramid. *American Journal of Public Health, 100*(4), 590–595.

Garrison, F. H. (1926). *History of medicine.* Philadelphia, PA: Saunders.

Glanz, K., & Rimer, B. K. (1995). *Theory at a glance: A guide to health promotion practice.* Bethesda, MD: National Cancer Institute.

Goldman, L., & Cook, E. F. (1984). The decline in ischemic heart disease mortality rates: An analysis of the comparative effects of medical interventions and changes in lifestyle. *Annals of Internal Medicine, 101*(6), 825–836.

Goodarz, D., Ding, E. L., Mozaffarian, D., Taylor, B., Rehm, J., Murray, C. J. L., & Ezzati, M. (2009). Preventable causes of death in the United States: Comparative risk assessment of dietary, lifestyle, and metabolic risk factors. *PLoS Medicine, 8*(1), e1000058. doi:10.1371/journal.pmed.1000058

Green, L. W. (1974). Toward cost-benefit evaluations of health education: Some concepts, methods, and examples. *Health Education Monographs, 2*(2), 34–64.

Green, L. W., & Kreuter, M. W. (1991). *Health promotion planning: An educational and environmental approach* (2nd ed.). Mountain View, CA: Mayfield.

Green, L. W., & Kreuter, M. W. (1999). *Health promotion planning: An educational and ecological approach* (3rd ed.). Mountain View, CA: Mayfield.

Green, L. W., & Kreuter, M. W. (2005). *Health promotion planning: An educational and ecological approach* (4th ed.). Mountain View, CA: Mayfield.

Green, L. W., Kreuter, M. W., Partridge, K., & Deeds, S. (1980). *Health education planning: A diagnostic approach.* Mountain View, CA: Mayfield.

Griffiths, W. (1972). Health education definitions, problems, and philosophies. *Health Education Monographs, 31*, 12–14.

Hunink, M. G. M., Goldman, L., Tosteron, A., Mittleman, M. A., Goldman, P. A., Williams, L. W., … Weinstien, M. (1997). The recent decline in mortality from coronary heart disease 1980–1990: The effect of secular trends in risk factors and treatment. *JAMA, 227*, 535–542.

Janz, N. K., & Becker, M. H. (1984). The Health Belief Model: A decade later. *Health Education Quarterly, 11*(1), 1–47.

Kamb, M. L., Fishbein, M., Douglas, J. M., Jr., Rhodes, F., Rogers, J., Bolan, G., … Project Respect Study Group. (1998). Efficacy of risk-reduction counseling to prevent human immunodeficiency virus and sexually transmitted diseases: A randomized controlled trial. *JAMA, 280*(13), 1161–1167.

Keusch, G. T. (2003). The history of nutrition: Malnutrition, infection and immunity. *Journal of Nutrition, 133*(1), 336S–340S.

Khaw, K., Wareham, N., Bingham, S., Welch, A., Luben, R., & Day, N. (2008). Combined impact of health behaviours and mortality in men and women: The EPIC-Norfolk prospective population study. *PLoS Medicine, 5*(1), E12.

Kinsler, J., Sneed, C. D., Morisky, D. E., & Ang, A. (2004). Evaluation of a school-based intervention for HIV/AIDS prevention among Belizean adolescents. *Health Education Research*, 19(6), 730–738.

Last, J. M. (2007). Miasma theory. In *A dictionary of public health*. Westminster College, PA: Oxford University Press.

McKeown, T. (1976). *The modern rise of population*. New York, NY: Academic Press.

McKinlay, J. B., & McKinlay, S. M. (1997). The questionable contribution of medical measures to the decline of mortality in the United States in the twentieth century. *Milbank Memorial Fund Quarterly: Health and Society*, 55(3), 405–428.

McLeroy, K. R., Bibeau, D., Steckler, A., & Glanz, K. (1988). An ecological perspective on health promotion programs. *Health Education Quarterly*, 15, 351–377.

Merrill, R. M. (2013). *Introduction to epidemiology* (6th ed.). Burlington, MA: Jones & Bartlett Learning.

Miller, K. (2005). *Communications theories: Perspectives, processes, and contexts*. New York, NY: McGraw-Hill.

Novick, L. F. (2008). The continuing first revolution in public health: Infectious disease. *Journal of Public Health Management and Practice*, 14(5), 418–419.

Preston, S. H., & Haines, M. (1991). *Fatal years: Child mortality in late nineteenth century American*. Princeton, NJ: Princeton University Press.

Prochaska, J. O., & DiClemente, C. C. (1983). Stages and processes of self-change of smoking: Toward an integrative model of change. *Journal of Consulting and Clinical Psychology*, 51(3), 390–395.

Prochaska, J. O., & DiClemente, C. C. (2005). The transtheoretical approach. In J. D. Norcross & M. R. Goldfried (Eds.), *Handbook of psychotherapy integration* (2nd ed., pp. 147–171). New York, NY: Oxford University Press.

Prochaska, J. O., Velicer, W. F., DiClemente, C. C., & Fava, J. (1988). Measuring processes of change: Applications to the cessation of smoking. *Journal of Consulting and Clinical Psychology*, 56(4), 520–528.

Riley, J. C. (2001). *Rising life expectancy: A global history*. New York, NY: Cambridge University Press.

Rogers, E. M. (1962). *Diffusion of innovations*. Glencoe, IL: Free Press.

Roggero, P., Mangiaterra, V., Bustero, F., & Rosuti, F. (2007). The health impact of child labor in developing countries: Evidence from cross-country data. *American Journal of Public Health*, 97(2), 271–275.

Rosen, G. (1993). *A history of public health* (Expanded ed.). Baltimore, MD: Johns Hopkins University Press.

Rosenstock, I. M. (1974). Historical origins of the health belief model. *Health Education Quarterly*, 2, 328–335.

Sigerist, H. E. (1956). *Landmarks in the history of hygiene*. London, UK: Oxford University Press.

Stokols, D. (1992). Establishing and maintaining healthy environments: Toward a social ecology of health promotion. *American Psychologist*, 47, 6–22.

Whitlock, E. P., Orleans, C. T., Pender, N., & Allan, J. (2002). Evaluating primary care behavioral counseling interventions: An evidence-based approach. *American Journal of Preventive Medicine*, 22(4), 267–284.

World Bank. (2001). Life expectancy. Retrieved from http://www.worldbank.org/depweb/english/modules/social/life/chart1.html

World Bank. (2014). Indicators. Retrieved from http://data.worldbank.org/indicator/

World Health Organization. (1948). Constitution of the World Health Organization. Retrieved from http://apps.who.int/gb/bd/PDF/bd47/EN/constitution-en.pdf

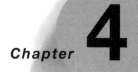

Determinants of Behavior

B ehavioral epidemiology is the study of personal behaviors (the manner of conducting oneself), how these behaviors influence health-related states or events in human populations, and how behaviors can be modified to prevent and control health problems. To modify behaviors that can influence health outcomes, it is necessary to understand the laws and principles that underlie a person's behavior (i.e., behaviorism). Basic research in the behavioral sciences attempts to understand causes and effects of human behavior. The causes of human behavior may be biological, psychological, and social. The focus of this chapter will be on the causes of human behavior. Specifically, this chapter will address some of the reasons why people behave the way they do, why people continue to engage in bad habits, even when trying to stop them, why it is easy to change some behaviors and very difficult to change others, why some behaviors seem to come automatically while others occur only with concentrated focus, and why some causes of behavior are easy to identify while others seem impossible to understand.

Cause and Effect

The definition of epidemiology includes the study of determinants (causes) of health-related states or events in human populations. This is because by identifying and understanding the process by which certain exposures, conditions, or behaviors are associated with adverse health outcomes, a strategy can be followed to prevent and control the health problem. Health education and promotion are ways to influence intentions and behaviors, which, in turn, can prevent disease, prolong life, and improve health. Thus, in behavioral epidemiology we are interested in not just studying the relationship between behaviors and health, but in understanding the factors that influence behavior. The connection among biological, psychological, and social factors to human health behaviors is based on causal inference. Whereas *statistical inference* involves reaching a conclusion about a population based on information from a sample and using probability to indicate the level of reliability of that conclusion, *causal inference* involves making conclusions about associations among variables based on lists of criteria or conditions applied to the results of scientific studies. Causal inference considers the totality of evidence in making a judgment about causality (Weed, 1995). Causal inferences provide a scientific basis for understanding behavior.

A statistical association that is not explained by bias, chance, or confounding does not mean an association is causal. For example, in the 1700s, life expectancy in the United States was less than 50 years. Today, life expectancy is about 80 years. Because people did not have the Internet in the 1700s, but today most people do, can we say that the Internet has extended life expectancy? No. The explanation is likely due to higher infant mortality, higher rates of women dying during childbirth, and higher rates of infectious disease in the 1700s.

For each of us, we infer that something is true or highly probable based on our expectations and experiences. We may exercise every day because we expect it will help our mental and physical health, or we may brush our teeth because we expect it will save us a painful experience at the dentist. Inference in epidemiology is similar to inference in daily life in that it also is based on expectations and experience; however, in science, expectations are referred to as hypotheses, theories, or predictions, and experiences are called results, observations, or data. Inference in everyday life serves as a basis for action (Weed, 1995). In a similar manner, causal inferences provide a scientific basis for human behavior.

The inferences we personally make are informal and based on expectations about a given event, reasons for its existence, and experience with similar situations. In contrast, scientists typically base their inferences on the application of formal methods. For instance, on the basis of sample data, we may draw certain conclusions about the population. Probability is used to indicate the level of reliability in the conclusion. Sample techniques are used to obtain a representative sample, and data are evaluated using statistical methods.

Some causes of our behaviors are engaged in consciously, easily identified, and clearly linked to expected outcomes. We push on gas pedals to accelerate a vehicle, we eat to satisfy hunger, and we hug someone to show affection. Behaviors with clear causal connections are readily understood and often easy to alter. To stop at a traffic light, we release the gas pedal and push on the brake pedal to decelerate a vehicle; to avoid heartburn, we stop eating when we are full; to express disapproval, we raise our voice.

Decision Making

The process of making a decision consists of the four elements shown in **Figure 4-1**. This figure illustrates the relationships among four elements, the individual, and the environment. Two of the elements that take place within a person's mind, behavioral intention and the decision to act, are therefore affected by personal factors, which describe traits of an individual during a specific time period. Personal factors are identified and measured by a wide range of physical, mental, emotional, and demographic variables. All four elements, along with the individual, will always be located within an identifiable environment that will have a complement of environmental factors. These factors describe the traits of the environment during a specified time frame and are measured by a wide range of physical, social, cultural, and political variables. Environmental factors may impact all four elements of behavioral decision making, as well as the relationships among the four elements.

The connection among intention, decision, behavior, and outcome is not always clear or easy to understand. In reference to Figure 4-1, negative outcomes can occur during any part of the causal

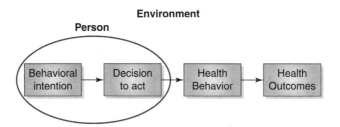

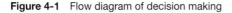

Figure 4-1 Flow diagram of decision making

connection. We can select a harmful intention, a poor decision, an unsafe health behavior, or a negative health outcome. For example, we may choose to get drunk or to hurt the feelings of someone we are angry with. However, we often select negative intentions, behaviors, or outcomes unconsciously. Habits often fall into this category. Anytime you ask yourself why you did something you are reflecting on a behavior with no clear intention. Buyer's remorse is an example of a negative intention that is realized after the fact. Why did I buy that when I did not have that money to spend?

We can also be mistaken or unaware of the association among intentions, decisions, behaviors, and outcomes. For example, we may select a vegetarian diet with the intention of reducing the risk of heart disease, but we end up gaining weight and increasing blood cholesterol if the diet is not undertaken correctly. To confuse things even further, decisions are often complicated by competing intentions and incomplete information. We may yell at a misbehaving child with the intention of making her stop, but yelling rarely makes a child more agreeable. When making behavioral decisions, we often must weigh a number of competing intentions and respond without much time to analyze expected outcomes. These behaviors are much more difficult to understand and to change in a conscious manner.

Behavioral decisions are never made in a vacuum. We must constantly weigh competing intentions and revise our information about behavioral effects. So how do we become better decision makers? Behavioral epidemiology identifies those factors that are most influential in the causal pathway from intention to outcomes. In this chapter, we will focus on behavioral determinants, which are defined as variables that influence where, when, how, and why people engage in specific behaviors. The purpose of behavioral epidemiology is to understand the causal connection among intention, decision, behavior, and outcome for improving health behaviors and, consequently, preventing disease, prolonging life, and contributing to the six dimensions of health. The remainder of this chapter describes common behavioral determinants that influence health behaviors.

What Is a Behavioral Determinant?

Many factors can exert an influence on health behaviors. As these factors are identified, they will naturally fall into one of two groups. The first group includes variables that influence behavior and are directly modifiable. These qualify as behavioral determinants because they can function as the catalyst that ultimately changes the health behavior pathway. The second group includes variables that influence behavior, but they are not directly modifiable. These variables cannot function as behavioral determinants because they cannot serve as the catalyst that alters the health behavior pathway.

The first group includes variables that are both *influential* and *directly modifiable* by health promotion activities. These are the most important variables because they have the potential to respond to health promotion interventions, and, therefore, they influence the Health Behavior Pathway. Think of the behavioral influence variable as the first in a series of dominoes that is knocked over to ultimately achieve a health outcome goal. As the behavioral influence is improved, it should create a cascade of effects, whereby behavior intention improves, decision to act improves, behavior improves, and finally outcomes improve. It is important to keep this causal pathway in mind when exploring behavioral influences.

The second group of variables will have some influence on the Health Behavior Pathway but will not be directly alterable by health promotion activities. These variables should not be targeted as behavioral influences in health promotion activities, but they can still be useful in intervention design. Physiological variables and demographic variables often fall into this category. These types of variables may influence the Health Behavior Pathway, but they cannot be directly altered by health education and promotion interventions. Physiological variables often relate to genetics, disease states, or biological systems. They might be changed indirectly, as the final result of an intervention, but that means they are functioning as outcome variables, not behavioral influence variables.

To illustrate, consider the following example, and refer to Figure 4-1. Stanley has diabetes and a mild form of autism. Both of these conditions could be considered physiological variables, and both affect his cognitive capacity to make informed, rational decisions about fruit and vegetable consumption. Providing Stanley with education about nutrition would have no impact on his autism, so despite that variable's impact on his cognitive ability, it would not be useful in our attempts to improve his nutritional status. In other words, targeting Stanley's autism would not produce the cascade of changes needed to improve his health outcomes. Providing Stanley with nutrition education may ultimately help him manage his diabetes, but only indirectly. Stanley's diabetes status could only be improved after some other factor was identified to improve his nutrition-related intentions, decisions, and behaviors. Therefore, even though his disease state may affect his cognitive abilities, it cannot function as a behavioral determinant for the purposes of behavioral interventions. It is only useful as a health outcome variable because it can only be improved indirectly through the Health Behavior Pathway, at the end of the line of dominoes. Since the whole point of identifying behavioral influences is to identify specific variables that can be directly altered by health promotion activities, most physiological factors would not be appropriate behavioral influences to target.

Demographic variables are similar to physiological variables in that they cannot be altered directly by health education or promotion. Continuing with our previous example, no education that we could provide would alter Stanley's age, gender, sexuality, or race. Education might have an impact on things Stanley can choose to alter, like religion, education, or income level, but these things are extremely difficult and time consuming to change. Raising a person's income above the poverty level, for example, requires considerable resources and, ultimately, it is unclear exactly how that would influence a desired change in health behavior. There are also ethical issues involved. Would it be appropriate to ask Stanley to change his religion in the name of changing his eating habits?

Table 4-1 explains in further detail the differences between unmodifiable and modifiable characteristics, and how these factors apply to research and behavioral interventions. It is important to note that behaviors, much like diseases, have multiple causes. There may be several factors in place before a behavior occurs, and there may be various combinations of risk factors for any one behavior to arise. For example, a person may be more likely to consume large quantities of cheeseburgers if they live in an environment with easy access to inexpensive fast food. The built environment, genetics, and the social environment all contain factors that influence behavior. Other factors include the way we were raised and our emotional state (McGraw-Hill, 2008).

Table 4-1		
Unmodifiable and Modifiable Types, Explanations, and Applications		
Type	**Explanation**	**Application to research**
Unmodifiable	Characteristics that cannot be changed about an individual, such as age and family history	Study of these factors can contribute to understanding etiology and identifying particular subgroups that may benefit, more or less, from interventions targeted at modifiable risk factors
Modifiable, but no prevention and control targets	Characteristics that can be changed, but are not targets for change, because recommending changes may be impractical or controversial, such as occupation, geographic residence, or parity	Study of these factors can contribute to understanding etiology and identifying particular subgroups that may benefit more or less from interventions targeted at modifiable risk factors
Modifiable, with prevention and control targets	Characteristics that can be realistically changed; the change is associated with an improvement in health or prevention of disease, such as smoking or condom use	Study of these factors can contribute to understanding etiology of disease and developing behavior-targeted interventions

If these types of variables are not as useful as behavioral influences, how are they useful in designing health promotion interventions? The answer is that they are often used as grouping variables to assess *health disparities* or *relative risk* among different groups of people. These groupings guide intervention planning strategies by identifying groups of people with shared identifiable traits that influence their relative risk for specified health outcomes. For example, recent research has found that women are more likely than men to engage in protected sex. To reduce this disparity, the appropriate action would not be to convince all men to be surgically altered to become women. Instead, we would conduct further research to identify the modifiable factors in men that lead to their lower use of safe sex practices. After they are identified, intervention strategies can be better tailored for men, in addition to women.

Taxonomy of Behavioral Determinants

What variables should be explored to identify behavioral determinants, which are both influential and modifiable? Identifying behavioral determinants is absolutely critical for ultimately changing behavior for the improvement of health outcomes. Without identifying behavioral determinants, we have no way of knowing how to change behaviors that adversely affect health. Why does Steve eat fried foods, even after balloon angioplasty with stents? Why does Betty still not exercise, even after joining a nearby gym? Why does Stan still refuse to use a condom, even after he contracted gonorrhea? To find answers to these questions, behavioral epidemiologists must first specify, identify, and measure variables that have potential for being important behavioral determinants. So how does a researcher know what variables to measure when trying to identify important behavioral determinants? In some cases, these variables may have been discovered by previous research or by experience. In other cases, important variables have yet to be identified. Either way, classifying common behavioral determinants will help the researcher narrow the field of variables to include in a given study.

Using the Health Behavior Pathway model, behavioral determinants can be grouped first into two primary categories: personal factors and environmental factors.

■ *Personal factors* are those person-related characteristics that vary from one individual to the next and can be measured or categorized. Epidemiologic studies usually concentrate on major demographic characteristics of the person (e.g., age, gender, race/ethnicity, marital and family status, occupation, and education). However, other variables that characterize persons that can be considered when assessing behavior include inherent factors (disease or injury status, organizational productivity, task orientation, recall memory, recognition memory, emotional status, spiritual traits, and achievement). Comparing health behaviors according to these characteristics, and their combinations, can help explain the behaviors.

■ From a practical point of view, the traits used to describe the person aspects of epidemiology are limited according to the purpose and resources of concern to a particular study or investigation. Information already available from common sources, such as public health departments and government agencies, and information gathered from the investigation should be used. Survey data and medical records are also good sources of person-related factors.

■ *Environmental factors* are external to the human host, such as physical and psychosocial conditions. Several physical and psychosocial environmental factors can influence behavior. For example, physical stresses, such as excessive heat or cold, or environmental disruptions (e.g., floods, droughts, earthquakes, fires, and tsunamis), can influence exercise, diet, and personal hygiene. Psychosocial environmental factors include socioeconomic status, social networks and social support, neighborhoods and communities, formal institutions, and public policy. Several studies have shown how these factors can influence health behaviors.

■ Environmental factors vary across geographic regions. Within regions, individuals share environmental factors, but their responses may differ. A single study may include more than one environment, and the researcher needs to be careful to define the environments being assessed. For example, suppose you want to measure the effects of cigarette availability and the enforcement of bans to sell cigarettes to minors in two small towns. Since each town has its own set of cigarette vendors and its own independent police force, each town should be defined as a distinct environment. One town would have one measure for availability and enforcement, and the other town would have another measure of availability and enforcement.

Each of these two major categories—personal factors and environmental factors—comprises other types of variables. The following sections describe many variables that often function as behavioral determinants. They can be used to help identify variables that can be explored in behavioral epidemiology research. They are not meant to be exhaustive; instead, they provide a starting point for effective research design.

Common Behavioral Determinants

PERSONAL FACTORS

Awareness and Knowledge

Awareness is knowledge or perception of a situation or fact. In relation to health behavior, it refers to a person's conscious recognition of the triggers, patterns, and consequences of engaging in a specified behavior. This conscious recognition is critical to promoting healthy behavior change because it is the first step for an individual to regain purposeful control over his or her behavioral patterns. When people are not aware of the where, when, how, or why, they may be more likely to engage in a behavior and not exercise control over the behavior. They may be on autopilot, which can contribute to being more susceptible to a host of negative health influences.

When exploring awareness as a behavioral influence, it must be defined as awareness of something, and there can be multiple awareness-related variables included in a single study. For example, if we want to discover why an individual refuses to cover her mouth when she coughs, we might ask if she is aware of where, when, or how often she engages in this behavior. We might ask if she is aware of the health risks posed to others because of her behavior. We might also ask if she is aware of other coughing response behaviors available to her. All of these awareness factors should be explored to determine the levels and types of awareness related to the coughing behavior. Awareness factors should be one of the first influences explored in any study focusing on behavior because they are influential and modifiable. In fact, awareness variables are often the easiest to modify through health education and promotion efforts.

Knowledge refers to facts, information, and skills acquired by a person through experience and education—the theoretical or practical understanding of a subject (Knowledge, 2014). Knowledge differs from other personal factors in its verifiable objectivity. In health behavior research, knowledge variables will usually reflect a person's understanding about the relationship between a given health behavior and its expected outcomes. After awareness in the cognitive process, the next step is behavioral decision making. A person may be aware of his or her behavioral triggers, patterns, and consequences, but that is rarely enough to alter behavioral patterns. Without specific knowledge of how and why a behavior relates to health outcomes, a person may not know how to adequately conceptualize behavioral alternatives. For example, suppose an individual is aware that eating fried foods is linked to increased risk of heart disease. However, he doesn't know how this relationship works. Because of this, he relies on food marketing messages for choosing heart-healthy foods. He purposefully avoids fried foods, but he continues to eat many other highly processed foods with low fat and high levels of sodium. He is surprised when his dietary change has actually increased his blood pressure. His lack of knowledge about why fried foods are unhealthy led him to make a poorly informed behavioral change, which failed to improve his health outcomes.

Testing health knowledge in this way helps to identify factors that are both influential to health behaviors and modifiable. In fact, after awareness, knowledge is the second easiest factor to change health education and promotion activities. Knowledge is essential for helping people make voluntary health behavior changes, and addressing knowledge is a necessary, albeit not sufficient, component of behavior change.

Beliefs and Perceptions

Belief refers to something one accepts as true or real, a firmly held opinion or conviction (Belief, 2014). Beliefs, like knowledge, reflect a person's understanding of the world and can be applied to a large variety of topics. Whereas knowledge is defined by content that is objective and verifiable, the content of beliefs is subjective opinion. Beliefs can be shared across groups of people and are often based on some degree of verifiable information, but they reflect conclusions that are subjective in nature. This lack of verifiability is what distinguishes a belief from knowledge.

In relation to behavioral epidemiology, beliefs are often measured in terms of expectations and perceptions about risk of harm or illness. For example, an individual believes that if he has dated the same woman for at least 6 months, he no longer has to wear condoms during sex to be protected from sexually transmitted infections. Another person believes that if a food is labeled with "100% natural ingredients" then it is nutritious. These examples, like many beliefs, reflect inaccurate conclusions that are based on a combination of both accurate and inaccurate information.

A perception is a belief or opinion. Perception is the ability to see, hear, or become aware of something through the senses (e.g., the perception of pain) (Perception, 2014). It may be thought of as a mental impression; an intuitive insight and understanding; or a way of regarding, understanding, or interpreting something. A perception constitutes a functional reality for the perceiver and must be accounted for when understanding health behavior. Suppose a woman has a perception (belief) that she will inevitably contract cancer because both her parents and three grandparents died from cancer. Because of her high level of perceived susceptibility to cancer, she takes no measures to protect herself against cancer risk.

Attitudes and Values

Attitude is a way of thinking or feeling about someone or something, often reflected in a person's behavior (Attitude, 2014). Value is the regard, importance, worth, or usefulness that is given to something (Value, 2014). Attitudes and values are subjective assessments of relative worth made by an individual. In behavior change theory, attitudes and values both reflect evaluations of whether a behavior or health outcome is good, bad, or neutral. These are usually expressed as an attitude toward something or the perceived value of something. In general, a positive attitude toward a behavior or health outcome indicates that it is highly valued, whereas a negative attitude indicates that it is poorly valued.

Values, when not applied to a specific thing, generally refer to an abstract set of ideals or principles that shape a person's character and guide decisions. This definition of values is not generally useful to health behavior research because it is too vague and broadly applied to be measured. Thus, for the purposes of behavioral epidemiology, value variables are defined in terms of how much something in particular is valued.

Readiness to Change

Readiness to change refers to a state of receptiveness of information or persuasion to alter one's behavioral patterns. Readiness to change variables are subjective in nature and require that a person self-reflect with a high degree of honesty. Although these variables are subjective, they are not useless. In other words, a person can be mistaken about, or insincere about, his or her self-reported readiness to change. Thus, measuring these variables requires the use of well-validated instruments.

Readiness to change is often conceptualized in stages, as defined in the Stages of Change Model. The levels span from precontemplation (before a person has even begun to consider a behavior change) to maintenance (when a person is trying to maintain a new behavioral habit). The level of readiness is important for understanding how and why a person engages in a particular health behavior (Prochaska & DiClemente, 1983).

Motivation

Motivation variables are distinct from other subjective personal variables in that they specifically describe desired future outcomes. Motivation variables almost always work in tandem with perceptions or beliefs; we choose to engage in a particular behavior because we believe the action will lead to a desired outcome. Motivation variables are not normative, but they often become more potent when connected to a normative perception or belief (Graham & Weiner, 1996). For example, a woman may perceive that she needs to be thin in order to be accepted by her peers. Consequently, she begins purging with the intention of losing weight. The normative belief that she should be thin, coupled with the desire to be accepted (motivation), influence her nutritional behavior. Since neither factor alone is enough to induce purging behavior, an intervention can have a positive impact by addressing either one.

Self-Efficacy

Self-efficacy theory was first described by Albert Bandura in 1977. Self-efficacy was defined as beliefs regarding one's ability to perform the tasks that one views as necessary for attaining valued goals (Bandura, 1977). He proposed that self-efficacy was among the most important determinants of human behavior. He further offered self-efficacy theory as a unifying theory for all types of behavior changes. Self-efficacy concerning the ability to perform behaviors was contrasted with the expected results of the performed behavior. According to Bandura, self-efficacy beliefs developed from four main sources: (1) performance attainments and failures—what we try to do and how well we succeed; (2) vicarious performances—what we see other people do; (3) verbal persuasion—what people tell us about what we are able or not able to do; and (4) imaginal performances—what we imagine ourselves doing and how well or poorly we imagine ourselves doing it.

Self-efficacy is usually expressed in terms of a subjective rating for a specified behavior, and it may be situational. For example, a man avoids going to bars because his self-efficacy for refusing alcohol in those settings is very low, but his self-efficacy for persuading his friends to go to other places for fun is very high. Self-efficacy appears in several prominent health behavior theories and is often considered an essential component of successful health behavior change strategies.

Skills

A skill is the learned ability to carry out a task and to do it well. Skill variables measure a person's physical and/or mental capabilities of engaging in a behavior. These capabilities can be defined in terms of know-how, physical ability, or expertise. (Opportunities and permissions for engaging in behavior are considered external factors, which are addressed in the following "Environmental Factors" section.) People cannot be expected to correctly engage in a behavior if they are physically or mentally unable to do so. Therapeutic noncompliance, for example, is often caused by a lack of skill, mainly related to health literacy and communication skills. A Spanish-speaking patient who receives medical advice in English will very likely not understand important prescription and dosage information. The ability to understand medical advice is a skill variable that will have an impact on health outcomes.

Personality Traits

Over many decades of psychological research, a number of personality traits have been found to influence health behaviors and outcomes. For example, type A personalities exhibit traits related to aggression, competitiveness, impatience, hostility, and holding grudges (Friedman & Rosenman, 1974). Type A personalities have been correlated with higher risk of high blood pressure and heart disease (Sparagon et al., 2001). Type D personalities exhibit traits of distress, worry, anxiety, social inhibition, and depression, all of which can also lead to heart disease and clinical mental health issues (Emons, Meijer, & Denollet, 2007). On the positive side, hardy personality types and survival personality types (e.g., flexible, committed to survival, stays cool, playful curiosity, sense of humor, and gets over it) tend to show increased resilience and problem-solving skills that can decrease risk for many health problems.

When studying personality traits as behavior influences, it is important to define the specific trait being explored, use validated psychometric instruments for measuring these traits, and identify the specific behavioral mechanism by which these traits impact behavior outcomes. For example, a behavioral epidemiologist would want to discover how the trait of aggression increases the risk of heart attacks. Is it because aggressive people engage in a riskier health behavior, or is it by some other mechanism? If there is no behavioral pathway, then the connection between the trait and the health outcome may or may not be responsive to behavioral interventions.

Variables in Behavior Theory

Along with personal factors described so far in this chapter, some behavior theories contain specific variables that help explain behavior. A summary of these variables is found in **Table 4-2**.

ENVIRONMENTAL FACTORS

Environmental determinants of health include physical, chemical, biological, social, and psychological factors. Many of these factors can influence health behavior, as previously discussed. To facilitate the identification, isolation, and measurement of these many factors, the Institute of Medicine groups them into five primary categories

Table 4-2			
	Theory-based Variables in Behavioral Research		
Health Belief Model	Theory of Planned Behavior and Reasoned Action	Stages of Change Model (Transtheoretical Model)	Social Cognitive Theory
Perceived susceptibility	Subjective norm	Consciousness raising	Knowledge about risks
Perceived severity	Perceived behavioral control	Counterconditioning	Benefits of change
Perceived benefits	Behavioral belief	Dramatic relief	Self-efficacy
Perceived barriers	Evaluation of behavioral outcome	Environmental reevaluation	Outcome expectations
Subjective norm	Normative beliefs	Helping relationships	Facilitators or barriers
	Control beliefs	Reinforcement management	
	Perceived power	Self-liberation	
		Self-reevaluation	
		Social liberation	
		Stimulus control	

(Institute of Medicine, 2001): social relationships, living conditions, neighborhoods and communities, institutions, and social and economic policies. Each of these groupings is further described in the following sections.

Social Relationships

Individuals are highly influenced by the people they interact with on a regular basis, such as family members, coworkers, friends, neighbors, and service providers of all kinds. Even more distal relationships—often called acquaintances—will exert a degree of social expectations. These relationships create emergent variables that describe the influence of social interactions on behavioral choices, such as norms, rewards, punishments, social capital, and social support.

Norms are a key construct to consider when studying human behavior. This construct appears in many forms in the health behavior theories, particularly in the Theory of Reasoned Action/Theory of Planned Behavior and the integrated belief model, as subjective norms and normative beliefs (Glanz, Rimer, & Lewis, 2002). Norms are the behaviors that are deemed acceptable by a particular group or society. Specific norms can vary among different societies, but almost all cultures have implicit and explicit rules that its members are expected to follow (Savarimuthu & Cranefield, 2011).

Punishments are negative consequences for practicing behaviors that are considered undesirable or unacceptable in a society. This construct is also extensively utilized in many current health behavior theories. Social Cognitive Theory describes punishment through its construct of incentive motivation (Glanz et al., 2002). However, punishment may be problematic if it violates human rights. For example, several countries in west and central Africa have attempted to punish the transmission of HIV by criminalizing or punishing individuals who refuse to reveal their HIV status to their spouses or sexual partners, regardless of their intent to transmit the virus. Although the law was initially put in place to protect the public, patients' human rights and their right to confidentiality has been seriously violated (Sanon, Kabore, Wilen, Smith, & Galvao, 2009).

Rewards are used to encourage behaviors that society or an individual might want repeated. Rewards can be given out in the form of self-rewards or by other individuals and groups. Some states have even begun to offer financial rewards for engaging in healthy behaviors. Florida has offered Medicaid receipts up to $125 for engaging in smoking cessation and weight management programs (Greene, 2007). Researchers have also found that although rewards can be useful for promoting short-term voluntary behavior change, it can still be difficult for some individuals to maintain long-term changes in their behavior through rewards (Donatelle et al., 2004).

Motivation can come from outside oneself, such as the motivation to receive a financial reward, get a good grade, gain attention and recognition from peers, or attract media attention. This is known as external (or extrinsic) motivation because it involves participation in something when the reward is external to the process of participation. A person may also be motivated to do something to avoid a negative outcome, which too is external motivation. When participation stems from the sheer enjoyment that comes from the process (i.e., participation is enjoyable, exciting, interesting) and is not preoccupied by external rewards, the process is internally (or intrinsically) motivated. Internally motivated behavior involves participation in the process for its own sake.

External rewards may be beneficial in attracting interest and participation in something when initially there was no interest, and it can be used to motivate people to acquire new skills or knowledge, which, in turn, may then become internally motivated. Extrinsic rewards may also be viewed as a source of feedback in which people are made aware of whether their performance was acceptable or attained a certain standard. Promoters may also get someone to accomplish a task when that person otherwise had no interest in doing it. External motivators may not be appropriate if the individual already is intrinsically motivated.

Internal motivation comes with a complete absence of any internal or external pressure to perform well. Most people can recall a time from their childhood when they were playing a game with friends that was so enjoyable that they were entirely engrossed in what they were doing; it didn't matter who won the game, and the time flew by because they were having such a great time. Internal motivation is closely related to a desire to become better, to feel competent, to excel in certain ways, and to develop meaningful relationships with other people. Internal motivation is about enjoyment and immersion in an activity.

Research has found that extrinsic rewards can influence intrinsic motivation in three ways: (1) unexpected external rewards tend to decrease intrinsic motivation; (2) praise can help increase internal motivation; and (3) intrinsic motivation will decrease if external rewards are given for completing a specific task or only doing minimal work (Plotnik & Kouyoumjian, 2011).

Behaviors that are characterized by persistence, a positive attitude, and unflinching concentration are likely both internally and externally motivated. If a behavior is predominantly externally motivated, and if a reward does not come, then the person is likely to get discouraged and the behavior is likely to stop. On the other hand, if behavior is predominantly intrinsically motivated, there might not be the competitive drive or determination to excel. Therefore, both internal motivation and external motivation are important for driving behavior.

Social capital is the idea that there is an intrinsic value to social networks and relationships. Social capital can affect everything from community safety to physical, emotional, and mental health. This concept has been recognized for nearly 200 years with the writing of *Democracy in America*, by Alexis de Tocqueville, in the early half of the 1800s (de Tocqueville, 1835). In this novel, de Tocqueville, a French native, observed the functionality and cohesiveness of the American people and government. Despite the recognition of this idea over the course of many decades, the formalization of the theoretical construct of social capital can be largely attributed to James S. Coleman's paper, "Social Capital in the Creation of Human Capital," which was published in 1988. Some simple and current examples of how we see social capital in our communities today are as follows: joining with others in the community to be a part of coalitions and the parent–teacher association; parents knowing their children's friends; having the expectation to live in a community for a long time; and creating an overall sense of community and belonging among members.

Living Conditions

An individual's living conditions often reflect the relative availability of resources and social power, which have an impact on behavioral choices. Living conditions are directly related to physical, safety, social, and esteemed needs. A single-family home that is secure, safe, roomy, organized, and comfortable and has a social support structure will have a very different impact on an individual's health than a home that is cramped, noisy, dirty, unsafe, disorderly, and the family is dysfunctional.

In 1943, Abraham Maslow proposed a theory in psychology known as Maslow's Hierarchy of Needs (Maslow, 1943, 1954). Paralleling many theories of human developmental psychology, Maslow used specific needs to describe the pattern of motivation that tends to be experienced in life. Maslow's theory focused on the development of healthy individuals. This theory is often shown as a pyramid (**Figure 4-2**).

In the pyramid, the strongest needs, physiological needs, which come first in a persons' exploration for satisfaction, is at the base. After the physiological needs are satisfied and no longer dominate thoughts and behaviors, the need for safety becomes relevant. After the physiological and safety needs are well satisfied, the needs of love, affection, and belonging can surface. To overcome feelings of loneliness and alienation, we seek friendships, family support, and companionship with a partner. Specifically, after the needs identified in the first three levels of the pyramid are satisfied, the need for self-esteem can be realized. Individuals have an intrinsic need for stability, self-respect, and respect from others. When this occurs, self-confidence

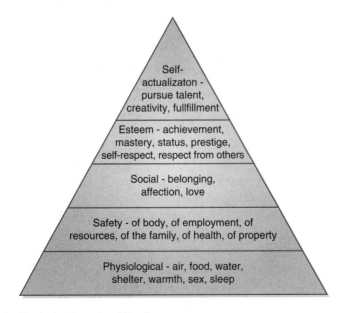

Figure 4-2   Maslow's Hierarchy of Needs

Data from Maslow, AH (1954). *Motivation and Personality*. New York, NY: Harper and Row; Maslow, AH (1943). A theory of human motivation. *Psychological Review, 50*(4), 370–396.

and personal value exists. Otherwise, there are feelings of inferiority, weakness, helplessness, and worthlessness. Finally, when all the other needs are satisfied, then needs for self-actualization can result. According to Maslow, self-actualization is doing what you are "fitted for" (Maslow, 1943, p. 382). It is an intrinsic desire, not a driving force, that results in a person realizing their potential, achieving self-fulfillment, seeking personal growth, and reaching peak experiences (Simons, Irwin, & Drinnien, 1987). Normally, functioning people have a desire to move up the hierarchy toward self-actualization. However, progress is frequently disrupted by failing to meet a lower need. Maslow thought that only one in a hundred people become fully self-actualized (Maslow, 1943, 1954).

Living conditions that satisfy physical, safety, and social needs provide a basis for seeking superior health, as well as esteem and self-actualization, all of which are interrelated. The definition of health suggests that it has six dimensions that carry aspects of esteem and self-actualization. Perhaps health education and promotion efforts are only effective when these initial needs are met.

The six dimensions of health are directly related to Maslow's Hierarchy of Needs. For physical health to occur, a person must have access to basic requirements that are vital to survival (**Table 4-3**). Security needs are also important, such as health care, safe neighborhoods, and shelter from the environment. For social and mental health to occur, physical, safety, and social needs must be met. Complete emotional health may require that physical, safety, social, emotional, and self-actualization needs be met. *Spiritual health* is a personal matter that involves religious faith, beliefs, values, ethics, principles, and morals that provide a purpose in our lives. All of Maslow's Hierarchy of Needs can contribute to spiritual health. Finally, like social and mental health, environmental health implies that physical, safety, and social needs are also met.

In a study of 18 people considered to be self-actualized (including Abraham Lincoln and Albert Einstein), Maslow identified 15 characteristics of a self-actualized person (Maslow, 1968, 1970). He observed that while the way people achieve self-actualization may be unique, they tend to have the following certain characteristics in common:

- Perceive reality efficiently and can tolerate uncertainty
- Accept themselves and others for what they are
- Spontaneous in thought and action
- Problem centered (not self-centered)
- Unusual sense of humor
- Able to look at life objectively
- Highly creative

Table 4-3

Relating the Six Dimensions of Health to Maslow's Hierarchy of Needs

Dimension	Definition	Physical	Safety	Social	Esteem	Self-Actualization
Physical	Ability of the human body to function properly; includes physical fitness and activities of daily living	✓	✓			
Social	Ability to have satisfying relationships; interaction with social institutions and societal mores	✓	✓	✓		
Mental	Ability to think clearly, reason objectively, and act properly	✓	✓	✓		
Emotional	Ability to cope, adjust, and adapt; self-efficacy and self-esteem	✓	✓	✓	✓	✓
Spiritual	Feeling as if part of a greater spectrum of existence; personal beliefs and choices	✓	✓	✓	✓	✓
Environmental	External factors (i.e., one's surroundings, such as habitat or occupation) and internal factors (i.e., one's internal structure, such as genetics)	✓	✓	✓	✓	

- Resistant to enculturation, but not purposely unconventional
- Concerned for the welfare of humanity
- Capable of deep appreciation of basic life experience
- Establish deep satisfying interpersonal relationships with a few people
- Peak experiences
- Need for privacy
- Democratic attitudes
- Strong moral and ethical standards

Experiencing all of these characteristics is not necessary for becoming self-actualized. On the other hand, people who are not self-actualized can possess some of these characteristics. However, self-actualized people tend to possess many of these characteristics. In addition, self-actualization is a continual process of becoming, not a perfect state attained toward happy ever after (Hoffman, 1988). Research is warranted that seeks to understand the interrelationship between characteristics of self-actualization and health.

Neighborhoods and Communities

Geographic and cultural communities also exert an influence on behavioral choices. The built environment that houses a neighborhood or geographic community determines what options are available for interacting with that environment. For example, a community with public tennis courts, running trails, basketball courts, swimming pools, and playgrounds will provide many more opportunities for residents to exercise than a community without these amenities. Likewise, a high availability of cigarette vendors, elevators (instead of stairs), liquor stores, and candy shops will likely increase a variety of risky health behaviors.

Climate can also be an important factor of a geographic location that influences health behaviors, especially physical activity and sociability. Availability of recreational equipment and opportunities may not be enough to counteract distempered climates. However, careful event planning can take advantage of comfortable climates as a motivator for participation in social and physical activities.

Cultural communities are often defined by common beliefs, heritage, or experiences and may or may not be colocated geographically. The gay and lesbian community, for example, shares a commonality of experience as a minority group, but members are distributed widely across geographic areas. Cultural communities do not share a common physical environment, but they will share some common values, beliefs, norms, expectations, and viewpoints—all of which can exert an influence on behavioral choices. Americans who live in the South are a quintessential example of a cultural community that does not have a specific or unique physical environment but shares commonality in values and culture among all Southerners.

Institutions

Institutions are formal organizations that have some degree of social power within a given community. An individual's relationship with an institution and the impact it has on his or her health behavior can vary greatly. Employees, owners, investors, customers, clients, and subjects are all very different roles. In behavioral epidemiology, identifying the nature of an institutional relationship can help identify the influence on health behavior. For example, a prison located within a community will have different impacts on inmates than it will on neighbors, workers, and suppliers. The prison may actually increase physical activity for an inmate because it provides time and facilities; it may reduce physical activity for neighbors because they don't feel safe walking nearby. Some institutions will have very obvious impacts on health behaviors, such as health departments, hospitals, grocery stores, and schools. Others may be less obvious, but they may be highly influential nonetheless, such as a corporate culture of safety.

Social and Economic Policies

Social and economic policies often have an indirect and complex influence on individual health behaviors, which can make them difficult to discover. The help of a trained policy or economic analyst may be beneficial when exploring this category of environmental factors. Economic incentives, such as government subsidies, taxation, or cheap importation can alter the cost of behavioral options with either positive or negative effects. For example, government subsidies of the corn industry have reduced the cost of high-fructose corn syrup in comparison to sucrose (table sugar), which has led most major food producers to switch to the cheaper product, greatly increasing its consumption in the United States.

Government policies can also be more direct, such as laws requiring the use of seat belts, helmets, and child seats. These laws target individuals' behaviors directly, instead of altering the incentives of intermediary organizations. These are the most obvious policies to consider in behavioral epidemiology, and they can be a good place to start any investigation of environmental influence.

Another common way in which policies affect health behaviors is through consumer protection programs, such as nutrition labeling, clean water standards, household product regulation, and approval of medicinal products.

Summary

1. To modify behaviors related to health outcomes requires an understanding of the laws and principles that underlie a person's behavior. The general causes of human behavior are biological, psychological, and social.

2. Statistical inference involves reaching a conclusion about a population based on information from a sample and using probability to indicate the level of reliability of that conclusion.

3. Causal inference involves making conclusions about associations among variables based on lists of criteria or conditions applied to the results of scientific studies.

4. The process of making a decision consists of four elements: behavioral intention, decision to act, health behavior, and health outcomes. Environmental factors may impact all four elements of behavioral decision making, as well as

the relationships among the four elements. The purpose of behavioral epidemiology is to understand the causal connections among intention, decision, behavior, and outcome for improving health behaviors and, consequently, preventing disease, prolonging life, and contributing to the six dimensions of health.

5. Factors that can exert an influence on health behaviors may be directly modifiable or not directly modifiable. These latter variables cannot function as behavioral determinants because they cannot serve as the catalyst that alters the Health Behavior Pathway. The first group includes variables that are both influential and directly modifiable by health promotion activities. These are the most important variables because they have the potential to respond to health promotion interventions and, therefore, influence the Health Behavior Pathway.

6. With a better understanding of the factors influencing behavior and the choices people make, one can better understand how to change behavior. Behavior is often dictated by behavioral determinants, which are the personal and environmental factors that influence a person every day.

7. Personal factors, knowledge, belief, attitudes, self-efficacy, and skills are commonly understood and examined through the context of several widely used theories including the Health Belief Model, Theory of Planned Behavior and Theory of Reasoned Action, and Social Cognitive Theory. These models attempt to identify the individual components of behavior. By looking at where a belief comes from or why it is held, as well as assessing an individual's belief that they can change, an intervention can be developed to address these determinants of behavior and facilitate behavior change.

8. Environmental factors include everything from social relationships to the communities and institutions with which an individual interacts. Environmental factors often define individual choices.

References

Attitude. (2014). In *Oxford dictionaries*. Retrieved from http://www.oxforddictionaries.com/us/definition/american_english/attitude

Bandura, A. (1977). Self-efficacy: Toward a unifying theory of behavior change. *Psychological Review, 84*(2), 191–215. doi:10.1037/0033-295X.84.2.191

Belief. (2014). In *Oxford dictionaries*. Retrieved from http://www.oxforddictionaries.com/us/definition/american_english/belief

Coleman, J. S. (1988). Social capital in the creation of human capital. *American Journal of Sociology, 94,* S95–S120. Retrieved from http://www.jstor.org/discover/10.2307/2780243?uid=2&uid=4&sid=21104273122757

de Tocqueville, A. (1835). *Democracy in America*. London, UK: Saunders and Otley.

Donatelle, R. J., Hudson, D., Dobie, S., Goodall, A., Hunsberger, M., & Oswald, K. (2004). Incentives in smoking cessation: Status of the field and implications for research and practice with pregnant smokers. *Nicotine and Tobacco Research, 6*(2), S163–S179. doi:10.1080/14622200410001669196

Emons, W. H., Meijer, R. R., & Denollet, J. (2007). Negative affectivity and social inhibition in cardiovascular disease: Evaluating type-D personality and its assessment using item response theory. *Journal of Psychosomatic Research, 63*(1), 27–39. doi:10.1016/j.jpsychores.2007.03.010

Friedman, M., & Rosenman, R. H. (1974). *Type A behavior and your heart.* New York, NY: Knopf.

Glanz, K., Rimer, B. K., & Lewis, F. M. (Eds.). (2002). *Health behavior and health education: Theory, research and practice* (3rd ed.). San Francisco, CA: Jossey-Bass.

Graham, S., & Weiner, B. (1996). Theories and principles of motivation. In D. C. Berliner & R. C. Calfee (Eds.), *Handbook of educational psychology* (pp. 63–84). New York, NY: Macmillan.

Greene, J. (2007). *Medicaid efforts to incentivize healthy behaviors.* Retrieved from http://www .chcs.org/media/Medicaid_Efforts_to_Incentivize_Healthy_Behaviors.pdf

Hoffman, E. (1988). *The right to be human: A biography of Abraham Maslow.* Los Angeles, CA: Jeremy P. Tarcher.

Institute of Medicine. (2001). *Health and behavior: The interplay of biological, behavioral, and societal influences.* Washington, DC: National Academy Press.

Knowledge. (2014). In *Oxford dictionaries.* Retrieved from http://www.oxforddictionaries .com/us/definition/american_english/knowledge

Maslow, A. H. (1943). A theory of human motivation. *Psychological Review, 50*(4), 370–396. Retrieved from http://psychclassics.yorku.ca/Maslow/motivation.htm

Maslow, A. H. (1954). *Motivation and personality.* New York, NY: Harper & Row.

Maslow, A. H. (1968). *Toward a psychology of being.* New York, NY: D. Van Nostrand.

Maslow, A. H. (1970). *Motivation and personality.* New York, NY: Harper & Row.

McGraw-Hill. (2008). PsychInteractive online: Multiple causes of behavior. Retrieved from http://highered.mheducation.com/sites/0073382736/student_view0 /perspectives_in_psychology/multiple_causes_of_behavior__/index.html

Perception. (2014). In *Oxford dictionaries.* Retrieved from http://www.oxforddictionaries .com/us/definition/american_english/perception

Plotnik, R., & Kouyoumjian, H. (2011). *Introduction to psychology.* Belmont, CA: Wadsworth.

Prochaska, J. O., & DiClemente, C. C. (1983). Stages and processes of self-change of smoking: Toward an integrative model of change. *Journal of Consulting and Clinical Psychology, 51*(3), 390–395. doi:10.1037//0022-006X.51.3.390

Sanon, P., Kabore, S., Wilen, J., Smith, S. J., & Galvao, J. (2009). Advocating prevention over punishment: The risk of HIV criminalization in Burkina Faso. *Reproductive Health Matters, 17*(34), 146–153. doi:10.1016/S0968-8080(09)34484-5

Savarimuthu, B. T. R., & Cranefield, S. (2011). Norm creation, spreading and emergence: A survey of simulation models of norms in multi-agent systems. *Multi-agent and Grid Systems, 7*(1), 21–54. doi:10.3233/MGS-2011-0167

Simons, J. A., Irwin, D. B., & Drinnien, B. A. (1987). *Maslow's hierarchy of needs.* New York, NY: West.

Sparagon, B. J., Friedman, M., Breall, W. S., Goodwin, M. L., Fleishmann, N., & Ghandour, G. (2001). Type A behavior and coronary atherosclerosis. *Atherosclerosis, 156*(1), 145–149. doi:10.1016/S0021-9150(00)00604-3

Value. (2014). In *Oxford dictionaries.* Retrieved from http://www.oxforddictionaries .com/us/definition/american_english/value

Weed, D. L. (1995). Causal and preventive inference. In P. Greenwald, B. S. Kramer, & D. G. Weed (Eds.), *Cancer prevention and control* (pp. 285–302). New York, NY: Marcel Dekker.

Chapter 5

Behavioral Epidemiologic Research

© Dmytro Humytskiy/ShutterStock, Inc.

Behavioral epidemiologic research is the study of personal behaviors, the factors that influence these behaviors, how these behaviors influence health-related states or events in human populations, and how behaviors can be modified to prevent and control health problems. Several behaviors (e.g., physical activity, diet, and safety precautions) and conditions (e.g., an unhealthy state, a state of fitness, something that is essential to the occurrence of something else) may directly influence disease states and events. Certain disease states and events can also impact behavior.

Research is "the systematic investigation into and study of materials and sources in order to establish facts and reach new conclusions" (Research, 2014). In behavioral epidemiology, our materials and sources consist of data related to human populations. Research may be viewed from two perspectives: the tangible elements of the study plan (i.e., research question, design, subjects, measurements, sample size, calculation, and so on), and how well it works (Hulley, Newman, & Cummings, 2013a). The purpose of this chapter is to present epidemiologic research from these two perspectives. The research approach outlined in this chapter applies to behavioral epidemiology.

Elements of the Study Plan

The systematic structure of a research project is presented in the study plan. This plan consists of the research questions, background and significance, design, subjects, variables, and statistical issues. In other words, it will address what questions the study will address, why these questions are important, how the study will be structured, who the subjects will be and how they will be selected, what measurements will be made, how many people will be included in the study, and how their data will be analyzed.

The Question

All epidemiologic investigations begin with a research question. There may be one question or a primary question and then secondary questions. The primary question sets out the main objective of the study. It presents an unknown issue or uncertainty that the study is intended to resolve. A research question can be motivated as an area of interest to the investigator, a response to public health concerns, or a response to a policy requirement.

The research question should be specific. Consider the question, Should people use more sunscreen? Before planning can begin, the question needs to be better focused. The question can be broken down into more specific questions, and one or two can be singled out for the focus of the study plan. Some examples are as follows:

- How often do individuals at outdoor swimming pools in the summer use sunscreen?
- Do some brands of sunscreen provide more protection than others while swimming?
- How frequently should sunscreen be applied?
- What sun protection factor (SPF) is sufficient?
- Is there any advantage of using sunscreen with an SPF above 50?
- What age groups are at greatest need for sunscreen?

For each of our questions, we need to consider whether it passes the so what test. In other words, why is answering the question important? If children who get sunburns are more susceptible to skin cancer later in life than older adults who get sunburns, answering the question is clearly important.

FINER criteria for a good research question and study plan have been presented by Cummings, Browner, and Hulley (2013). They suggest that a good research question and study plan will be Feasible, Interesting, Novel, Ethical, and Relevant (FINER). *Feasible* means that there will be a sufficient number of subjects; the investigators will have the skills, equipment, and expertise necessary for designing the study, recruiting the subjects, measuring the variables, managing and assessing the data; sufficient resources, in time and money, are available for the different components of the study; the investigators are not attempting too much, and the study is focused on the most important goals; and the study is fundable.

An investigator may be motivated to conduct a study for several reasons, such as financial support, career building, or a genuine desire to understand a process or situation. It may be that this last reason is most likely to help the investigators see the study through, despite the challenges and frustrations that often accompany the research process. Nevertheless, what is *interesting* to you may not be interesting to others. For this reason, it is useful to seek advice from experts in the area you are studying.

Novel research provides new findings; confirms, refutes, or extends previous research; and may produce new concepts, methods, or interventions. However, it is not always necessary for the research question to be completely novel. In some cases, it is useful to confirm other studies, determine whether the results previously found in one population applies to another, or if a new approach can help us better understand an association between a risk factor and an outcome.

A research question that involves human subjects must maintain respect for persons, do no harm, and be fair. Otherwise, the research question needs to be modified. The purpose of institutional review boards (IRBs) is to protect the rights of human subjects. If there is uncertainty about whether a research question is *ethical*, it should be discussed with the IRB as early in the research process as possible. More will be said about ethics in public health research later in this chapter.

Finally, the *relevance* of the question may be determined by considering if answering the question will advance scientific knowledge, influence health policy and services, change concepts and methods, or have a meaningful effect on future research. Again, consulting with experts in the field can help establish whether a research question is relevant.

Background and Significance

This is the section of the study plan in which the rationale for the study is established. A thorough understanding of the existing research is needed to establish what is already known. This information should help form the research question and identify where gaps in knowledge exist and where the proposed research question fits in with previously conducted research. A literature review and synthesis of existing knowledge on a topic will often result in refining the research question.

Research Design

The research design represents the purpose of the investigation, whether analytic, descriptive, or exploratory. It is an approach that describes how we will address the research question; it is a formal approach of scientific investigation. The analytic study design is used to identify associations between variables linked to the research question. This type of study is very structured and involves a comparison group. The descriptive study design aims to provide an accurate and valid representation of the variables that are relevant to the research question. It is less structured than the analytic design but more structured than the exploratory study design. In an exploratory study design, there is a high level of uncertainty, or little is known about the health problem. Questions and examples associated with the different study designs are shown in **Table 5-1**.

Table 5-1		
Types of Study Designs and Corresponding Research Questions		
Type of design	**Question**	**Examples**
Analytic	Why? What are the causes of the health problem?	Is smoking the primary cause of heart disease? Will a new antibiotic lower the risk of a given disease in a specific population?
Descriptive	How many cases? What is the incidence rate of the disease? What is the prevalence proportion for the disease? Are selected variables related?	How many students visited the health center in the past week complaining of flu symptoms? What is the rate of depression among heart transplant patients? What is the prevalence of arthritis in the adult population? Has the prostate cancer screening program produced a decline in prostate cancer mortality? Is there an association between fruit and vegetable intake and family income?
Exploratory	What is a case? What are the key factors involved?	What reasons are there for the high percentage of children absent from school today? What reasons are there for the increased mortality in a given area?

Study designs commonly used in epidemiology to describe or explore data include case reports, case series, cross-sectional surveys, and ecologic studies. Analytic designs assess associations between variables, which include case-control, cohort, case-crossover, and experimental designs. There are also methods from other fields of study that may be helpful to understanding behavior outcome relationships in human populations. A field of network epidemiology uses social networks to evaluate the spread of infectious diseases. This field can also be useful to evaluate ways that information is spread through a population based on human behavior and relationships.

A description of ecologic designs, case studies, and cross-sectional surveys is presented in **Table 5-2**. The ecologic design involves making comparisons between variables where the unit of analysis is aggregated data on the population level rather than on the individual level. This study design is susceptible to *ecologic fallacy*, which is an error that results if the researcher mistakenly assumes that because the majority of a group has a characteristic, the characteristic is definitively associated with those experiencing the health-related state or event in the group. Ecologic studies are perhaps more appropriate when group-level interventions are involved (modifications to physical, social, technological, political, economical, and organizational environments), rather than efforts to change individual behaviors (Stevenson & McClure, 2005).

A case study design (i.e., case report or case series) is useful for identifying new, emerging health problems. It is a useful approach for obtaining qualitative data. A case report is a profile of a single individual, and a case series involves a small group of patients with a similar diagnosis.

A cross-sectional survey is a detailed inspection or investigation of a population at a snapshot in time. It is often referred to as a prevalence survey and is useful for estimating the prevalence of the health-related state or event being investigated. Cross-sectional surveys that are routinely conducted are referred to as serial surveys. They are useful for showing changing patterns of health behaviors or disease outcomes over time.

Descriptions of case-control, case-crossover, nested case-control, and cohort study designs are presented in **Table 5-3**. These are each observational analytic studies because the researchers observe relationships between variables. In analytic experimental studies, each subset of the study participants is assigned the intervention. Alternatively, the participants are grouped according to their receipt of different levels of the intervention.

Key features of the case-control study design are as follows:

■ Enrolls a group with disease (cases) and an appropriate group without disease (controls) and compares their patterns of previous exposures

Table 5-2

Descriptive Epidemiologic Studies

	Description	Strengths	Weaknesses
Ecologic	Aggregate data are involved (i.e., no information is available for specific individuals). The prevalence of a potential risk factor is compared with the rate of an outcome condition.	• Takes advantage of preexisting data • Relatively quick and inexpensive • Can be used to evaluate programs, policies, or regulations implemented at the ecologic level • Allows estimation of effects not easily measurable for individuals	• Susceptible to confounding • Exposures and disease or injury outcomes not measured on the same individuals • Ecologic fallacy (i.e., an error that occurs if one mistakenly assumes that because the majority of a group has a characteristic, the characteristic is associated with those experiencing the outcome)
Case study	A snapshot description of a problem or situation for an individual or group is provided. Qualitative descriptive research of the facts are provided in chronological order.	• In-depth description • Provides clues to identify a new disease or adverse health effect resulting from an exposure or experience • Identifies potential areas of research	• Conclusions limited to the individual, group, and/or context under study • Cannot be used to establish a cause–effect relationship
Cross-sectional	Variables are measured at a point in time. There is no distinction between potential risk factors and outcomes.	• Control over study population • Control over measurements • Several associations between variables can be studied at same time • Short time period required • Complete data collection • Exposure and injury/disease data collected from same individuals • Produces prevalence	• No data on the time relationship between exposure and injury/disease development • Potential bias from low response rate • Potential measurement bias • Higher proportion of long-term survivors • Not feasible with rare exposures or outcomes • Does not yield incidence or relative risk

Reproduced from Jones & Bartlett Learning, "Reproductive Epidemiology" Merrill, 2010.

Table 5-3

Description, Strengths, and Weaknesses of Observational Analytic Study Designs

	Description	Strengths	Weaknesses
Case-control	The presence of risk factor(s) for people with a condition is compared with presence of risk factor(s) for people without a condition.	• Effective for rare outcomes • Compared with the cohort study, it requires less time and money • Yields an odds ratio (when the outcome condition is rare, it is a good estimate of the relative risk)	• Limited to one outcome condition • Does not provide incidence, relative risk, or natural history • Less effective than a cohort study at establishing time sequence of events • Potential recall and interviewer bias • Potential survival bias • Does not yield incidence or prevalence
Case-crossover	The exposure frequency during a window immediately prior to an outcome event is compared with exposure frequencies during a control time or times at an earlier period.	• Controls for fixed individual characteristics that may otherwise confound the association • Effective when studying the effects of short-term exposures on the risk of acute events	• Does not automatically control for confounding from time-related factors
Nested case-control	A case-control study is conducted within a cohort study. To carry out a nested case-control study, samples or records of interest must be available from before the outcome condition occurred.	• Has the scientific benefits of a cohort design • Less expensive to conduct than cohort studies • Smaller sample size required than for a cohort study • Less prone to recall bias than a case-control study	• Nondiseased persons from whom the controls are selected may not be representative of the original cohort because of death or loss to follow-up among cases
Cohort	People are followed over time to describe the incidence or the natural history of a condition. An assessment can also be made of risk factors for various conditions.	• Establishes time sequence of events • Avoids bias in measuring exposure from knowing the outcome • Avoids Berkson's bias and prevalence–incidence bias • Several outcomes can be assessed • Number of outcomes grows over time • Allows assessment of incidence and the natural history of disease • Yields incidence, relative risk, attributable risk	• Large samples often required • May not be feasible in terms of time and money • Not feasible with rare outcomes • Potential bias caused by loss to follow-up

- Generally used to explore rare diseases
- Useful for exploring several risk factors for a given outcome
- Retrospective
- Ratio of cases to controls may be up to 1:4; larger number of controls to cases typically occurs to increase power in studies where only a small number of cases are available

Key features of the cohort study design are as follows:

- Categorize subjects on the basis of exposure and then follow-up to see if they develop the health condition being studied
- After some time compare the disease rate for the exposed with that of the unexposed
- Period of follow-up varies from a few days for acute diseases to several decades for chronic diseases (e.g., cancer, heart disease)
- Generally used when the exposure is rare
- Useful when there are several outcomes related to a given exposure
- Generally prospective, although may be retrospective

A cohort study design may be *prospective* or *retrospective*, which is determined by when the investigators come on the scene to evaluate the data. If they participate in classifying the cohort according to exposure status and then follow the cohort into the future to evaluate health outcome status, this is called a *prospective cohort study*. Alternatively, if data on exposure and outcome variables are available for a cohort of people, and the investigator evaluates existing exposure and outcome data for the given cohort, this is a *retrospective cohort study*. Do not confuse a retrospective cohort study design with a case-control study design. Although a case-control study is also considered retrospective, the word *retrospective* is used in a different way than in the context of a cohort study.

In case-crossover studies, individuals serve as their own controls. The analytic unit is time—where the time just before the acute event is the case time compared with some other time, referred to as the control time. This design assumes there are no confounding time-related factors or that they are adjusted for in the analysis. The simplest case-crossover design is similar to a matched-pair case-control design. To illustrate, suppose 150 cardiac events are identified, and you are interested in measuring whether cardiac events are associated with particulate matter in the air. The case period is designated as the 24 hours preceding the cardiac event, and the control period is designated as 1 week prior to the case period. Now suppose particulate

Table 5-4			
Exposure to Particulate Matter of 150 Cardiac Patients			
		Control	
		High	Low
Case	High	45	30
	Low	15	60

matter is classified as high versus low levels, and assume the data are as presented in **Table 5-4**.

Among the cardiac patients, 45 experienced high particulate matter during the case and control periods; 30 experienced high particulate matter during the case period but not during the control period; 15 experienced low particulate matter during the case period but high particulate matter during the control period; and 60 experienced low particulate matter during both the case and control periods. An odds ratio can be estimated by taking the ratio of discrepant pairs, which is 2 (= 30/15).

Study Participants

Study participants are selected who can best answer the research question. In a therapeutic trial, selection is based on already having a disease or condition, usually based on inclusion and exclusion criteria. People are excluded from a study if they are likely to bias the results. In a prophylactic trial, the selection of participants typically involves healthy volunteers with a range of exposures and possible outcomes. Recruitment often involves incentives to ensure an adequate number of participants in the study. Probabilistic (random) sampling is a useful way to get a representative group of the target population. However, when random selection is not feasible, convenience sampling is often used, yet the goal is to minimize sampling bias where a systematic error causes the sample of persons in the study to not represent the target population.

Variables

A *variable* is a characteristic, number, or quantity that varies from one observation to the next and can be measured or counted. A numerical variable is continuous or discrete. A *continuous variable* has an infinite number of values (e.g., time), whereas a *discrete variable* reflects fixed units, usually integer values (e.g., number of days exercised). These types of variables are often described using means and standard deviations. Categorical variables are nominal (unordered categories) or ordinal (ordered categories with intervals that are not quantifiable). In epidemiology, we often consider two level nominal data (e.g., exposed or not exposed, or alive or dead). These data are described using counts and proportions. Nominal data with more than two levels are also described using counts and proportions. Ordinal data are described using counts, proportions, medians, and ranges.

On the basis of observation and experience, variables are classified as exposure (predictor) and outcome variables. An exposure may be a behavior (e.g., longboarding), and an outcome can be a health-related state or event (e.g., injury) that the behavior is believed to influence. The predictor may be a prophylactic trial that evaluates whether a preventive measure is efficacious.

Statistical Issues

Statistical issues involve hypotheses, sample sizes, and analytic techniques. We begin with hypotheses because they influence the required sample size. Sample size is the required number of subjects needed to attain a certain level of power. In descriptive studies, the required sample size is what we need to attain a certain level of precision in our estimates and the width of a confidence interval for a mean, proportion, or other descriptive statistic that is considered acceptable.

HYPOTHESIS

A *statistical hypothesis* is a belief about a population parameter. A *hypothesis* is a proposed explanation for a phenomenon in one or more populations. *Hypothesis testing* is a procedure based on sample information and probability that is used to test statements regarding a characteristic of one or more populations; it is a statement about the population parameter called the null hypothesis H_0. After formulating the null hypothesis we then make a statement that contradicts H_0, called the alternative or research hypothesis, H_1. A set of six steps is used in hypothesis testing:

1. Formulate the null hypothesis in statistical terms. A parameter is used in expressing the null hypothesis.
2. Formulate the alternative hypothesis in statistical terms. A parameter is used in expressing the alternative hypothesis. Together, the null and alternative hypotheses cover all

possible values of the population parameter in that one of the two statements is true.

3. Select the level of significance for the statistical test and the sample size. By convention, the level of significance is 0.05. However, if a more conservative test is desired, 0.01 may be used. On the other hand, in exploratory studies, or if stepwise model selection procedures are used, the level of significance may be 0.1 or higher.

4. Select the appropriate test statistic and identify the degrees of freedom and the critical value.

5. Collect the data and calculate the statistic.

6. Reject or fail to reject the null hypothesis. If we fail to reject, we are not saying the null hypothesis is true but that there is insufficient evidence from our sample to reject it.

We conduct research despite knowledge that human measurement is imperfect. Although research is about pursuing truth, it can never verifiably prove truth because there is always the possibility of error. Probability is employed in statistical inference (i.e., the process of drawing conclusions about the population based on a representative sample of the population) to capture the chance of error. *Type I error* refers to rejecting the null hypothesis given it is true. *Type II error* refers to failing to reject the null hypothesis given it is false. Without actually knowing the true characteristics of a population from which we obtained our sample, our aim is to minimize the chance of committing either type of error. Hence, if our null hypothesis is in fact true, we can limit the probability of rejecting it to the value we select for α. This value is typically 0.05, but it may be smaller if we want to be particularly cautious against committing a type I error, or it may be higher if we are doing exploratory work. If the null hypothesis is in fact false, we will limit the probability of accepting it to a value β, which is typically specified as 0.2. The *power* of a test is $1-\beta$, or rejecting H_0 when H_1 is true. A valid conclusion assumes that the study is sufficiently powered to result in statistical significance for the main hypothesis.

The *p-value* is the probability that an effect as large or larger than that observed in a given study could have occurred by chance alone, given that there is truly no relationship between the exposure and the outcome. The p-value is essentially a measure of chance. When analyses are based on sample data, it is possible to obtain a result that is merely due to the luck of the draw, and it does not represent the overall population. The p-value is obtained from the table that corresponds with a hypothesis test statistic. As the sample size increases, the value of the test statistic increases, and the corresponding probability of a chance finding represented by the p-value decreases.

A confidence interval is similar to a p-value in that it helps us understand how confident we are that our findings reflect the larger population. However, the two measures are distinct in that a p-value is a single number between 0 and 1, and a confidence interval is a range of values represented by the low and high on a range of possible values and is scaled according to the variable of interest. Confidence intervals can be developed for any statistic (e.g., means, ratios, proportions, and rates; correlation coefficient, regression slope estimate, odds ratio, and relative risk). A confidence interval is used to express the precision and uncertainty related to a given sampling method. Confidence intervals have a level of confidence threshold and a measurement error.

SAMPLE SIZE

A good research study has an adequate number of subjects to address the research question and evaluate the corresponding hypotheses. A study with a sample size that is too small can result in a study with no realistic chance of being statistically significant. A study with a sample size that is too big can waste resources and expose more participants than necessary to risks related to the study. Hence, the study plan must show that the sample size has been well thought out.

Several approaches are available for calculating the sample size, depending on the study design and the nature of the data involved. These sample size formulas depend on whether the study design is descriptive or analytic and whether the exposure and outcome variables are continuous or binary. The general steps for estimating the sample size of descriptive and analytic study designs, along with their objectives and framework, are presented in **Table 5-5**. Thus, the steps for estimating the sample size differ between descriptive studies that do not involve hypotheses and analytic studies. It should be emphasized that even if some of the steps involve uncertainties, it is important that the sample size be estimated in the design phase of the study.

STATISTICAL TECHNIQUES

Statistics can be divided into four general areas: descriptive (methods of organizing, summarizing, and describing numerical data); probability (random variables, probability distributions, sampling methods, sampling distributions, etc.); inferential (drawing a conclusion about a characteristic of the population from information obtained from a sample; hypothesis testing); and statistical techniques. There are many statistical techniques employed in epidemiology. The measures used for assessing exposure and outcome data depend on the type of data involved and specific assumptions about the distribution of the variables involved. *Data* are numerical information from selected variables; they are pieces of information and are obtained from observation,

Table 5-5	
Criteria for Estimating Sample Size for Descriptive and Analytic Study Designs	
Descriptive design	**Analytic design**
Objective: Estimate a parameter	Objective: Evaluate a hypothesis
Framework: Sampling distribution	Framework: Power analysis
Select the primary study variable and identify whether it is continuous or binary.	State the null hypothesis and the alternative hypothesis (one or two sided).
Identify the population of interest, based on the study objectives.	Select an appropriate statistical test. This is based on the type of exposure and outcome variables (continuous or binary).
Derive the expected population value and standard deviation of the estimate.	Identify the anticipated difference or effect size of the exposure (or intervention).
Decide on a desired confidence level (e.g., 95%).	
Decide on an acceptable range of error in the estimate (precision). Precision × 2 = width.	Estimate the standard deviation of the difference.
Estimate the sample size using the appropriate formula, based on the study assumptions.	Select a tolerable level of error (alpha) and the desired level of power for rejecting the null hypothesis when it is false (power).
	Estimate the sample size using the appropriate formula, based on the study assumptions.

measurement, or experiment of the phenomenon of interest. Data may be nominal, ordinal, discrete, or continuous. Common statistical techniques used for describing data are presented in **Table 5-6**.

In addition to the statistical methods presented in the table, nominal data are often described using ratios, proportions, and rates. Identifying the frequency of cases is a primary focus in epidemiology,

Table 5-6		
Types of Data and Methods of Description		
	Description	**Statistics**
Nominal (dichotomous is two levels; multichotomous is more than two levels)	Unordered categories	Number of cases
		Frequency distribution
		Relative frequency
Ordinal	Ordering of categories is informative	Number of cases
		Frequency distribution
		Relative frequency
Discrete	Integers (whole numbers)	Geometric mean
	Ordering and magnitude are important	Arithmetic mean
		Median
		Mode
		Range
		Variance
		Standard deviation
		Coefficient of variation
Continuous	Values on a continuum	

particularly in assessing and monitoring the health of communities and populations at risk of developing health-related states or events.

There are many approaches for evaluating the association between variables. A complete presentation of these various methods is beyond the scope of this text, but it involves both parametric and nonparametric methods.

Validity

The goal of epidemiologic research is to design the study so that correct conclusions are drawn and the conclusions are appropriately generalized. To draw correct conclusions, the study needs to be internally valid. *Internal validity* is an indication of the quality of the study itself, usually manifested by sound methodology and a lack of bias. *Bias* is a deviation of the results from the truth. For a study involving sample data to be representative of the larger population requires random selection of subjects. *Selection bias* occurs when participants in a study are selected nonrandomly, which can invalidate the results. *Information bias* is any form of bias that involves the collection, handling, or analysis of data. For example, a survey might have misleading or double-barreled questions or be incorrectly coded. *Confounding* occurs when factors outside those that the researchers study influence the study outcomes. A valid measure of association must control for the threat of confounding. *External validity* is related to the applicability of study sample findings to the larger population. High external validity means that the study results reflect the larger population. For example, a study of randomly selected college students from a church school may produce high external validity for the students at that school. However, external validity may be low in terms of the results based on these students being applicable to all college students.

Precision is the degree to which something is reproducible, reliable, and consistent. Precision is directly associated with random error and, in statistics, is generally measured using the standard deviation. Precision can be improved by increasing the size of the study or by modifying the study design to increase the efficiency of obtaining information from the study participants; poor precision can result from observer variability, instrument variability, or subject variability. Strategies to improve precision include standardizing the measurement methods in an operations manual; training and certifying the observer; refining the instrument; automating the instrument; and repeating the measurement (Hulley, Newman, & Cummings, 2013b). The accuracy of a variable is the extent to which it represents the true value. Accuracy is a function of *systematic error* (also called measurement error). Systematic error occurs when variables are incorrectly collected or measured. This type of error can occur when the outcome is subjective and the measurement techniques are untested or invalid. Poor accuracy may result from observer bias, instrument bias, or subject bias. Strategies to minimize measurement error to improve accuracy include standardizing the measurement methods in an operations manual; training and certifying the observer; refining the instrument; automating the instrument; making unobtrusive measurements; calibrating the instrument; and blinding (Hulley et al., 2013b).

A valid measure is both precise and accurate. However, a precise measurement is not necessarily valid because it is possible for a measure to be consistently wrong. On the other hand, it is possible for an accurate measure to lack precision to the point that it is not useful. Hence, validity reflects accuracy and takes into account its reproducibility, reliability, and consistency. In survey research, we often evaluate the validity of an instrument by whether it satisfies certain criteria, such as the following:

- *Face validity*, which refers to the reasonableness of an assessment method to measure what it is supposed to measure. Commonsense criteria are used to determine the suitability of a data source for study investigation.
- *Content validity*, which refers to the extent to which a measure represents all aspects of the phenomena that should be covered.
- *Construct validity*, which refers to the extent to which a measure agrees with a construct.
- *Criterion-related validity*, which refers to the degree to which a new measurement correlates with a measure already held to be valid.

In comparing a new test against a gold standard, we often use measures of sensitivity, specificity, predictive value positive, predictive value negative, and likelihood ratio test.

In summary, the study should be implemented to reflect the study plan. We want to avoid getting a misleading answer to our research question merely because of a lack of precision and/or accuracy as we carry out the study. Strategies to improve precision and accuracy were given by Hulley and colleagues (2013b).

Communicating the Results

To conclude this chapter, some guidelines will be presented on communicating the research results. The meaningful transfer of study results can shape public health practice and influence the need for further research. By meaningful transfer we mean that the information we communicate must be done in a convincing manner. The following guidelines have been suggested for communicating epidemiologic information through writing: develop your findings logically; consider friendly persuasion in the discussion; make your style as simple as possible; use plenty of transition devices; and avoid being wrong, talking down to the reader, and mixing opinion with fact (Gregg, 2008). He also suggests the following guidelines for oral communication of scientific papers: do not take more time than allotted; use high-quality visual aids that can be easily read and are not too busy; be sure you are familiar with the location where you will be presenting; know about the media capabilities in the room; do not talk down to the audience; and control your emotions (e.g., do not get upset or angry) (Gregg, 2008).

The dissemination of results is a primary source of feedback that can be used in defining new research questions and hypotheses to add to the body of existing knowledge. A summary of selected outlets for disseminating study results is presented in **Table 5-7**. For each of these outlets, the suggested communication guidelines presented by Gregg (2008) are applicable.

Research Ethics

There are several historical research studies that were considered to have been completed under controversial research ethics, such as withholding known effective treatment, exposure to potentially harmful

Table 5-7	
Selected Outlets for Disseminating Research Findings	
Method	**Likely recipients**
Scientific journals that are not discipline specific	Scientists across many research areas, usually within a broad field (e.g., public health or medicine)
Discipline-specific journal articles	Scientists within the related discipline (e.g., cancer epidemiology)
Research summaries (briefs or reports)	Scientists across many research areas, usually within a broad field (e.g., public health or medicine)
Press releases	Scientists and nonscientist individuals
Online or print news media	Scientists and nonscientist individuals
Social media	Scientists and nonscientist individuals
Scientific seminars or conferences	Scientists across many research areas, usually within a broad field (e.g., public health or medicine)
Newsletters	Varies depending on who the newsletters are sent to, but they can be used to inform research study participants
Letter to study participants	Research study participants

chemicals or illnesses, and research in vulnerable populations. In one example, the Stanford Prison Experiment, 24 research subjects were assigned to roles as "guards" or "prisoners" in a mock prison situation (Haney, Banks, & Zimbardo, 1973).The research subjects were chosen from a pool of college-age men who tested psychologically stable prior to the study. The goal of the study was to evaluate situational factors and behavior. The prisoners were informed that some basic rights would be curtailed, but they would receive adequate food, clothing, and medical care. The guards were instructed to maintain a reasonable degree of order but were forbidden from inflicting physical punishment. During the course of the study, five prisoners had to be released early due to severe psychological symptoms. The 2-week study was halted after 6 days because, as noted by the researchers in an article 25 years later,

> Several of them [guards] devised sadistically inventive ways to harass and degrade the prisoners, and none of the less actively cruel mock-guards ever intervened or complained about the abuses they witnessed. Most of the worst prisoner treatment came on the night shifts and other occasions when the guards thought they could avoid the surveillance and interference of the research team. Our planned two-week experiment had to be aborted after only six days because the experience dramatically and painfully transformed most of the participants in ways we did not anticipate, prepare for, or predict. (Haney & Zimbardo, 1998, pp. 1-2)

In work published in 1970, a sociologist named Laud Humphreys studied characteristics of men who engaged in sexual activities in tearooms, a general slang term believed to refer to public restrooms (Humphreys, 1970).The findings of the study, referred to as the Tearoom Trade Study, indicated that many of the men were not bisexual or homosexual and that many were of higher socioeconomic status, which was counter to the stereotypes at that time. An early element of the study was to serve as a lookout for tearoom participants and record sexual encounters on a systematic observation sheet. Humphreys then engaged participants in conversations outside the restroom and disclosed his role as a researcher to some of the men. For other men, he covertly recorded the license plate number and description of the car. Then, using another research position, he added his sample developed from covert tracking to the sample for a social health survey that was designed to be a random selection of men in the community. For the interviews, he changed his physical appearance so as not to be recognized by the men. Overall, the means by which the research was conducted and data were collected is of considerable ethical debate. It interesting to note Humphrey's own conclusion regarding the data collection: "At each level of research, I applied those measures that provided maximum protection for research subjects and the truest measurement of persons and behavior observed" (Plummer, 2002, p. 365).

There is considerable debate regarding whether what was learned from these behavior-related experiments for society was appropriately balanced with adverse participant effects, given the knowledge at the time. However, these experiments and research studies would be considered out of balance in terms of participant protections and gained scientific knowledge, and such studies would not be considered ethical today. At the least, the Stanford Prison Experiment would violate beneficence, and the Tearoom Trade Study would violate respect for persons. In light of these and other research studies and events, the National Research Act was established in 1974 (Fischbach, 1992). As part of this act, the National Commission for the Protection of Human Subjects of Biomedical and Behavioral Research was created, and a requirement was put in place for the establishment of IRBs at institutions that receive funding from the U.S. Department of Health and Human Services (HHS) for research. The commission was charged to identify basic ethical principles that underlie research conduct in human populations and to develop guidelines for the conduct of such research. An IRB is a review body comprised of at least five members "with varying backgrounds to promote complete and adequate review of research activities commonly conducted by the institution" (U.S. Department of Health and Human Services [USDHHS], 2009, §46.107). The function of the IRB is to review research to evaluate whether it meets basic principles of ethical human subjects research. The need for this type of review is underscored by Humphrey's interpretation of his own research.

In 1979, the commission published the *Belmont Report*, which describes three basic principles that underlie all human subject research: respect for persons, beneficence, and justice. These are described in **Table 5-8**. The principles are considered to have equal moral force, and no one principle outweighs another.

Additional issues that need to be taken into consideration when conducting research on human subjects include the need for independent, objective review and public trust. Because individuals cannot be wholly objective about their own research, it is important that an independent, objective review is conducted to evaluate the risks and benefits of the research. Conducting research is a privilege, not a right, and loss of the public trust can result in the public's withdrawal of the privilege to conduct research.

The federal government provides minimum standards for protecting research subjects. Additional and more stringent regulations

Table 5-8	
Ethical Principles in Research from the *Belmont Report*	
Principle	**Description**
Respect for persons	This principle incorporates at least two ethical convictions: (1) individuals should be treated as autonomous agents; and (2) persons with diminished autonomy are entitled to protection. The principle is thus divided into two moral requirements: (1) the requirement to acknowledge autonomy; and (2) the requirement to protect those with diminished autonomy.
Beneficence	Persons are treated in an ethical manner, not only by respecting their decisions and protecting them from harm, but also by making efforts to secure their well-being. Beneficence in the *Belmont Report* is understood as an obligation in which two general rules have been formulated as complementary expressions of beneficent actions: (1) do not harm; and (2) maximize possible benefits, and minimize possible harm.
Justice	The principle of justice may be conceived that equals ought to be treated equally in the question of who ought to receive the benefits of research and bear its burdens. An injustice occurs when some benefit to which a person is entitled is denied without good reason or when some burden is imposed unduly.

Data from U.S. Department of Health & Human Services. (1979). The Belmont Report. Retrieved July 29, 2014, from http://www.hhs.gov/ohrp/humansubjects/guidance/belmont.html

may be in place at the state, local, and institutional levels. The federal regulations were first written by the HHS and are labeled 45 CFR 46 (USDHHS, 2009). There are four subparts to the federal regulations. Subpart A (also referred to as the Common Rule) provides the basic HHS policy for the protection of human research subjects. The additional subparts provide additional safeguards for populations identified as vulnerable, namely pregnant women, fetuses, and neonates (subpart B); prisoners (subpart C); and children (subpart D). The regulations cover what research must be reviewed, who must review it, what questions should be addressed in the review process, and what kinds of review need to take place during the life of a project.

A key part of establishing what research needs to be reviewed is in defining *research* and *human subject*. As stated in 45 CFR 46, "Research means a systematic investigation, including research development, testing and evaluation, designed to develop or contribute to generalizable knowledge" (USDHHS, 2009, §46.102). Also as stated in 45 CFR 46, "Human subject means a living individual about whom an investigator (whether professional or student) conducting research obtains (1) data through intervention or interaction with the individual, or (2) identifiable private information" (USDHHS, 2009, §46.102).

Some activities meet the definition of research with human subjects but, are not covered by the provisions of the Common Rule. This research may be eligible for exemption. Whether research is exempt is not determined by the researcher, but by the institution at which the research is being conducted. Research may be eligible for exemption if all the activities associated with the research fall into one of six categories, which are described in detail in 45 CFR 46 (USDHHS, 2009); relevant to this course is "research involving the collection or study of existing data, documents, records, pathological specimens, or diagnostic specimens, if these sources are publicly available or if the information is recorded by the investigator in such a manner that subjects cannot be identified, directly or through identifiers linked to the subjects" (USDHHS, 2009, §46.101).

Summary

1. Epidemiologic research consists of a set of tangible elements that are presented in the study plan: the research question; the design (analytic, descriptive, or exploratory); study participants (entry criteria, sampling design, and data collection); measurement approaches (what variables to assess, what associations to consider, the exposure and outcome variables); and statistical issues (sample size, management, and assessment methods of the study data). In general, the study plan tells what the study is designed to do and should be devised so it can be feasibly implemented with reasonable internal and external validity.

2. Internal validity refers to the degree to which the study has applied sound methodology such that the results represent the truth. External validity refers to the investigator's ability to correctly generalize the results to an external population. Larger samples are more representative of the population of interest than smaller samples or convenience samples.

3. A good research question and study plan will be Feasible, Interesting, Novel, Ethical, and Relevant (FINER).

4. The study design is an approach that describes how the research question will be addressed.

5. The direction of the research question is formulated using hypotheses. The null hypothesis reflects the status quo or what is commonly believed. The alternative (research) hypothesis reflects what we expect to find, which is contrary to the null hypothesis. Analytic study designs are used to evaluate hypotheses.

6. A good study plan will specify an adequate number of subjects to address the research question and evaluate the corresponding hypotheses.

7. Statistical techniques are used to describe variables and assess associations between variables. The techniques employed depend on the type of data involved and whether specific assumptions are satisfied about the distribution of the variables. Data are numerical information from selected variables and are obtained from observation, measurement, or experiment of the phenomenon of interest.

8. A valid measure is both precise and accurate. Precision is the degree to which something is reproducible. It is directly associated with random. Poor precision can result from observer variability, instrument variability, or subject

variability. Accuracy is a function of systematic error and occurs when variables are incorrectly collected or measured. Poor accuracy may result from observer bias, instrument bias, or subject bias.

9. When communicating study results in writing, develop the findings logically; consider friendly persuasion in the discussion; use as simple a style as possible; use plenty of transition devices; and avoid being wrong, talking down to the reader, and mixing opinion with fact. When conveying study results orally do not take more time than allotted; use high-quality visual aids that can be easily read and are not too busy; be sure you are familiar with the location where you will be presenting; know about the media capabilities in the room; do not talk down to the audience; and control your emotions (e.g., do not get upset or angry).

10. Three principles set out in the *Belmont Report* for guiding research involving human subjects are respect for persons (e.g., informed consent, confidentiality, compensation), beneficence (do no harm), and justice (moral rightness in action or attitude).

References

Cummings, S. R., Browner, W. S., & Hulley, S. B. (2013). Conceiving the research question and developing the study plan. In S. B. Hulley, S. R. Cummings, W. S. Browner, D. G. Grady, & T. B. Newman (Eds.), *Designing clinical research* (4th ed., pp.14–22). Philadelphia, PA: Lippincott Williams & Wilkins.

Fischbach, R. L. (1992). The Tuskegee legacy. *Harvard Medical Alumni Bulletin, 93*, 24–28.

Gregg, M. B. (2008). Communicating epidemiologic findings. In M. Gregg (Ed.), *Field epidemiology* (3rd ed., pp. 249–261). New York, NY: Oxford University Press.

Haney, C., Banks, W., & Zimbardo, P. (1973). Interpersonal dynamics in a simulated prison. *International Journal of Criminology and Penology, 1*, 69–97.

Haney, C., & Zimbardo, P. (1998). The past and future of U.S. prison policy twenty-five years after the Stanford prison experiment. *American Psychologist, 53*(7), 709–727.

Hulley, S. B., Newman, T. B., & Cummings, S. R. (2013a). Getting started: The anatomy and physiology of clinical research. In S. B. Hulley, S. R. Cummings, W. S. Browner, D. G. Grady, & T. B. Newman (Eds.), *Designing clinical research* (4th ed., pp. 2–13). Philadelphia, PA: Lippincott Williams & Wilkins.

Hulley, S. B., Newman, T. B., & Cummings, S. R. (2013b). Planning the measurements: Precision, accuracy, and validity. In S. B. Hulley, S. R. Cummings, W. S. Browner, D. G. Grady, & T. B. Newman (Eds.), *Designing clinical research* (4th ed., pp. 32–42). Philadelphia, PA: Lippincott Williams & Wilkins.

Humphreys, L. (1970). Tearoom trade: Impersonal sex in public places. *Trans-action, 7*(3), 10–25. Retrieved from http://link.springer.com/article/10.1007%2FB F02812336?LI=true

Merrill, R. M. (2010). *Introduction to epidemiology* (5th ed.). Sudbury, MA: Jones and Bartlett Publishers.

Plummer, K. (2002). *Sexualities: Some elements for an account of the social organisation of sexualities.* New York, NY: Routledge.

Research. (2014). In *Oxford dictionaries*. Retrieved from http://www.oxforddictionaries .com/us/definition/american_english/research

Stevenson, M., & McClure, R. (2005). Use of ecological study designs for injury prevention. *Injury Prevention*, 11, 2–4.

U.S. Department of Health and Human Services. (1979). The *Belmont Report*. Retrieved from http://www.hhs.gov/ohrp/humansubjects/guidance/belmont.html

U.S. Department of Health and Human Services. (2009). Code of federal regulations: General requirements for informed consent. Retrieved from http://www.hhs.gov/ohrp/humansubjects/guidance/45cfr46.html#46.116

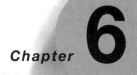
Frequency Measures in Epidemiology

There are many subfields of public health. Epidemiology, biostatistics, health services, and other fields make it possible for the three core areas of public health to be carried out. These core function areas of public health involve assessment, policy development, and assurance (Institute of Medicine, 1988). *Assessment* involves monitoring health status to identify and solve community health problems. *Surveillance* is the process of observing or monitoring. Assessment also involves diagnosing and investigating health problems and health hazards in the community. Monitoring, diagnosing, and investigating disease and health-related events are primary functions of epidemiology that assist in decisions about appropriate action and identify whether progress is being made in prevention and control efforts.

Assessment in behavioral epidemiology includes monitoring and investigating personal health behaviors and related disease. In the United States, assessment of health behaviors is the primary function of the Behavioral Risk Factor Surveillance System (BRFSS) (Centers for Disease Control and Prevention [CDC], 2014a), the Youth Risk Behavior Surveillance System (YRBSS) (CDC, 2014d), State Tobacco Activities Tracking and Evaluation (STATE) (CDC, 2014c), National

© Dmytro Hurnytskiy/ShutterStock, Inc.

Household Travel Survey (U.S. Department of Transportation, 2014), Total Diet Study (TDS) (U.S. Food and Drug Administration, 2013), the National Health and Nutrition Examination Survey (CDC, 2014b), and others. Health outcomes related to health behaviors and other factors are also obtained from a number of sources (e.g., vital statistics registration systems, hospitals, and disease registries).

The purpose of this chapter is to describe direct and indirect measures of exposure (e.g., health behaviors) and outcome data and present measures of frequency used in epidemiology. Measures of association will be assessed for dichotomous exposure and outcome variables, and confidence intervals will be presented for evaluating precision in our frequency estimates and the measures of association.

Data

Data obtained from study subjects are numerical measurements on one or more variables of interest from the target population. There are several methods for collecting numerical (quantitative) data, including observing and recording well-defined events, surveys with close-ended questions, experiments, program evaluations, and relevant data from management information systems. Results from quantitative data collection methods can be summarized, compared, and generalized in a straightforward manner. On the other hand, qualitative data collection techniques include in-depth interviews, observation methods, and document reviews. Such data are often useful for improving the quality of survey-based quantitative evaluations by helping to generate new hypotheses, strengthen the design and quality of survey questionnaires, and clarify and expand quantitative research findings.

Data may involve collecting new information (i.e., primary data) or reviewing and synthesizing existing data (i.e., secondary data). Both types of data are commonly used in epidemiology to answer specific research questions. In the research process, an important consideration is whether the available information and data will appropriately answer the research question or whether there is a need for new data. Some research questions can be answered with existing data, and other research questions require the collection of new data.

If existing data are available to answer the research question, the study can be done more quickly and at lower cost. Often secondary data from large organizations' or governments' data sets may be of high quality, based on rigorous standards. However, a common downside of secondary data is that it may not directly represent the population of interest, and the sample size may be insufficient to represent subgroups of the population. These strengths and limitations are factors to consider in the research process.

There are many sources of existing, available data, some of which were mentioned in the introduction of this chapter. These sources tend to provide information in aggregate form. After existing data are aggregated, they can be qualitatively or quantitatively summarized and evaluated for associations. Two common ways to qualitatively summarize data are narrative and systematic. A narrative review typically consists of a description of the studies and findings. Narrative reviews do not necessarily follow a particular structure. Systematic reviews typically start with a predefined structure, and specific information is collected from each paper and summarized. A common way to summarize aggregated results from research studies is to conduct a meta-analysis. A quantitative assessment of ecologic data is the same as conventional analyses involving individual level data.

Exposure Data

The investigator decides what variables will be treated as the exposure and the outcome variables. *Exposure* refers to having come in contact with a cause or possessing a characteristic that is a determinant of a given health problem. It may represent an actual exposure (e.g., a toxic chemical or microorganism), an individual attribute (e.g., age, gender, race/ethnicity), or a behavior (e.g., alcohol consumption, cholesterol awareness, screening practices, exercise, fruit and vegetable consumption, healthcare access, immunization, oral health, weight management, physical activity, and tobacco use). Linking an exposure to a health-related state or event requires an accurate assessment of exposure. Measuring the intensity and duration of exposure is often necessary for supporting causal inference. Exposure may involve an intense dose over a relatively short period of time or a low-level, prolonged dose over a period from weeks to years. Identifying an association between dose and an adverse health outcome provides support for causality. The quality of the exposure measurements influences the validity of the study. A challenge in measuring behavior is that we often rely on individual responses to questionnaire data, which is susceptible to bias. If we are interested in measuring behavior that occurred in the distant past, accurate recall becomes an area of concern. In addition to limited recall, incomplete measurements, inaccurate records, and variability of exposure from person to person are important issues to consider. A direct measure of the past exposure may not be possible and can require estimation through modeling.

An exposure may be a specific event and relatively easy to measure. Other exposures can be subdivided into dose or duration (e.g., number of glasses of water, number of years worked in a coal mine, and average number of cigarettes smoked per day and for how many years). A disease may require a minimal level of exposure and increase in probability with longer exposure. Such a relationship between exposure and disease may be missed with a dichotomous measure characterizing the presence or absence of the exposure. In many cases it is more appropriate to use ordinal or continuous measures of the exposure, especially when trying to assess a dose–response relationship, such as tobacco smoking and lung cancer. It may be useful to restrict the study group to those who are most likely exposed or to those with the most years of exposure. This may increase the probability of finding a dose-related effect while increasing the efficiency of the study by requiring fewer participants.

Measurement of an exposure variable on a continuous scale is the most informative for evaluating associations. Continuous scaled data allows us to measure dose–response between variables. In some cases, however, exposure information is only available on a nominal scale (e.g., exposed versus unexposed). This may be the only alternative when only perceived exposure versus documented exposure is available or when the exposure occurred in the past and cannot be directly measured. There is also the basic question as to what to measure (e.g., average exercise, peak exercise, or cumulative exercise).

Both direct and indirect measures of data can be used to estimate exposure. Direct measures of exposure may occur through personal monitoring and the use of biologic markers. Personal measurement allows for assessment of the contaminant. Biological markers are useful for representing total dose to the body from multiple routes of exposure. These data can provide exposure measures on a continuous scale, which is ideal for identifying adverse health outcomes, according to dose and whether a threshold exists. Indirect measurements of dose are easier to obtain but are clearly less precise. Limited resources may cause us to rely on indirect measures of exposure such as estimates of drinking water use and food use.

DIRECT MEASURES

Direct measures of exposure include personal monitoring and use of biologic markers. Personal monitoring involves quantitative measurements of personal exposure. Individuals wear personal monitoring devices while they perform their normal activities. For example, an individual may wear a pedometer to indicate steps taken; a dosimeter to estimate total exposure to radiation in the workplace through air, water, and food; or a personal air monitor may be worn to measure exposure to air pollutants in the home. There are currently many other direct monitoring devices available on the market. For example, Phillips activity monitor is a small device that can be put in a person's pocket to track body motion and energy expenditure (Phillips, 2014). The device can then be connected to a computer to monitor activity data. Withings blood pressure monitor measures blood pressure via an iPhone, iPod touch, or iPad, with graphs, charts, and readings to help gauge the impact of fitness efforts (Withings, 2014). Heart rate monitors are also widely available for directly measuring a person's heart rate during various activities (Polar, 2014).

A *biomarker* is a biological molecule found in blood, other body fluids, or tissues that indicates normal or abnormal process, or conditions or diseases (National Cancer Institute, 2014). The approach to measuring pollutant levels in tissue or fluid samples is called *biomonitoring* (U.S. Environmental Protection Agency, 2014). Biologic markers are those specific anatomic, physiologic, biochemical, or molecular characteristics used to measure the presence and severity of a disease or condition. Biological monitoring can involve measurements of concentrations in human tissues (blood lead), metabolic products (dimethylarsenic acid in urine after arsenic exposure), or markers of physiologic effects (e.g., protein adducts induced by beta-naphthylamine in cigarette smoke) (Hertz-Picciotto, 1998). For example, heavy metals and some pesticides can accumulate in the body and can be identified through biologic markers.

INDIRECT MEASURES

Although personal monitoring and use of biologic markers can reflect certain behaviors and various environmental factors, indirect methods for obtaining exposure information are often more common, particularly in the behavioral sciences (e.g., questionnaires, surrogates, existing records, and diaries). Questionnaires translate the research objectives into specific questions. Answers to these questions provide the data used in data analysis. Questionnaire data rely on individual recall and knowledge and are thus subject to error. Bias may be introduced by the interviewer's inflections, expressions, gender, and appearance. Telephone interviews are becoming more difficult to conduct because of caller identification, cell phones, and a decreasing tolerance of telemarketing in the population. Mailed questionnaires avoid interviewer influences but are subject to low response rates. (As a general rule of thumb, a response rate of 80% or better is ideal in epidemiologic studies. However, a 60% response rate or better is good for a mail study.) In addition, they exclude individuals who cannot read, and they do not allow the responder to obtain item clarifications. Email questionnaires are becoming an increasingly popular way to obtain information because of their relative speed, low cost, and ability to attach pictures and sound files; they often stimulate higher response levels than snail mail surveys. However, some challenges to email surveys include obtaining (or purchasing) a list of email addresses, nonresponse to unsolicited email (which may be higher than unsolicited regular mail), and obtaining a representative sample of the general population.

Some exposures may be represented by surrogate measures. For decedents who committed suicide or who died from an accidental drug overdose, their next of kin or close friends may be asked questions about potential behaviors that may have caused the adverse health outcome. However, such measures are more prone to errors. It may also be possible to obtain exposure information from existing records, such as hospital admission or discharge records, pathology records, and crisis assessment prevention intervention services. This approach avoids the problems of interviewer bias, recall bias, and response bias.

Several studies have used diaries to identify exposure. For example, in one study, daily diaries were used to record exposure to environmental tobacco smoke until the occurrence of clinical pregnancy or for up to 1 year. Environmental tobacco smoke was defined as "the mean number of cigarettes smoked per day at home by household members over an entire menstrual cycle before the menstrual period" (Chen, Cho, & Damokosh, 2000, p. 1019). The results of the study showed an increased risk of dysmenorrhea, or excessive menstrual pain, among women exposed to environmental tobacco smoke, and more so with higher levels of exposure.

Outcome Data

An *outcome* is any result that came from an exposure to a causal factor or from an intervention. Outcome status is typically measured as a dichotomous variable (e.g., present versus not present; alive versus dead), but it may also be measured on an ordinal scale (e.g., severe, moderate, mild, no disease), a discrete scale (e.g., number of events), or as a continuous variable (e.g., concentrations of lead in the blood). The type of data considered is often determined by accessibility. The outcome status should be based on a standard case definition with an adequate level of reporting. A standard case definition will minimize misclassification and consequential bias.

The clinical criteria of a case, particularly in the setting of an outbreak investigation, may be restricted by person (e.g., children or the elderly), place (e.g., a certain work site), and time (e.g., cases occurring in the past 48 hours) variables. The clinical criteria may include laboratory confirmation. However, obtaining the biological media and having the available expertise and resources for assessment may be complicated. Clinical criteria often include specific signs, symptoms, and other information. Examinations and tests are used by clinicians to characterize disease. The validity of a test is determined by the test's sensitivity (proportion of patients with a given outcome who have a positive test) and specificity (proportion of individuals without a given outcome who have a negative test), as well as its reliability (performance over time).

In some situations the outcome is not a disease characterized by a specific case definition, but it involves an outcome that is more subjectively based. For example, suppose the outcome of interest is general health. The BRFSS routinely asks, "How is your general health?" with the possible responses of "excellent," "very good," "good," "fair," and "poor." In 2012, the percentages corresponding to these responses were 18.8, 33.4, 30.9, 12.5, and 4.4, respectively (CDC, 2012). A challenge with these results is that they are based on personal responses among people who may view health much differently. Classifying someone as healthy or not, or anywhere on a continuum of health, requires an agreed-upon definition and interpretation of health. The World Health Organization proposed six dimensions of health. It is unlikely that many of the people who completed the BRFSS survey were fully aware of or considered this definition of health as they responded to the question. Herbert Spencer defined health as "the perfect adjustment of an organism to its environment" (1861–1919). At the population level, the concept of perfect adjustment can be illustrated by herd immunity in which a population adjusts to the presence of a pathogen by containing the individuals that cannot be protected via inoculation within a pool of immune individuals. Under Spencer's definition, health on an individual level would be measured by the ability to adapt to new threats in the environment without a change in their health state. For example, the body has the ability to metabolize a newly introduced toxin without changing other aspects of overall health. Is this how some people interpreted health as they responded to the BRFSS questionnaire? Some might merely have interpreted health as the ability to resist disease, while others might base it on how they currently feel, rather than how they feel on average.

It would be ideal to count the number of healthy people in a population and attempt to maintain or increase this level of health, but because of the aforementioned challenges, measuring health is less straightforward than measuring, say, disease in a population. When one thinks about how to count the number of healthy people in a population, it becomes apparent that it is difficult to know how an individual defines health when asked about his or her general health.

Asking people about their general health, as was done in the BRFSS survey, may be a good approach to reflect overall health, but it may be improved if respondents were given a specific definition of health to think about prior to answering the question. In practice, there are several health indicators available. Instruments have been developed that focus on several aspects of health (e.g., physical fulfill-ment, psychosocial comfort and closeness, family planning, opportu-nities for choice, satisfaction with and perceived quality of services, community involvement, trust in others, perceived enabling factors, community participation, peace, safety, and factors associated with poor reproductive health such as abuse, exploitation, unwanted preg-nancy, disease, death, and more).

Many of the health outcomes that are regularly monitored and reported in public health tend to involve data that are required by law (e.g., death certificates, hospital discharge information, and notifi-able disease). The advantage of using these data is that it generally involves high standards for data quality and collection methods. Thus, summary statistics of these data are more likely to be complete and reliable. When considering health indicators, one should know that they can be potentially misleading if based on small sample sizes, nonrepresentative samples, poor response rates, changes in reporting over time, differential response, changes in procedures for data col-lection, changes in dentitions and values related to health, changes in socioeconomic characteristics of the population, and more (World Health Organization, 2006).

Ratios, Proportions, and Rates

Exposure and outcome variables measured on a dichotomous scale are typically described using ratios, proportions, and rates. Ratios, proportions, and rates can all be expressed using the same general formula,

$$\text{Ratio, proportion, rate} = \frac{x}{y} \times 10^n$$

A ratio is a part divided by another part, a proportion is the number of observations with the characteristic of interest divided by the total number of observations, and a rate is a number of cases of a particular outcome divided by the size of the population in that period. A ratio is multiplied by $10^0 = 1$, a proportion is multiplied by $10^2 = 100$, and if we desire to express it as a percentage, a rate is multiplied by 10^n, where n is a number between 0 and 6, depending on what it takes to make the results more interpretable. The base rate is 10^n. For example, suppose the rate of Hodgkin's disease in the United States in 2014 is 0.00003. This rate reflects the number of cases (x) divided by the midyear population. Thus, rather than trying to communicate this rate in this form, we could multiply the rate base by 100,000 and say the rate of Hodgkin's disease in the United States in 2014 is 3 per 100,000. You may agree that this latter way of expressing information is preferable.

There are four common measures of incidence, described in **Table 6-1**. The first three measures represent rates, but the last measure is a proportion because it reflects all existing cases at a given point in time.

Cohort data are used in calculating incidence rates. Sometimes the incidence rate reflects the risk of a chronic condition over a year. In this situation, we typically use the midyear population to estimate the person years at risk. For example, in 2011 the number of female malignant breast cancer cases reported to 18 tumor registries in the Surveillance, Epidemiology, and End Results (SEER) Program of the National Cancer Institute was 57,004 (SEER, 2014). The female population on July 1 of that year was 43,955,802. Thus, the incidence rate of female breast cancer was $\frac{57,004}{43,955,802} \times 100,000 = 129.7$ per 100,000 person years.

The incidence rate (sometimes called the person-time rate), attack rate, and secondary attack rate are measures of risk and are associated with certain factors. Several studies have linked reproductive behaviors with cancer risk. Cancer risk associated with early and late maternal age at first birth has been widely studied. For example, first childbirth at age 35 or older may be at increased risk for breast and brain cancers, and birth occurring at age 19 or younger may increase the risk for cervical and endometrial cancers (Merrill, 2010). High parity and breastfeeding have also been associated with reduced risk of female breast cancer (Daniels, Merrill, Lyon, Stanford, & White, 2004). This research provides information that can be useful in family planning, and it can serve as a guide in establishing and reorienting existing healthcare services to better meet the needs of specific age groups.

Point prevalence is a measure that is useful for describing the magnitude of a public health problem at a point in time. The measure is sometimes referred to as an indicator of burden and is used instead of incidence for assessing diseases when it is difficult to identify the exact time a person became a case (e.g., arthritis or diabetes). Prevalence is a dynamic measure in that it reflects the influences of incidence, mortality, and cure. Prevalence is often obtained from cross-sectional survey data. For this reason, cross-sectional surveys are sometimes called prevalence surveys.

Historically, mortality data have been more readily available than incidence data. For this reason, disease risk was typically estimated using mortality rates. However, in recent decades the number of disease registries has increased, and risk estimates of disease can be more directly measured. Yet mortality measures are still widely used in epidemiology to monitor and compare health statuses throughout

Table 6-1

Measures of Incidence

Measure	Numerator (x)	Denominator (y)	Expressed per number at risk	Example
Incidence rate	Number of new cases of a specified disease reported during a given time interval	Estimated time individuals in the population are at risk	Varies	Three injuries occurred among 48 employees who worked a total of 1,824 hours in the past month. Incidence rate = $\frac{3}{1,824} \times 1,000 = 1.64$ injuries per 1,000 hours worked.
Attack rate	Number of new cases of a specified disease reported during an epidemic period	Population at start of the epidemic period	Usually 100	In a small community of 460 residents, 88 attended a social event that included a meal prepared by several individuals. Within 3 days, 37 of those who attended the event became ill with a condition diagnosed as salmonella enterocolitis. Attack rate = $\frac{37}{88} \times 100 = 42\%$.
Secondary attack rate	Number of new cases of a specified disease among contacts of known cases	Size of contact population at risk	Usually 100	In a community of 908 households (population 4,520), public health authorities found 120 persons with condition X in 80 households. A total of 400 persons lived in the 80 affected households. Assuming that each household had only one primary case, the secondary attack rate is $\frac{120-80}{400-80} \times 100 = 12.5\%$.
Point prevalence	Number of existing cases at a specified point in time	Estimated population at the same point in time	Usually 100	Among 172 adults who completed a survey, 38 indicated that a doctor had told them they have arthritis. The point prevalence is $\frac{38}{172} \times 100 = 22.1\%$.

the world (**Table 6-2**). The first and most basic measure of death is the mortality rate. However, different measures of mortality are often used, each conveying a specific type of information. For example, the maternal mortality rate says something about the overall health of a population. It further represents family planning; antenatal care coverage; births attended by skilled health personnel; availability of basic essential obstetric care; and availability of comprehensive essential obstetric care. In 2013, the maternal mortality was 28 per 100,000

Table 6-2

Measures of Mortality

Measure	Numerator (x)	Denominator (y)	Expressed per number at risk
Mortality rate	Total number of deaths reported during a given time interval	Estimated midinterval population	1,000 or 100,000
Cause-specific death rate	Number of deaths assigned to a specific cause during a given time interval	Estimated midinterval population	100,000
Proportional mortality ratio	Number of deaths assigned to a specific cause during a given time interval	Total number of deaths from all causes during the same time interval	100
Death-to-case ratio	Number of deaths assigned to a specific disease during a given time interval	Number of new cases of that disease reported during the same time interval	100
Neonatal mortality rate	Number of deaths younger than 28 days of age during a given time interval	Number of live births during the same time interval	1,000
Postneonatal mortality rate	Number of deaths from 28 days to, but not including, 1 year of age during a given time interval	Number of live births during the same time interval	1,000
Infant mortality rate	Number of deaths younger than 1 year of age during a given time interval	Number of live births reported during the same time interval	1,000
Maternal mortality rate	Number of deaths assigned to pregnancy-related causes during a given time interval	Number of live births during the same time interval	100,000
Maternal mortality ratio	Number of deaths of women during or shortly after a pregnancy	Number of live births	100,000
Fetal mortality rate	Number of fetal deaths after at least 20 weeks of gestation	Number of live births plus fetal deaths	1,000
Abortion rate	Number of abortions done during a given time interval	Number of women ages 15–44 years during the same time interval	1,000

live births in the United Sates (World Bank, 2014). Other selected rates were 8 in the United Kingdom; 470 in Zimbabwe; 23 in Ukraine; 4 in Sweden; 140 in South Africa; 850 in Somalia; 24 in the Russian Federation; 3 in Poland; 49 in Mexico; 4 in Iceland; 140 in Guatemala; 420 in Ethiopia; 22 in Chile; and 6 in Australia.

Measures of natality are shown in **Table 6-3**. A number of factors have been associated with the decision to have children: governmental policies (e.g., incentives and restrictions); social beliefs (e.g., male children valued more than female children); religious beliefs (e.g., may influence use of contraception); abortion rates; poverty or economic prosperity; literacy; infant mortality rate (higher infant mortality rates generally equate to higher birth rates); conflict (e.g., war, security, safety); and urbanization. A related measure to the fertility rate is the total fertility rate, which is the total number of children a woman would have by the end of her reproductive period if she experienced the currently prevailing age-specific fertility rates throughout her childbearing life (ages 15–49 years). In other words, it is the average number of births per woman. In contrast, the fertility rate represents the number of live births per 1,000 females of childbearing age. A total fertility rate equal to 2 means that each pair of parents is replacing themselves. However, because some children will die before they grow up to have their own children, the replacement rate is actually 2.1 or 2.2. In countries with low life expectancies, the replacement rate might be even higher. The United States has the highest total fertility rate among major wealthy countries (**Figure 6-1**).

STANDARDIZING RATES

Rates provide a more meaningful comparison among groups than raw numbers. This is because the number of cases is expressed relative to

Table 6-3			
Measures of Natality			
Measure	Numerator (x)	Denominator (y)	Expressed per number at risk
Birth rate	Number of live births reported during a given time interval	Estimated total population at midinterval	1,000
Fertility rate	Number of live births reported during a given time interval	Estimated number of women aged 15–44 years at midinterval	1,000
Rate of natural increase	Number of live births minus the number of deaths during a given time interval	Estimated total population at midinterval	1,000

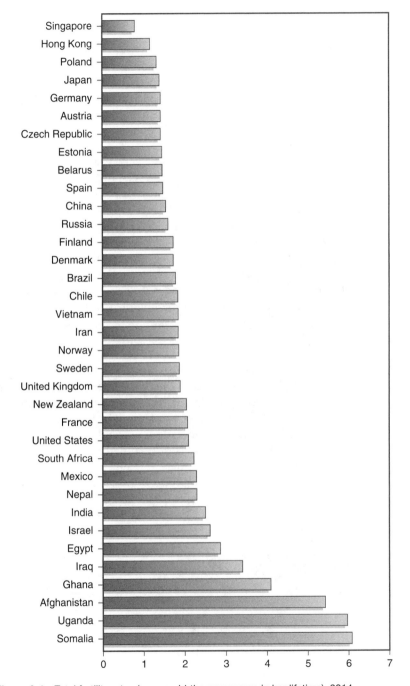

Figure 6-1 Total fertility rates (average births per woman in her lifetime), 2014

Data from Central Intelligence Agency. (2014). Total Fertility Rate by Country. Retrieved July 25, 2014, from https://www.cia.gov/library/publications/the-world-factbook/rankorder/2127rank.html.

the size of the populations. A *crude rate* is a single number computed as a summary measure for an entire population. A *specific rate* is derived in comparatively small, well-defined subgroups. A problem that can occur when crude rates for different groups are compared is when the populations vary substantially with respect to characteristics such as age and gender. For example, if two populations have vastly different age distributions, differences in incidence and mortality rates may be due to location or differences in the age distributions that influence incidence or mortality.

When a health outcome of interest is related to age, if the age distribution differs between or among the groups being compared, the rates should be adjusted to avoid bias from confounding. Similarly, if a disease rate is being monitored over time within a group, and that disease is associated with age, the rates should be adjusted. If there is no difference in the age distribution between groups being compared or within a group being monitored over time, even though the health outcome of interest may be associated with age, age adjustment is not necessary.

There are two methods for age adjusting rates: the direct method of standardization and the indirect method of standardization.

DIRECT METHOD OF STANDARDIZATION

An *age-standardized rate* (also called an *age-adjusted rate*) is a weighted average of the age group specific rates. The weights are the proportions of persons in the corresponding age groups of a selected population, which we call the standard population. To illustrate, data are shown for two hypothetical populations in **Table 6-4**. First, select a standard population. Let us choose Population A, although the choice is arbitrary. Second, calculate the age group specific rates in Population B, which are $120/5,000 = 0.024$, $20/2,000 = 0.01$, and $20/500 = 0.04$. Third, weight these rates using the age group specific populations in A: $0.024 \times 1,500 = 36$, $0.01 \times 4,500 = 45$,

---

Table 6-4

Age, Population, and Deaths of Populations A and B

Population A			Population B		
Ages (years)	Population	# Deaths	Ages (years)	Population	# Deaths
15–19	1,500	30	15–19	5,000	120
20–24	4,500	16	20–24	2,000	20
25–29	6,000	121	25–29	500	20
Total	12,000	167	Total	7,500	160

and $0.04 \times 6,000 = 240$. Fourth, sum the weighted rates and divide by the total population in A: $(36 + 45 + 240)/12,000 = 0.02675$. We can multiply this age-adjusted rate by a rate base of, say, 100,000 to get 2,675 per 100,000. Therefore, if Population B had the same age distribution as Population A, then we would expect a rate of 2,675 per 100,000. In comparison, the rate in Population A is 1,392 per 100,000. The rate in Population B is 1.92 times (or 92%) higher than in Population A, after adjusting for differences in the age distribution.

INDIRECT METHOD OF STANDARDIZATION

The indirect method is used when age group specific rates are unstable because of small numbers or when there are missing numbers. The indirect method of age adjustment involves selecting a standard population, calculating the age-specific rates for the standard population, multiplying the age-specific rates by the age-specific population values in the comparison populations to obtain the expected number of health-related states or events in each age group, then dividing the total number of health-related states or events observed in the comparison population by the total number of expected health-related states or events. We call this ratio the standardized morbidity (or mortality) ratio (SMR), which is expressed as follows:

$$SMR = \frac{Observed}{Expected}$$

Interpreting SMR

SMR = 1: The health-related states or events observed were the same as expected from the age-specific rates in the standard population.

SMR > 1: More health-related states or events were observed than expected from the age-specific rates in the standard population.

SMR < 1: Fewer health-related states or events were observed than expected from the age-specific rates in the standard population.

To illustrate the indirect method of standardization, assume we have the data shown in **Table 6-5**. First, we will choose Population A as the standard. Second, the age group specific rates for Population A are as follows: $30/1,500 = 0.02$, $16/4,500 = 0.003556$, and $121/6,000 = 0.020167$. Third, multiply these rates by the age group specific population values in Population B to get the expected number of deaths in Population B, assuming they had the same age distribution as Population A: $0.02 \times 5,000 = 100$, $0.003556 \times 2,000 = 7$, and 0.020167

Table 6-5					
Age, Population, and Deaths of Populations A and B					
Population A			**Population B**		
Ages (years)	Population	# Deaths	Ages (years)	Population	# Deaths
15–19	1,500	30	15–19	5,000	
20–24	4,500	16	20–24	2,000	
25–29	6,000	121	25–29	500	
Total	12,000	167	Total	7,500	160

$\times$ 500 = 10. The total expected number is 117. The observed number of deaths was 160. Therefore,

$$\text{SMR} = \frac{160}{117} = 1.37$$

This ratio indicates that more deaths occurred in Population B than would be expected if they had the same age group specific rates as Population A.

USES OF STANDARDIZED RATES

Standardized rates, particularly age-adjusted rates, are commonly used for monitoring trends in vital statistics and chronic diseases and conditions. In practice, we should adjust the rates only if there is a confounding factor such as age or gender. It is important to remember that the adjusted rates are hypothetical constructs and do not represent the actual frequency in the population of interest. For this reason, the choice of the standard population is arbitrary, although it should reflect the time period and the populations being studied. Applying the direct method of age adjustment to rates over time assumes that the age-specific rates have a similar trend over time. If age-specific trends are not approximately parallel, then an age-adjusted rate can mask important information. In the situation of nonparallel trends in age-specific rates, reporting age-specific rates is more appropriate.

In practice, the direct method of standardizing rates is more common than the indirect method. With computer software such as Excel, it is fairly easy to compute age-adjusted rates using either the direct or indirect methods. A good rule of thumb is to use the direct method when subgroup-specific rates are available for all the groups being compared. If not, or if the subgroup rates are based on small numbers and are therefore unstable, the indirect method should be used.

CONFIDENCE INTERVALS

If our study is based on sample data, it is appropriate to use confidence intervals. A *confidence interval* represents the level of confidence we have that our estimate reflects the truth; it is the range of values in which the true population value is likely to fall. Assuming a normal distribution, the 95% confidence interval for the true population mean is given by

$$\bar{X} \pm 1.96\frac{s}{\sqrt{n}}$$

where $\bar{X}$ is the sample mean, s is the standard deviation, and n is the sample size. For example, suppose mean body mass index in a sample of 50 adults is 27.3, with standard deviation of 2. The 95% confidence interval is

$$27.3 \pm 1.96\frac{2}{\sqrt{50}} \rightarrow 26.7 - 27.9$$

The 95% confidence interval for the true population proportion is given by

$$p \pm 1.96\sqrt{\frac{p(1-p)}{n}}$$

where p is the estimated proportion based on data from a sample. For example, suppose in a sample of 100 people, 25 indicated eating 5 or more servings of fruit and vegetables per day. The 95% confidence interval is

$$0.25 \pm 1.96\sqrt{\frac{0.25(1-0.25)}{100}} \rightarrow 0.165 - 0.335$$

The 95% confidence interval for the true population rate is given by

$$Rate \pm 1.96\sqrt{\frac{Rate(1 - Rate)}{Population\ at\ risk}}$$

For example, let us calculate the 95% confidence interval death rate for individuals aged 15–19 years in Population A:

$$0.02 \pm 1.96\sqrt{\frac{0.02(1 - 0.02)}{1,500}} \rightarrow 0.0129 - 0.0271$$

At this point we can multiply by a rate base, such as 1,000, yielding a 95% confidence interval for 20 per 1,000 of 12.9–27.1.

The 95% confidence interval for the SMR is given by

$$\frac{\left(\sqrt{\text{Observed}} \pm 1.96 / 2\right)^{2}}{\text{Expected}}$$

For the SMR $= \frac{160}{117} = 1.38$ previously shown, that corresponds to the data in Table 6-5, and applying the formula gives a 95% confidence interval of 1.16–1.59.

MEASURES OF ASSOCIATION

There are many approaches for evaluating the association between variables. A thorough discussion of these various methods is well beyond the scope of this text. In the remainder of this chapter, we will present ways to measure the association between dichotomous exposure and outcome variables.

Epidemiologic data tend to represent count data, which are combined with the at-risk population to calculate proportions and rates (see Tables 6-1, 6-2, and 6-3). A cohort refers to people who are followed over time to describe the incidence or the natural history of a health-related state or event. If an incidence rate is involved wherein the denominator reflects person time, then the ratio of two incidence rates is referred to as a rate ratio and is expressed as follows:

$$\text{Rate Ratio} = \frac{\text{Incidence Rate (Exposed)}}{\text{Incidence Rate (Unexposed)}}$$

This statistic is useful for assessing the relationship between an exposure and an outcome. For example, suppose the incidence rate of disease x is 200 per 100,000 person years for people who currently smoke cigarettes and 100 per 100,000 person years for people who do not. Then the rate ratio $= 2$; that is, current smokers are 2 times (or 100%) more likely to develop the disease.

When the ratio of two attack rates are being compared according to exposure status, we call it a risk ratio, which is expressed as follows:

$$\text{Risk Ratio} = \frac{\text{Attack Rate (Exposed)}}{\text{Attack Rate (Unexposed)}}$$

For example, suppose that following a picnic, several people developed gastrointestinal problems. The attack rate for those who ate the chocolate pudding pie was 5 per 100 people, and the attack rate for those who did not eat the chocolate pudding pie was 1 per 100 people. The risk ratio was 5, meaning that those who ate the chocolate pudding pie were 5 times (or 400%) more likely to become ill.

Although cohort data are useful because they allow us to calculate incidence and attack rates, in some epidemiologic studies we do not have the entire cohort of interest included in our study, which is true in case-control studies. In a case-control study, the presence of an outcome of interest is identified. Then a control group is selected of persons who look like the cases in terms of age, sex, race, and so forth, but who do not have the disease. Next we investigate whether the cases are more or less likely to have been exposed. Because the entire cohort is not available, incidence rates or attack rates cannot be calculated. However, an appropriate measure of association for these data is the odds ratio. The odds ratio is the odds of exposure among the cases divided by the odds of exposure among the controls. The following 2 × 2 table (**Table 6-6**) illustrates this point. The letters represent count data. The odds of exposure among cases is a/c. The odds of exposure among noncases is b/d. Then,

$$\text{Odds Ratio} = \frac{a/c}{b/d} = \frac{a \times d}{b \times c}$$

If sample data are involved, then a 95% confidence interval for the odds ratio may be used, which is computed as

$$\exp\left[\ln(\text{Odds Ratio}) \pm \left(1.96 \times \sqrt{\frac{1}{a} + \frac{1}{b} + \frac{1}{c} + \frac{1}{d}} \; \right) \right]$$

For example, in a case-control study, researchers explored whether a benign tumor that develops on the hearing and balance nerves near the inner ear is associated with exposure to loud noise (Fisher et al., 2014). One of the loud noise exposures assessed was attendance at concerts, clubs, or sporting events. Of those with the tumor, 62 attended concerts, clubs, or sporting events and 188 did not. Of those without the tumor, 60 attended these events and 315 did not. The odds ratio is calculated as follows:

$$\text{Odds Ratio} = \frac{62 \times 315}{60 \times 188} = 1.73$$

Because the odds ratio is the ratio of two odds, not probabilities, we should not use *likely*, which implies probability. Rather, we say something like the odds of having been exposed to loud noise among

Table 6-6		
2 × 2 Table		
	Outcome	
Exposed	Yes	No
Yes	a	b
No	c	d

tumor cases is 1.73 (95% confidence interval [CI] = 1.16–2.58) times greater than the odds of having had meningitis in the past, among controls.

If the data in the table came from a cohort study involving person-time data, the rate ratio would be calculated as follows:

$$\text{Rate Ratio} = \frac{a\,/\,(\text{person - time, exposed group})}{c\,/\,(\text{person - time, unexposed group})}$$

If sample data are involved, then a 95% confidence interval for the rate ratio can be reported with the estimated rate ratio. It is calculated as follows:

$$\exp\left[\ln(\text{Rate Ratio}) \pm \left(1.96 \times \sqrt{\frac{1}{a} + \frac{1}{c}}\right)\right]$$

For example, let's return to the 2011 female malignant breast cancer data from the SEER program (SEER, 2014). Lower breast cancer incidence rates of women of Hispanic origin, compared with not of Hispanic origin, have been previously identified, with some of the difference attributed to dietary, reproductive, and screening behaviors (Merrill, Harris, & Merrill, 2013). The 2011 female malignant breast cancer rate, age adjusted to the U.S. 2000 population, was 122.3 (50,878 cases; 95% CI 121.2–123.3) for non-Hispanic origin and 88.6 (6,126 cases; 95% CI: 86.4–91.0) for Hispanic origin. The rate ratio is 1.38 (95% CI: 1.34–1.42). Thus, non-Hispanic women were 1.38 times (or 38%) more likely than Hispanic women to be diagnosed with breast cancer, after adjusting for differences in the age distribution.

If the data in the table came from a cohort study involving attack rates, the risk ratio would be calculated as follows:

$$\text{Risk Ratio} = \frac{a\,/\,(a + b)}{c\,/\,(c + d)}$$

The 95% confidence interval for the risk ratio that is relevant when sample data are involved is calculated as follows:

$$\exp\left[\ln(\text{Risk Ratio}) \pm \left(1.96 \times \sqrt{\frac{b\,/\,a}{a+b} + \frac{d\,/\,c}{c+d}}\right)\right]$$

For example, suppose a dietary intervention was assigned to 174 individuals, with another 174 people instructed to maintain their current diet. After 6 months, 138 of those in the intervention group lowered their body mass index (BMI), and 98 of those in the comparison group lowered their BMI. Applying the previous formulas, the risk ratio was 1.41 and the 95% CI = 1.21–1.64. That is, the dietary intervention group was 1.41 times (41%) more likely to lower their BMI.

For cross-sectional data, the prevalence ratio is calculated the same way as the risk ratio, namely,

$$\text{Prevalence Ratio} = \frac{a / (a + b)}{c / (c + d)}$$

The 95% confidence interval for the prevalence ratio that is relevant when sample data are involved is calculated as follows:

$$\exp\left[\ln(\text{Prevalence Ratio}) \pm \left(1.96 \times \sqrt{\frac{b / a}{a + b} + \frac{d / c}{c + d}} \right) \right]$$

For example, a sample of middle school and high school students was asked whether they had ever felt sad or hopeless for 2 weeks or more. They were also asked if they had ever smoked marijuana. In the sample, 5,644 said they had felt sad or hopeless for 2 weeks or more, among which 963 said they had used marijuana, and 26,478 said they had not felt sad or helpless for 2 weeks or more, of which 1,260 said they had used marijuana. Applying the previous formulas gives a prevalence ratio of 3.60 (95% CI: 3.33–3.90). Thus, the prevalence of marijuana use is 3.60 times (or 260%) more likely among those with a history of feeling sad or hopeless than those who do not have such a history.

For matched data, such as in a case-crossover study or a matched case-control study, the odds ratio is estimated by taking the following ratio of discrepant pairs:

$$\text{Odds Ratio} = \frac{b}{c}$$

The 95% confidence interval for the odds ratio that is relevant when sample data are involved is calculated as follows:

$$\exp\left[\ln(\text{Odds Ratio}) \pm \left(1.96 \times \sqrt{\frac{1}{b} + \frac{1}{c}} \right) \right]$$

For example, a matched case-control study in Casablanca, Morocco, investigated whether candle lighting in the home increased the risk of lung cancer (Sasco et al., 2002). Controls were matched to cases according to smoking status, age, and sex. The data appear in **Table 6-7**.

Applying the formulas for matched case-control data gave an odds ratio of 2.5 (95% CI: 1.20–5.21). Thus, there is a significant positive association between candle lighting in the home and lung cancer.

Table 6-7		
Matched Case-Control Data from Casablanca, Morocco		
	Controls	
Cases	Candle lighting	No candle lighting
Candle lighting	25	25
No candle lighting	10	100

If data on a possible confounding factor were collected, to adjust for confounding at the analysis level of the study we can stratify or use multiple regression. Stratification eliminates the association between the confounder and exposure within the strata. In a case-control study, the Mantel-Haenszel method is useful for estimating a pooled (or summary) odds ratio across i homogeneous strata. It is computed as follows:

$$OR_{MH} = \frac{\sum \left(a_i d_i / n_i \right)}{\sum \left(b_i c_i / n_i \right)}$$

The 95% confidence interval for the pooled odds ratio that is relevant when sample data are involved is calculated as

$$OR_{MH} \left(1 \pm 1.96 / \sqrt{\chi_{MH}^2} \right)$$

For example, suppose we are interested in assessing whether smoking is associated with ovarian cancer. In a hypothetical case-control study to examine the association between smoking and ovarian cancer among nulliparous women, the results are as shown in **Table 6-8**.

The odds ratio = 0.498 (95% confidence interval = 0.261–0.950).

Now, suppose we stratify by oral contraceptive use (never versus ever) (**Table 6-9** and **Table 6-10**, respectively).

Table 6-8			
Hypothetical Case-Control Study Data			
	Cases	Controls	
Smoker	26	58	84
Nonsmoker	36	40	76
Total	62	98	160

Table 6-9

	Never Used Oral Contraceptives		
	Cases	Controls	
Smoker	9	8	17
Nonsmoker	32	28	60
Total	41	36	77

Table 6-10

	Ever Used Oral Contraceptives		
	Cases	Controls	
Smoker	17	50	67
Nonsmoker	4	12	16
Total	21	62	83

The odds ratio = 0.984 (95% confidence interval = 0.335–2.896).
The odds ratio = 1.02 (95% CI = 0.290–3.590).
The Mantel-Haenszel pooled (or summary) odds ratio across i homogeneous strata is

$$OR_{MH} = \frac{(9 \times 28)/77 + (17 \times 12)/83}{(32 \times 8)/77 + (4 \times 50)/83}$$

$$= 0.999 \ (95\% \ CI = 0.441 - 2.266)$$

Therefore, the odds ratio adjusted for contraceptive use is 0.999, which contrasts the crude odds ratio of 0.498. This suggests that the supposed protective effect from smoking was an artifact due to confounding with oral contraceptive use. Note that oral contraceptive use was a potential confounder because it was associated with smoking and, independent of that relationship, was also associated with uterine cancer. This can be shown by rearranging the data and estimating odds ratios for these associations.

It was appropriate to pool the stratified odds ratios in the previous example because they were homogeneous. Small differences in the odds ratios are likely explained by random error. If the stratified odds ratios were different, we would refer to the stratified variable as an effect modifier (**Table 6-11**). The same ideas also apply to cohort studies involving risk ratios or rate ratios.

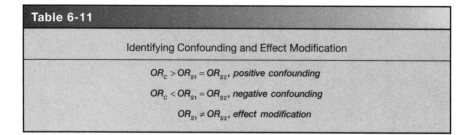

Table 6-11
Identifying Confounding and Effect Modification
$OR_C > OR_{S1} = OR_{S2}$, *positive confounding*
$OR_C < OR_{S1} = OR_{S2}$, *negative confounding*
$OR_{S1} \neq OR_{S2}$, *effect modification*

The Mantel-Haenszel risk ratio is

$$RR_{MH} = \frac{\sum (a_i(c_i + d_i)/n_i)}{\sum (c_i(a_i + b_i)/n_i)}$$

The 95% confidence interval for the pooled risk ratio that is relevant when sample data are involved is calculated as

$$RR_{MH}\left(1 \pm 1.96/\sqrt{\chi^2_{MH}}\right)$$

The Mantel-Haenszel rate ratio is

$$RR_{MH} = \frac{\sum (a_i \times \text{Time(not exposed group)}/\text{Time}_i)}{\sum (c_i \times \text{Time(exposed group)}/\text{Time}_i)}$$

The 95% confidence interval for the pooled risk ratio that is relevant when sample data are involved is calculated as

$$RR_{MH}\left(1 \pm 1.96/\sqrt{\chi^2_{MH}}\right)$$

Additional Epidemiologic Measures for Describing Cohort Data

It is unlikely that an exposure will be a necessary and sufficient cause of a health-related state or event, but it will likely explain a portion of the incidence rate in the exposed group. That is,

$$I_1 = \text{Incidence due to exposure} + I_0$$

If $I_1 > I_0$, the *excess incidence rate* (*rate difference* or *excess risk*) among those exposed to the risk factor, which is called the *attributable risk* (AR), is

$$AR = I_1 - I_0$$

AR is typically multiplied by a rate base.

The proportion of the incidence rate in the exposed group due to association with the risk factor is calculated as

$$AR\% = \frac{I_1 - I_0}{I_1} \times 100$$

The AR% can be expressed in terms of the risk ratio (or rate ratio) as follows:

$$AR\% = \frac{I_1 - I_0}{I_1} \times 100 = \frac{\frac{I_1 - I_0}{I_0}}{\frac{I_1}{I_0}} \times 100 = \frac{RR - 1}{RR} \times 100 \text{ given } RR \geq 1$$

If the outcome of interest is sufficiently rare such that relative odds (odds ratio [OR]) ≈ risk ratio [RR], then, if a case-control study is being conducted, AR% can be estimated using the odds ratio

$$AR\% = \frac{OR - 1}{OR} \times 100 \approx \frac{RR - 1}{RR} \times 100 \text{ given } OR \geq 1$$

Excess risk of the health-related state or event in the population that is attributed to the exposure is called the population attributable risk (PAR). It is calculated as

$$PAR = I - I_0$$

The PAR% measures the percentage of the health-related state or event in the population that can be attributed to the exposure and is calculated as

$$PAR\% = \frac{I - I_0}{I} \times 100$$

To illustrate, consider the data presented in Table 6-8, which involves a large cohort of Japanese American men examined from 1965 through 1968 and followed for 22 years (Chyou, Nomura, & Stemmermann, 1992). The purpose of the study was to assess the effect of cigarette smoking on cancer. From the data shown in **Table 6-12**, selected statistics were computed and are shown in **Table 6-13**. Assuming a causal association exists between cigarette smoking and cancer, any cancer risk for current smokers is 1.62 (62%) greater than for never smokers; the excess risk of cancer for current smokers attributed to their smoking is 84.59 (per 1,000); for cancer cases that are current smokers, the percentage of cases attributed to their smoking is 38.33%; the excess risk of cancer in the population attributed to current smoking is 34.61 (per 1,000); the percentage of cancer in the population that is attributed to current smoking is 18.60%. The results are interpreted in a similar manner for past cigarette smokers versus never smokers.

Table 6-12				
Smoking and Cancer Cohort Data Reflecting 8006 Japanese American Men				
	Any cancer			
	Yes	No	Total	Rate per 1,000
Current smokers	747	2,638	3,385	220.68
Never smokers	319	2,025	2,344	136.09
Total	1,066	4,663	5,729	186.07
Past smokers	323	1,708	2,031	159.03
Never smokers	319	2,025	2,344	136.09
Total	642	3,733	4,375	146.74

Table 6-13		
Summary Measures from the Japanese American Men Cohort Study		
	Any cancer	Any cancer
	Current versus never smokers	Past versus never smokers
Rate ratio	1.62	1.08
Attributable risk (AR)	84.59	22.94
AR%	38.33	14.43
Population AR	34.61	12.29
Population AR%	18.60	8.38

Summary

1. The core function areas of public health involve assessment, policy development, and assurance. Assessment in behavioral epidemiology includes monitoring and investigating personal health behaviors and related disease.

2. Primary data require collecting new information. Secondary data consist of reviewing and synthesizing existing data. Some research questions can be answered with existing data, and other research questions require the collection of new data. The strengths and limitations of both types of data should be considered in the research process.

3. An exposure variable represents a cause or a characteristic that is a determinant of a given health state. The measurement of an exposure variable on a continuous scale is the most informative for evaluating associations. However, in some cases exposure information is available only on a nominal scale (e.g., exposed versus unexposed). Both direct and indirect measures of data can be used to estimate exposure. Direct measures of exposure include personal monitoring and use of biologic markers. Indirect methods for obtaining exposure information are often more common, particularly in the behavioral sciences (e.g., questionnaires, surrogates, existing records, and diaries).

4. An outcome is any result that came from an exposure to a causal factor or from an intervention. It is usually measured on a dichotomous scale. Clinical criteria, often according to person, place, and time factors, are generally required to be a case.

5. Exposure and outcome variables measured on a dichotomous scale are typically described using ratios, proportions, and rates.

6. Four common measures of incidence data are the incidence rate, attack rate, secondary attack rate, and prevalence proportion.

7. A crude rate is a single number computed as a summary measure for an entire population. A specific rate is derived in comparatively small, well-defined subgroups. An age-standardized rate (also called an age-adjusted rate) is a weighted average of the age group specific rates. The weights are the proportions of persons in the corresponding age groups of a selected population, which we call the standard population.

8. The indirect method is used when age group specific rates are unstable because of small numbers or when there are missing numbers.

9. A confidence interval represents the range of values in which the true population value is likely to fall.

10. Measures of association between dichotomous exposure and outcome data include the rate ratio (for cohort data involving person-time rates), risk ratio (for cohort data involving attack rates), odds ratio (for case-control data), and prevalence ratio (for cross-sectional prevalence survey data).

11. Additional measures that are useful for describing cohort data include attributable risk, attributable risk percentage, population attributable risk, and population attributable risk percentage.

References

Centers for Disease Control and Prevention. (2012). Prevalence and trends data: Health status—2012. Retrieved from http://apps.nccd.cdc.gov/brfss/list.asp?cat=HS&yr=2012&qkey=8001&state=All

Centers for Disease Control and Prevention. (2014a). Behavioral risk factor surveillance system (BRFSS). Retrieved from http://www.cdc.gov/brfss/

Centers for Disease Control and Prevention. (2014b). National health and nutrition examination survey. Retrieved from http://www.cdc.gov/nchs/nhanes.htm

Centers for Disease Control and Prevention. (2014c). State tobacco activities tracking and evaluation (STATE) system. Retrieved from http://apps.nccd.cdc.gov/statesystem/Default/Default.aspx

Centers for Disease Control and Prevention. (2014d). Youth risk behavior surveillance system (YRBSS). Retrieved from http://www.cdc.gov/HealthyYouth/yrbs/index.htm

Central Intelligence Agency. (2014). Country comparison: Total fertility rate. Retrieved from https://www.cia.gov/library/publications/the-world-factbook/rankorder/2127rank.html

Chen, C., Cho, S., & Damokosh, A. I. (2000). Prospective study of exposure to environmental tobacco smoke and dysmenorrhea. *Environmental Health Perspectives*, 108, 1019–1022.

Chyou, P. H., Nomura, A. M., & Stemmermann, G. N. (1992). A prospective study of the attributable risk of cancer due to cigarette smoking. *American Journal of Public Health, 82*(1), 37–40.

Daniels, M., Merrill, R. M., Lyon, J. L., Stanford, J. B., & White, G. L., Jr. (2004). Associations between breast cancer risk factors and religious practices in Utah. *Preventive Medicine, 38*(1), 28–38.

Fisher, J. L., Petterson, D., Palmisano, S., Schwartzbaum, J. A., Edwards, C. G., Mathiesen, T, … Feychting, M. (2014). Loud noise exposure and acoustic neuroma. *American Journal of Epidemiology, 180*(1), 58–67.

Hertz-Picciotto, I. (1998). Environmental epidemiology. In K. Rothman & S. Greenland (Eds.), *Modern epidemiology* (pp. 555–584). Philadelphia, PA: Lippincott-Raven.

Institute of Medicine. (1998). *The future of public health.* Washington, DC: National Academy Press.

Merrill, R. M. (2010). *Reproductive epidemiology: Principles and methods.* Sudbury, MA: Jones and Bartlett Publishers.

Merrill, R. M., Harris, J. D., & Merrill, J. G. (2013). Differences in incidence rates and early detection of cancer among non-Hispanic and Hispanic whites in the United States. *Ethnicity and Disease, 23*(3), 349–355.

National Cancer Institute. (2014). Biomarker. Retrieved from http://www.cancer.gov/dictionary?cdrid=45618

Phillips. (2014). DirectLife. Retrieved from http://www.directlife.philips.com/

Polar. (2014). Heart rate monitoring. Retrieved from http://www.polar.com/us-en/b2b_products/physical_education/heart_rate_monitoring

Sasco, A. J., Merrill, R. M., Dari, I., Benhaim-Luzon, V., Carriot, F., Cann, C. I., & Bartal, M. (2002). A case-control study of lung cancer in Casablanca, Morocco. *Cancer Causes Control, 13*(7), 609–616.

Spencer, H. (1919). *Education.* London, UK: Williams and Norgate. (Original work published 1861)

Surveillance, Epidemiology, and End Results Program. (2014). Incidence—SEER 18 Regs Research Data + Hurricane Katrina Impacted Louisiana Cases, Nov 2011 Sub, Vintage 2009 Pops (2000–2009) <Katrina/Rita Population Adjustment>. Retrieved from http://seer.cancer.gov/data/seerstat/nov2011/

U.S. Department of Transportation. (2014). National household travel survey. Retrieved from http://nhts.ornl.gov/

U.S. Environmental Protection Agency. (2014). Biomonitoring. Retrieved from http://www.epa.gov/ace/biomonitoring/biomonitoring.html

U.S. Food and Drug Administration. (2013). Total diet study. Retrieved from http://www.fda.gov/food/foodscienceresearch/totaldietstudy/default.htm

Whithings. (2014). Withings blood pressure monitor. Retrieved from http://www.withings.com/us/blood-pressure-monitor.html

World Bank. (2014). Maternal mortality ratio (modeled estimate, per 100,000 live births). Retrieved from http://data.worldbank.org/indicator/SH.STA.MMRT

World Health Organization. (2006). *Reproductive health indicators: Guidelines for their generation, interpretation and analysis for global monitoring.* Retrieved from http://whqlibdoc.who.int/publications/2006/924156315X_eng.pdf

Chapter 7

Sources and Uses of Available Population-Based Behavior Data

Many research questions in behavioral epidemiology can be answered quickly and efficiently using data that have already been collected. Three general approaches are available for utilizing existing information: secondary data analysis, ancillary studies, and systematic reviews. *Secondary data analysis* involves assessing data that has already been collected to investigate questions other than the one you are currently addressing. *Ancillary studies* add additional measurement(s) to a study in order to answer a separate question. *Systematic reviews* are overviews of primary research on a specific research question from multiple previous studies. The primary advantages of studies that use existing data are that they save time and resources. The primary disadvantages are that they may represent populations that may not ideally answer the research question, the measurement approach may not be preferred, the quality of the data may be poor, and important confounders and outcomes may not have been measured.

The purpose of this chapter is to describe these three types of data for creatively making use of existing data.

Secondary Data Analysis

There are many sources of secondary data, including national surveys, vital statistics registration systems, healthcare billing files, insurance claims databases, medical records, research studies, and many other sources. A number of research studies collect more data than are initially assessed, which can be studied later by other investigators. Large, nationally funded surveys provide a rich source of secondary data. Tumor registries, such as the Surveillance, Epidemiology, and End Results (SEER) Program of the National Cancer Institute, are valuable sources of cancer incidence and survival data.

Secondary data are very useful for studies that evaluate patterns of utilization and clinical outcomes of medical treatment. While clinical trials may establish the efficacy of an intervention, the intervention may not be effective (efficacious and widely adopted in practice). Secondary data can help us understand the level of adoption and whether utilization varies across age groups, regions, and so on. In other words, secondary data are often a useful resource for identifying the efficiency of an intervention.

Secondary data may consist of individual-level information, or it may involve aggregated data. Aggregated data have been summarized for groups of persons, such as the incidence rate of prostate cancer in France or the percentage of current smokers in Russia. With such data, we can compare group information on a risk factor, such as comparing per capita meat consumption to the incidence of colon cancer among countries. When studies are based on aggregated data we refer to them as ecologic studies. For example, one study linked data on physical activity obtained from 355 counties in the Behavior Risk Factor Surveillance System (BRFSS) with seven weather classifications from 255 corresponding weather stations to show that season and climate significantly influence physical activity in the United States (Merrill, Shields, White, & Druce, 2005). Ecologic studies are susceptible to a special type of bias referred to as ecologic fallacy.

As the previous example illustrates, it is sometimes useful to link databases, including secondary databases. For example, SEER data have been linked with Medicare records to create a SEER–Medicare database for research purposes (National Cancer Institute, 2014; Warren, Klabunde, Schrag, Bach, & Riley, 2002). Research has also linked cancer data with insurance databases (Merrill et al., 1999; Potosky et al., 1997; Potosky et al., 1999), church records (Merrill & Lyon, 2005), sociodemographic data with cause of death information (National Cancer Institute, 2013), and many other databases. This merely expands our ability to address certain research questions.

In recent decades, the availability of secondary data related to health has proliferated. Data that are available in the public domain through U.S. surveys include the Medicare Current Beneficiary Survey; the National Ambulatory Medical Care Survey; the National Health and Nutrition Examination Survey; the National Health Interview Survey; the National Hospital Ambulatory Medical Care Survey; the National Hospital Discharge Survey; the National Nursing Home Survey; the National Vital Statistics System; and population estimates (Centers for Disease Control and Prevention [CDC], 2014b). Other sources include the BRFSS; the Youth Risk Behavior Surveillance System (YRBSS); State Tobacco Activities Tracking and Evaluation (STATE); the National Household Survey; and the Total Diet Study (TDS). Some other U.S.-based secondary data sources include the National Youth Physical Activity and Nutrition Study (NYPANS) (CDC, 2014a); the National Survey of Sexual Health and Behavior (Herbenick et al., 2010); the Youth Tobacco Survey (CDC, 2014d); and the National Survey of Family Growth (CDC, 2014c).

As a general rule, utilizing secondary data is possible only when they meet four criteria:

1. Available: The data set must exist, which means someone has collected and organized the data in a usable format.
2. Accessible: The data set must be accessible to the people who want to use it. Data sets may be accessed through personal or professional contacts, attendance at professional meetings, web-based searches, or local libraries.
3. Appropriate: The data set must include valid and reliable measures of the primary variable or variables under investigation. Measures that are close enough will most likely lead to specious results.
4. Adequate: The data set must include enough variables to capture the impact of additional influences. Behavioral studies that establish a relationship only between behavior and health outcomes are incomplete because they provide no guidance on how to intervene. After establishing an initial relationship, these studies should also explore contributing, mediating, and moderating factors that can form the basis of effective intervention strategies.

ACCESSING AVAILABLE DATA

Some secondary data sources are not directly available to the public, and a request must be submitted to obtain access. These data sets are not conducive to exploratory data analysis, but a well thought-out description of how the data will be used is necessary. Requests generally require a specific description of the variables required, the method of analysis, the aims and purpose of the study, and more.

For example, microdata from the National Health Interview Survey, which include sensitive information such as geocoded locations, require a proposal and time request for supervised analysis. Knowing which variables to include requires a clear research question and an understanding of the ways in which the exposure, confounder, or outcome variables can be related. A classic example is smoking. Smoking can be evaluated in several ways, including (but not limited to) the following:

- Yes or no
- Yes (at least 100 cigarettes) or no
- Current, former, never
- Amount smoked currently
- Greatest amount smoked ever
- Years smoked
- Age started smoking
- Years since last smoke
- Pack years

Each variable answers a different research question. For example, "age started smoking" may address the question of whether smoking started during a particular etiologically relevant window, which is associated with the disease outcome, whereas "pack years" may address the question of whether the dose of smoking over a lifetime is associated with the disease outcome.

Contextualizing research questions into variables is a helpful exercise to identify the required variables and guide the study. This involves considering the research question with respect to the following types of variables: exposure, outcome, confounder, and effect modifier. After each variable is identified, the corresponding question(s) from a data set can be identified. An example of this conceptualization is presented in **Table 7-1** for an analysis of bone health and fruit and vegetable consumption using data from the National Health and Nutrition Examination Survey (NHANES).

DATA ANALYSIS PLAN

Studies involving secondary data should include an initial data analysis plan. An analysis plan involves outlining the planned data analytic steps, writing a draft of the text for the data analytic procedures, and developing dummy tables. The data analysis plan should be as complete and accurate as possible. An outline of the planned data analytic steps should include all the planned analyses and how these analyses will be performed. The outline can be used as a quick guide when executing the data analysis plan. An example of a planned data analysis is presented for NHANES data in **Table 7-2**.

Table 7-1

Conceptualization of the Research Question "Is Dietary Intake of Fruits and Vegetables Correlated with Bone Mineral Density in Adults?" into Variables

Exposure	Dietary intake of fruits and vegetables	Examination: Dietary interview—first day	All variables
Outcome	Bone mineral density	Examination: DXX	All variables
Confounders	Weight	Examination: Body measurements	BMXWT
	Height		BMXHT
	Age	Examination: Body measurements	RIDAGEYR
	Energy intake	Demographics	DR1TKCAL
		Examination: Dietary interview—first day	
Effect modifiers	Sex	Demographics	RIAGENDR
Other descriptive	Race/ethnicity	Demographics	RIDRETH1
	Education	Demographics	DMDEDUC, DMDEDUC2, DMDEDUC3

It is helpful to then write a draft text for the data analytic procedures that can be described in a manner that is understandable to others. The draft text will be refined and updated for the final paper if any data analytic procedures are changed or eliminated. This is helpful because for some analyses it can take many months to complete the work, and having a foundation of analytic steps simplifies writing the final report. At the outset, this is just a summary of the data analysis procedures; details regarding the data set and measurement

Table 7-2

Steps for Data Analysis

1. Data cleaning (described in an upcoming section)
2. Create necessary categorical variables (quartiles of age, categories of education) or other calculated variables (BMI)
3. Create summary exposure variables: Total fruit and vegetable, total fruit, total vegetable, botanical groupings
4. Description of population stratified by sex: Frequencies, race/ethnicity, quartiles of age, education (less than high school, high school or more)
5. Description of confounders by sex: Means and standard deviations of caloric intake, weight, height, and BMI
6. Description of exposure by sex: Frequencies and percentages of categories of fruits and vegetables (total, groupings)
7. Description of outcome by sex: Means and standard deviations of BMD (total and site specific)
8. Association between exposure and outcome by sex, adjusted for age: Odds ratios for categorical exposures
9. Association between exposure and outcome by sex, adjusted for age, calorie intake, and body size: Odds ratios for categorical exposures

of variables will be included in other sections of the Methods section for the final paper. An example of draft text is presented here:

> Data from the National Health and Nutrition Examination Survey (NHANES) were analyzed. Data years included were 2003–2004. Fruit and vegetable intake variables were categorized into quartiles. Means and standard deviations were calculated to describe continuous variables. Frequencies and percentages were calculated to describe categorical variables. The correlation between dietary intake and BMD above and below the median was evaluated using logistic regression across the quartiles of dietary intake, adjusted for age and sex. Confounding by calorie intake and body size was evaluated using multiple logistic regression. Additional linear regression models were fit to evaluate the relationship between dietary variables and continuous BMD.

It is helpful to create dummy tables for the planned analyses. In the final write-up of the paper, only the key analyses will be presented in tables and figures, but putting analyses into tables (or figures, if appropriate) will help organize the results that may later be described in text. Example dummy tables for the description of the study population and for exposure/outcome relationships are included (steps 4 and 8 in Table 7-2). Other tables that would be created in the preliminary data analysis plan for this example include description of exposure variables and description of outcome variables, as illustrated in **Tables 7-3** and **7-4**.

There are many statistical analysis or database packages that analyze data, and individuals should choose what they are comfortable using or that best suits the data. The first steps toward data analysis include the following:

1. Obtaining data sets from the source (e.g., website or request to an agency for a CD or other medium)
2. Converting files to the format of the chosen statistical software, if necessary (e.g., this step may not be necessary because some newer files on the NHANES website can be directly exported to SAS)
3. Merging data files
4. Selecting variables and creating the data set
5. Saving the data set to a CD or other medium that can be used as the primary data location

DATA QUALITY, CLEANING, AND CODEBOOK

Data Quality

Evaluating the quality of data and cleaning the data are processes that may take a few iterations to complete. A codebook should be created after the data are evaluated for quality and are cleaned. Depending on

Table 7-3

Example Dummy Table for the Distribution of Demographic Factors in ### Adults, NHANES, 2003–2004

Characteristic	Males No. (%)	Females No. (%)
Age		
Q1: [range]	N (%)	N (%)
Q2: [range]	N (%)	N (%)
Q3: [range]	N (%)	N (%)
Q4: [range]	N (%)	N (%)
Race/ethnicity		
Non-Hispanic White	N (%)	N (%)
Non-Hispanic Black	N (%)	N (%)
Mexican American	N (%)	N (%)
Other Hispanic	N (%)	N (%)
Other	N (%)	N (%)
Education		
Less than high school	N (%)	N (%)
High school or more	N (%)	N (%)

Note: Notations in brackets (e.g., [range]) or symbols (e.g., ###) indicate a place where data from the analysis would be documented.

the number of variables, this process of data preparation can seem tedious and repetitive, but it is an important step in the preparation of data for analysis.

Evaluating the quality of data involves checking the data for errors, missing data, and outlying variables. A useful place to start in the data evaluation process is to create a table (e.g., **Table 7-5**) with the following information:

1. Variable name
2. Description
3. Variable type (date, character, categorical numerical, continuous numerical, etc.)
4. Valid values (range for continuous numbers or dates, appropriate text or numbers for categories, etc.)
5. Notes (used to indicate if and what changes need to be made in data cleaning)

Data errors are usually apparent as invalid numbers. For example, in the 2005–2006 data cycle, the variable for sex (RIAGENDR) can be coded as 1 (male), 2 (female), or . (missing). In older data cycles, missing values may be indicated by 9. Thus, a value of 3 for RIAGENDR would be considered an error to fix, if possible based on

Table 7-4

Example Dummy Table for Total Bone Mineral Density (Above and Below the Median) in ### Adults in Relation to Fruit and Vegetable Intake, NHANES, 2003–2004

Dietary intake	Males odds ratio, 95% CI	Females odds ratio, 95% CI
Total fruit and vegetable		
Q1: [range]	1.0 (reference)	1.0 (reference)
Q2: [range]	[OR, 95% CI]	[OR, 95% CI]
Q3: [range]	[OR, 95% CI]	[OR, 95% CI]
Q4: [range]	[OR, 95% CI]	[OR, 95% CI]
p-trend	[p-trend]	[p-trend]
Total fruit		
Q1: [range]	1.0 (reference)	1.0 (reference)
Q2: [range]	[OR, 95% CI]	[OR, 95% CI]
Q3: [range]	[OR, 95% CI]	[OR, 95% CI]
Q4: [range]	[OR, 95% CI]	[OR, 95% CI]
p-trend	[p-trend]	[p-trend]
Total vegetable		
Q1: [range]	1.0 (reference)	1.0 (reference)
Q2: [range]	[OR, 95% CI]	[OR, 95% CI]
Q3: [range]	[OR, 95% CI]	[OR, 95% CI]
Q4: [range]	[OR, 95% CI]	[OR, 95% CI]
p-trend	[p-trend]	[p-trend]

Note: Notations in brackets (e.g., [range]) or symbols (e.g., ###) indicate a place where data from the analysis would be documented.

Table 7-5

Data Evaluation Table of Selected Variables from NHANES

SEQN	Respondent sequence number	Character	Any	No changes needed
RIAGENDR	Gender	Categorical numerical	1 or 2	No changes needed
RIDAGEYR	Age at screening adjudicated— recode	Continuous numerical	0–84, 85	No changes needed
INDFMINC	Total family income	Categorical numerical	1–13, 77, 99	Need to combine categories 1 and 2 due to small numbers (will represent $0–$9,999); need to decide what to do with categories 12 (under 20k) and 13 (above 20k); need to replace categories 77 (refused) and 99 (don't know) to missing
DR1TKCAL	Energy (kcal)	Continuous numerical	500– 4,000	Need to exclude values below 500 and above 4,000

other information. For example, gender may be ascertained from other responses, such as age at first menstrual cycle. As a general note regarding errors, NHANES has been thoroughly checked for errors prior to public release; for this and other similar databases, one should not expect to find a substantial number of errors, but there could be some. However, if an error in the data is not obvious (e.g., income of category 5 coded as category 8), you may not be able to detect it.

Missing data are complex problems and are addressed in other resources (Pigott, 1994). Missing data are always sources of bias. The concern is the degree of bias. There are some basic options for handling missing data: (1) attempt to figure out a missing value (e.g., if sex is missing but the respondent answered questions about menstrual cycle, you can assume the respondent is female); or (2) exclude respondents with missing values from the analysis. For most, if not all, variables you will not be able to make such assumptions, and it may be best to exclude those respondents from analyses involving the relevant variable. If missing data for a variable is substantial (e.g., more than 10% of respondents who should have data do not have it), it may be best not to include the variable in the analysis due to the loss of power and generalizability that will occur.

Outlying values are those that are beyond a reasonable expectation for the variable. Sometimes an outlying value is an obvious error because of data entry. For example, a value of 110 for age is obviously an outlier, and it may be an error. It may be possible to figure out what the error might be and correct it, especially if original completed questionnaires are available, but this is not true in every situation. In dietary data, extreme values of caloric intake may be considered outliers, although whether they are errors or just extreme values is not always clear. In nutrition, the rule of thumb is to exclude individuals with less than 500 kcal per day or more than 4,000 kcal per day of energy intake. While it is physiologically possible to have people with such levels of consumption, these individuals are likely quite different from the underlying population (e.g., an elite athlete with high intake or a sick individual), and exclusion of these people will not affect external validity.

Data Cleaning

Data cleaning involves correcting errors in the data and making the data set ready for analysis. After data have been evaluated, the errors and outliers have been identified, and needed changes have been noted, it is helpful to create a command file in the statistical package. In many packages, this command file can be created in a data editor and saved for future use. It is advisable to create and use an initial command file to call data into the program at the beginning of each analysis. This is recommended so that key aspects of the data (variables or values) are not overwritten in the raw data file.

The most common data cleaning procedures include changing numerical codes for missing or other similar values (such as those for "don't know"), recoding categories to change the reference category, recoding categories to combine categories with small numbers of observations, and categorizing continuous variables. It is also helpful to label variables. In the case of NHANES, for newer data cycles, most of the variables are labeled. However, for older data cycles, the variables are unlabeled.

There are particular commands within each software program that can be helpful in the data cleaning process. For example, useful SAS commands for data cleaning are IF/THEN statements, LABEL, and PROC FORMAT.

- IF/THEN statements are used to recode variables—for example, changing energy values less than 500 (use IF statement) to missing (use THEN statement).
- LABEL is used to label the variable with an understandable name—for example, the variable INDFMINC has the label "Total family income."
- PROC FORMAT is used to assign labels to variables that are numerical categories—for example, the category "1" of INDFMINC could be formatted as "$0–$4,999." This is an optional step to help in the interpretation of data analysis output, but it is sometimes unnecessary (for example, if it is documented in a codebook that 1 = male and 2 = female, it may be helpful but not necessary).

Creating a Codebook

Codebooks provide the information needed to evaluate the data. They provide information about the structure, contents, and layout of a data file. Although codebooks of data files vary, they typically include column information and width for each variable, definitions of different record types, response codes for each variable, codes used to indicate nonresponse and missing data, exact questions and skip patterns used in a survey, and other indications of the content and characteristics of each variable. They may also contain frequency of response, survey objectives, concept definitions, a description of the survey design and methodology, a copy of the survey questionnaire (if applicable), and information on data collection, data processing, and data quality (Inter-university Consortium for Political and Social Research, 2014).

Surveys begin with a codebook that contains the format and labels of each variable. The codebook defines the variables used in the study. Five components of a variable are variable format, variable name, variable label, value labels (including valid codes and skip codes), and data entry control parameters. A codebook may contain some or all of these components.

The variable format describes the structure of the variable using the following syntax:

< Variable Type> <Number of Columns>.<Decimal >

Variable types are numeric or categorical, the number of columns represents the width allocated to the variable, and decimal format is the number of decimal places that will be used. The variable name must be unique. In some statistical software packages such as SAS, it must begin with a letter; cannot contain blanks; cannot contain special characters such as $, #, or @; and cannot exceed 32 characters. A variable label is a description of the variable. Value labels are used for the response categories of the variable. For example, $1 = 0\text{--}49$, $2 = 50\text{--}79$, $3 = 80\text{--}110$, or $M = Male$ and $F = Female$. An example of valid codes ranges for a variable may be $1 = Yes$, $2 = No$, $7 = Refused$, and $9 = Don't\ Know$. Skip codes can let you pass over certain variables under specific conditions. Data entry control parameters have to do with how the data entry will operate. In some situations, a variable will be mandatory (e.g., identification number), and the program will not allow you to continue entering data until a value is entered into the field. Other variables may not be mandatory, and leaving a field blank is acceptable. The program can also skip variables by advancing you to a specific variable, depending on the response of a certain variable. An example of a codebook entry from the NHANES 2011–2012 codebook is given in **Figure 7-1**.

Ancillary Studies

In some situations, a researcher can add one or more measurements to an existing study to address his or her research question. An ancillary study involves the collection of additional information such as studies requiring collection of data through additional questionnaires or additional questions added to a survey. An ancillary study has the same advantages as a secondary data analysis, but the research can also add a few key measurements to better address the research question. Ancillary studies can be added to any type of epidemiologic study, but they may be best suited for large prospective cohort studies and randomized trials that include either a predictor or outcome variable for the new research study (Grady, Cummings, & Hulley, 2013).

Systematic Reviews

Whenever more than one study has addressed the same research question, research synthesis can be performed from a systematic review. A systematic review is an overview of identified, completed studies that used explicit and reproducible methods to address a particular research

DMQMILIZ—served active duty in U.S. Armed Forces

Variable Name:

DMQMILIZ

SAS Label:

Served active duty in U.S. Armed Forces

English Text:

{Have you/Has SP} ever served on active duty in the U.S. Armed Forces, military Reserves, or National Guard? (Active duty does not include training for the Reserves or National Guard, but does include activation, for service in the U.S. or in a foreign country, in support of military or humanitarian operations.)

Target: Both males and females 17 YEARS–150 YEARS

Code or Value	Value Description	Count	Cumulative	Skip to Item
1	Yes	551	551	
2	No	5,456	6,007	DMDBORN4
7	Refused	0	6,007	DMDBORN4
9	Don't Know	0	6,007	DMDBORN4
.	Missing	3,749	9,756	

Figure 7-1 Selected variable entry from the 2011–2012 NHANES codebook

question. Systematic reviews apply scientific strategies that minimize bias in the collection, synthesis, and appraisal of the results of studies to draw conclusions on a specific topic. Meta-analyses are often part of a systematic review in which mathematical synthesis of the results of primary studies that consider the same hypotheses are assessed in the same way. Systematic reviews and meta-analyses are an effective way to communicate what is known about a body of research.

A systematic review begins with a protocol, which consists of the research question, literature search, description of data extraction, quality appraisal, data analysis and results, and interpretation of results.

PROTOCOL

The study plan (protocol) is a detailed written plan for a study. The Institute of Medicine of the National Academies provides criteria for developing a systematic review protocol, as shown in **Table 7-6**. The protocol provides direction and focus and can help minimize bias.

RESEARCH QUESTION

Formulating the primary research question is the first step in a systematic review. Questions may include phenomena associated with a certain behavior; behavior frequency; disease etiology and/or risk factors; frequency of the behavior-related outcome; and intervention effects. The goal of the systematic review is to then summarize the literature; identify strengths and weaknesses of the literature related to the question; increase the statistical power and improve the precision of smaller studies; and improve the generalizability of research findings on the study question.

LITERATURE SEARCH

There are several sources that are available in the literature search (**Table 7-7**). Two or more reviewers are typically involved at the first stage of screening to identify titles and abstracts, based on the research question and other possible factors (e.g., population, intervention, study design, and outcome of interest). The second stage of screening involves selecting full-text articles.

Table 7-6
Standards for Systematic Reviews: The Protocol
• Describe the context and rationale for the review from both a decision-making and research perspective.
• Describe the study screening and selection criteria (inclusion/exclusion criteria).
• Describe precisely which outcome measures, time points, interventions, and comparison groups will be addressed.
• Describe the search strategy for identifying relevant evidence.
• Describe the procedures for study selection.
• Describe the data extraction strategy.
• Describe the process for identifying and resolving disagreements among researchers in study selection and data extraction decisions.
• Describe the approach to critically appraising individual studies.
• Describe the method for evaluating the body of evidence, including the quantitative and qualitative synthesis strategies.
• Describe and justify any planned analyses of differential treatment effects according to patient subgroups, how an intervention is delivered, or how an outcome is measured.
• Describe the proposed timetable for conducting the review.
Modified from Institute of Medicine of the National Academies. (2011). Standards for Systematic Reviews. Retrieved July 31, 2014, from http://www.iom.edu/Reports/2011/Finding-What-Works-in-Health-Care-Standards-for-Systematic-Reviews/Standards.aspx.

Table 7-7
Sources for Literature Search
Bibliographies and references available in primary sources
CINAHL – Cumulative index to nursing and allied health.
Cochrane Library – Database of systematic reviews of research on evidence-based health care.
Cochrane Handbook appendix – Contains information on unpublished primary clinical trials.
Conference proceedings and abstracts.
DARE – Database of abstracts of reviews of effects of interventions.
Entrez – Cross-database search system of many health sciences databases.
Global Health – Database on public health research and practice.
Medline – National Library of Medicine journal citation database.
MedlinePlus – Online information on health and drug issues. It also provides a dictionary of medical services.
PubMed Central – Contains journal literature provided by participating publishers and author manuscripts that have been submitted in compliance with the Public Access Policy required by the National Institutes of Health and other research funding agencies.
PubMed – Includes the Medline database, PubMed Central database, and the National Center for Biotechnology Information book shelf plus other types of citations. It includes in-process citations, out-of-scope citations from certain Medline journals, ahead of print citations, citations to some additional life sciences journals.
PsychINFO – Database of peer-reviewed literature in behavior science and mental health.
Scopus – A large collection of multidisciplinary abstracts and citations of peer-reviewed research literature.
Unpublished academic literature (grey literature), ongoing studies, and raw data from published studies – These types of data are obtained through personal communication.

DATA EXTRACTION

Data extraction involves items like study objectives, study design, population, intervention, outcome, references, and details about the quality of the study.

QUALITY APPRAISAL

A quality appraisal is used to assess internal and external validity of the studies. Internal validity reflects the extent the study represents systematic errors (bias) and random errors (precision). Precision is typically depicted using confidence intervals. External validity is assessed to determine the extent to which results are applicable to a given target population.

DATA ANALYSIS

The rationale for including studies in the systematic review should be described in the protocol. A study may be excluded because of poor quality. Some inclusion and exclusion criteria may be studies conducted during a certain time frame, with a specific design, involving a given population, involving a certain intervention or risk factor, with an acceptable level of loss to follow-up, a minimum length of follow-up, an acceptable control group, acceptable outcomes, and, for certain designs, require blinding, randomization, and control of confounding factors (Grady et al., 2013).

The quality appraisal will result in narrowing the eligible studies for evaluation. After the studies have been chosen, each study may be described based on selected information, such as identified in **Table 7-8**. The information can then be summarized. Some measures

Table 7-8	
Potential Items to Include in a Description of Each Study	
Authors	List all the authors on the article
Title	List the title of the article
Citation	List the citation (journal, date) of the article
Date reviewed	State the date the article was reviewed
Reviewer	State the name of the individual who reviewed the article
Aims of the study	Summarize the aims of the study as stated or implied by the authors
Type of study	Note the type of study (prospective cohort, case-control, etc.)
Number of participants (number of cases and controls; number exposed and unexposed)	List the total number of participants and the participants by case status (case-control) or exposure status (cohort or intervention)
Sampling and inclusion criteria	Summarize the subjects that were sampled and what the inclusion/exclusion criteria for the study were
Participation rate	Note the participation rate (i.e., of those recruited, what proportion participated); if possible and appropriate, indicate the participation rate by case status
Number of individuals not retained in the final sample	Summarize any information on individuals who were lost to follow-up, dropped out, or were lost from the study for other reasons
Main exposure variables	List the main exposure variables
Definition and measurement of exposures	Describe how the exposure variables were defined and measured
Main outcome variables	List the main outcome variables
Definition and measurement of outcome variables	Describe how the outcome variables were defined and measured
Confounders and effect modifiers considered	List any confounders or effect modifiers that were considered
Data analysis	Summarize the data analysis techniques used
Unadjusted associations observed	If provided, summarize the unadjusted associations for the relevant analyses
Adjusted associations observed	If provided, summarize the adjusted associations for the relevant analyses
Major conclusions by the authors	Summarize the major conclusions provided by authors
Strengths of the study	Summarize the strengths of the study as discussed by the authors and the strengths that you perceive
Limitations of the study	Summarize the limitations of the study as discussed by the authors and the limitations that you perceive
Other notes	Make any notes about the study that you want to document

will require a qualitative assessment, and some measures can be analyzed statistically (e.g., sample size, population size, rates, length of follow-up, and quality score). A summary of important characteristics of each study that are included in the review can be presented in a table. An analytic assessment of the findings (e.g., measures of association such as odds ratios, risk ratios, rate ratios, prevalence proportions) from the individual studies is also performed and presented in a table or figure. Sensitivity and subgroup analysis is often performed for data in systematic reviews. A *sensitivity analysis* shows how robust the results of a meta-analysis are to certain aspects of the review design or according to the inclusion of given studies (Grady et al., 2013).

Meta-analyses combine information from a group of eligible studies, with a summary estimate of effect having greater precision than estimates in the individual studies. After the data have been extracted from the original studies, a summary estimate (summary odds ratio, summary risk ratio, summary rate ratio, summary risk difference, and so on) and confidence interval are generally calculated. Meta-analyses increase the power for answering a specific research question. There are several excellent sources of methods for assessing synthesized data (Cooper & Hedges, 1994).

Combining the results of several studies in a meta-analysis assumes that the studies are similar with respect to population, intervention, outcome, control condition, blinding, and so on. To determine homogeneity among studies, the individual studies need to be assessed for whether substantial differences exist in population, intervention, and so forth. Whether there is sufficient homogeneity to combine studies requires judgment. Every meta-analysis should include a discussion of homogeneity of the studies and how this may have affected the results.

A disadvantage of meta-analyses is that they do not contain individual-level data and, consequently, are unable to control for confounding factors. Meta-analyses are also unable to perform individual subgroup analyses. In some situations, data can be obtained from individual studies, and the data can be pooled and analyzed. This approach has the advantage of being able to control for confounding factors and assess subgroup effects (Grady et al., 2013).

INTERPRETATION

Correct data interpretations are critical, along with acknowledgement of potential limitations (e.g., publication bias, poor quality of data) and the potential effects these may have on the results. *Publication bias* exists if published studies do not represent all studies done. Studies with significant results tend to be published more than those with null findings. Hence, care should be given to not overgeneralize the results of a systematic review. In addition, interpreting the results should be based on the best scientific evidence available. In many situations, a systematic review will generate new hypotheses and yield direction for further research.

Summary

1. Three conventional approaches are used to assess existing information: secondary data analysis, ancillary studies, and systematic reviews. Secondary data analysis involves assessing data that have already been collected to investigate questions other than the one you are currently addressing. Ancillary studies add an additional measurement to a study in order to answer a separate question. Systematic reviews are overviews of primary research on a specific research question from multiple previous studies.

2. The use of existing data has the advantage of saving time and resources. However, the use of such data has the disadvantage that it may not represent populations that are ideally suited to answer the research question, the method of measurement may not be preferred, the quality of the data may be poor, and potential confounders and effect modifiers may not have been measured.

3. Sources of secondary data include national surveys such as NHANES and BRFSS, tumor registries, vital statistics registration systems, healthcare billing files, insurance claims databases, medical records, research studies, and many other sources. Secondary data are often useful in evaluating utilization rates and regional variations, as well as effectiveness of programs.

4. We call studies of association involving aggregated data ecologic studies. These types of studies are often used in descriptive epidemiologic studies and are useful for generating hypotheses, but they may be susceptible to ecologic fallacy.

5. Utilizing secondary data requires that it be available, accessible, appropriate, and adequate. Begin with a data analysis plan detailing the analytic steps to be taken.

6. Evaluating the quality of data involves checking the data for errors, missing data, and outlying variables. This can be done by creating a table that contains the variable name, variable description, variable type (date, character, categorical numerical, continuous numerical, etc.), valid values (range for continuous numbers or dates, appropriate text or numbers for categories, etc.), and notes (used to indicate if and what changes need to be made in data cleaning).

7. Data cleaning involves correcting errors in the data and making the data set ready for analysis.

8. Codebooks provide the information needed to evaluate the data. It provides information about the structure, contents, and layout of a data file. All surveys begin with a codebook that contains information such as variable format, variable name, variable label, value labels (including valid codes and skip codes), and data entry control parameters.

9. An ancillary study is a secondary data analysis that involves making one or more new measurements to address a new research question with comparatively little cost or effort.

10. A systematic review is an overview of identified completed studies that used explicit and reproducible methods to address a particular research question. Meta-analyses are often part of a systematic review in which mathematical synthesis occurs of the results of primary studies that consider the same hypotheses, assessed in the same way.

11. A systematic review begins with a protocol, which consists of the research question, a literature search, a description of data extraction, quality appraisal, data analysis and results, and interpretation of results.

References

Centers for Disease Control and Prevention. (2014a). Adolescent and school health. Retrieved from http://www.cdc.gov/healthyyouth/yrbs/nypans.htm

Centers for Disease Control and Prevention. (2014b). Health data interactive. Retrieved from http://www.cdc.gov/nchs/data_access/hdi/hdi_data_sources.htm

Centers for Disease Control and Prevention. (2014c). National survey of family growth. Retrieved from http://www.cdc.gov/nchs/nsfg.htm

Centers for Disease Control and Prevention. (2014d). Youth tobacco survey. Retrieved from http://www.cdc.gov/tobacco/data_statistics/surveys/YTS/

Cooper, H., & Hedges, L. V. (1994). *The handbook of research synthesis*. New York, NY: Russell Sage.

Grady, D. G., Cummings, S. R., & Hulley, S. B. (2013). Research using existing data. In S. B. Hulley, S. R. Cummings, W. S. Browner, D. G. Grady, & T. B. Newman (Eds.), *Designing clinical research* (4th ed., pp. 192–207). Philadelphia, PA: Lippincott Williams & Wilkins.

Herbenick, D., Reece, M., Schick, V., Sanders, S. A., Dodge, B., & Fortenberry, J. D. (2010). Sexual behavior in the United States: Results from a national probability sample of men and women ages 14–94. *The Journal of Sexual Medicine, 7*(5), 255–265.

Institute of Medicine of the National Academies. (2011). Standards for systematic reviews. Retrieved from http://www.iom.edu/Reports/2011/Finding-What -Works-in-Health-Care-Standards-for-Systematic-Reviews/Standards.aspx

Inter-university Consortium for Political and Social Research. (2014). What is a codebook? Retrieved from http://www.icpsr.umich.edu/icpsrweb/ICPSR /support/faqs/2006/01/what-is-codebook

Merrill, R. M., Brown, M., Potosky, A. L., Riley, G. F., Taplin, S. H., Barlow, W., & Fireman, B. H. (1999). Survival and treatment for colorectal cancer Medicare patients in two group/staff health maintenance organizations and the fee-for-service setting. *Medical Care Research and Review, 56*, 177–196.

Merrill, R. M., & Lyon, J. L. (2005). Cancer incidence among Mormons and non-Mormons in Utah (United States) 1995–1999. *Preventive Medicine, 40*(5), 535–541.

Merrill, R. M., Shields, E. C., White, G. L., Jr., & Druce, D. (2005). Climate conditions and physical activity among adults in the United States. *American Journal of Health Behavior, 29*(4), 371–381.

National Cancer Institute. (2013). National longitudinal mortality study (NLMS) and linked SEER–NLMS databases. Retrieved from http://surveillance.cancer.gov /disparities/nlms/

National Cancer Institute. (2014). SEER–Medicare linked database. Retrieved from http://appliedresearch.cancer.gov/seermedicare/

National Center for Biotechnology Information. (n.d.). PubMed clinical queries. Retrieved from http://www.ncbi.nlm.nih.gov/pubmed/clinical

Pigott, T. D. (1994). Methods for handling missing data in research synthesis. In H. Cooper & L. V. Hedges (Eds.), *The handbook of research synthesis* (pp. 163–176). New York, NY: Russell Sage.

Potosky, A. L., Merrill, R. M., Riley, G. F., Taplin, S. H., Barlow, W., & Fireman, B. H. (1997). Breast cancer survival and treatment in health maintenance organization and fee-for-service settings. *Journal of the National Cancer Institute, 89,* 1683–1691.

Potosky, A. L., Merrill, R. M., Riley, G. F., Taplin, S. H., Barlow, W., & Fireman, B. H. (1999). Prostate cancer survival and treatment in HMO and fee-for-service settings. *Health Services Research, 34*(2), 525–546.

Simons, M. (2011). Guidelines for writing systematic reviews. Retrieved from http://www.library.mq.edu.au/libguides/Guidelines%20for%20writing%20systematic%20reviews.pdf

Warren, J. L., Klabunde, C. N., Schrag, D., Bach, P. B., & Riley, G. F. (2002). Overview of the SEER–Medicare data: Content, research applications, and generalizability to the United States elderly population. *Medical Care, 40*(Suppl. 8), IV3–IV18.

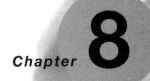
Data Collection, Misclassification, and Missing Data

In many situations it is necessary to collect original data to address our research questions. Much of the information used in behavioral epidemiology is based on original data, involving direct or indirect measures. Original direct measures of behavior include personal monitoring (quantitative measurements of personal behavior) and biological markers. Original indirect measures of behavior include questionnaires, interviews, and online surveys.

Personal monitoring devices are available to assess steps taken, track body motion and energy expenditure, estimate total exposure to radiation and air quality, and measure blood pressure and heart rate during various activities.

A biomarker is a biologic specimen that can indicate exposure to some substance, or it may reflect host characteristics. It can be measured from a biosample (blood, urine, tissue) or a recording obtained from a person (blood pressure, electrocardiogram, or Holter), or it can be an imaging test (computer tomography scan, echocardiogram) (Vasan, 2006). Biomarkers can indicate several health and disease characteristics (e.g., environmental exposure, genetic susceptibility, genetic responses to exposures, markers of disease, or indicators of

163

response to therapy). For example, nicotine and cotinine levels in the blood or urine can be used to study tobacco smoking behavior; low-density lipoprotein cholesterol, triglycerides, and glucose in the blood, as well as blood pressure, can reflect certain dietary behaviors; and certain biomarkers can indicate a predisposition toward addictive-related behaviors, aggressive tendencies, and suicidal tendencies. Dietary intake has traditionally been based on self-reported measures. However, it is possible to measure dietary intake more objectively through nutritional biomarkers. A nutritional biomarker can indicate nutritional status and the integration of intake and metabolism, but this is a new area of research, and biomarkers are not yet available for some dietary constituents (National Cancer Institute, 2013).

Many common behaviors are more practically measured by eliciting information from participants through a questionnaire, interview, or online survey. These instruments indirectly collect behavior data from the study subjects. The reliability and validity of these instruments should be determined prior to administration. Some instruments are easily validated, while others require sophisticated validation procedures. For example, variables such as beliefs, perceptions, or values are subjective in nature. A person is generally not wrong when describing his or her own beliefs, perceptions, or values. Knowledge variables are more objective, but they can be compared to verifiable information to determine the accuracy of measurement tools. Affective variables, such as self-efficacy, are difficult to measure because they reflect constructs that have no verifiable objective standard.

The study protocol needs to include a description of the data collection process. The steps of developing an instrument for collecting data must be carefully thought out. Designing questionnaires, interviews, and online surveys must take into account several issues such as location, accessibility, literacy, language, cultural acceptability, and much more. Designing the instrument involves both science, wherein valid and reliable questions are selected, and art—when the questionnaire is created, the visual presentation of the questions and supporting material is appropriate and interesting, not distracting. The purpose of this chapter is to provide a detailed discussion of questionnaires, interviews, and online surveys, as well as sample size and data issues involving management, misclassification, and sources of error.

Sampling

The number of people who meet the criteria for selection into a study is often so large that it is not feasible to assess everyone. Hence, it is necessary to choose a sample from the population. The primary aim is to select this sample so it is representative of the overall population.

From our evaluation of the sample, we infer or generalize to the larger population.

There are many reasons for studying a sample rather than the entire population. First, a sample can be studied more quickly than a large population. Second, examining a sample rather than the entire population is less expensive, particularly in studies with long follow-up involved. Third, for large populations, it is typically impossible to study everyone. Fourth, sample results may be more accurate than population results, if greater attention and precision can go into measuring fewer numbers. Fifth, probability methods can be used to estimate error in the statistics. Sixth, a sample can be selected to reduce variability in the group. Hence, a smaller sample may be preferred to studying the entire population, but a sufficient sample size is also needed for there to be sufficient power to evaluate the hypotheses.

Methods of Sampling

Probability samples are the best approach to ensure reliable and valid inferences. There are four common probability sampling methods used in epidemiology: simple random sampling, stratified sampling, systematic sampling, and cluster sampling. Each of these approaches involves a random process.

A *simple random sample* means that each subject in the population has an equal chance of selection. This approach of data selection is the most basic and the easiest to assess. Simple random samples have been used in numerous studies. To draw a random sample requires that you have a list of all members of the population from which the sample will be drawn. This is called a *sampling frame*. Such studies may be expensive, and some variables may be poorly distributed across the sampling frame.

A *stratified sample* divides the population by a specific variable of interest and conducts random samples within each level of the variable to obtain an even sample. The strata should not overlap; it should be homogeneous within strata, albeit heterogeneous among strata. A random sample is then taken within each stratum. This method assures better representation from each stratum. For example, if you wanted to conduct a survey comparing perceptions of mammography among different races, you would probably want to get a representative sample of each race. However, if you were to conduct this study in a location where few African American individuals live, the likelihood of selecting enough people to make valid statements about association would be low. Conducting a stratified analysis allows you to include enough individuals of each race in your study and develop balanced evaluations of the situation.

A *systematic sample* involves selecting subjects from an ordered sampling frame, most commonly using an equal-probability method. This method selects every k^{th} case number from an ordered set of records, and k is determined by dividing the number of items in the sampling frame by the desired sample size. For example, if we wanted to conduct a systematic sample of 200 medical records from 5,000 records, $5,000/200 = 25$, so every 25th record is selected. To make this approach random, we randomly select a number between 1 and 25, then select every 25th record beyond that; that is, if the first randomly selected number was 10, we would next select 35, then 60, and so on. This approach is appropriate when elements (e.g., individuals, households, medical records) can be ordered in some manner.

Cluster sampling is a technique that can be used if there are natural, relatively homogeneous groups in the target population. A random selection of clusters is taken from the population, not the individual elements we are ultimately interested in assessing. Then everyone is assessed within the selected clusters or, if a sampling frame is available, a random selection within the cluster is obtained. For example, schools in a district are the clusters. Following a random selection of schools, all the children in the randomly selected schools are evaluated. This approach tends to have less precision than simple random sampling. As a general rule, the sample size should be twice as large as in simple random sampling to achieve the same level of precision.

The second type of sampling is called nonprobability sampling. In a nonprobability sample, the probability that a subject will be selected is unknown. Two types of nonprobability sampling methods are convenience samples or quota samples. A *convenience sample* is a type of nonprobability sampling in which a sample population is selected because it is readily available and convenient. For example, if one city has fluoridated water, another city without fluoridated water may serve as a control, and dental caries from both groups could be used to evaluate the efficacy of fluoridation. Similarly, if one state requires seat belt use and another does not, the death rate from motor vehicle accidents or some other seat belt–related outcome measure between the two states could be compared to determine the efficacy of seat belt use.

Quota sampling is the nonprobability equivalent of stratified sampling. A certain number of subjects are selected from each stratum according to a nonprobability approach (e.g., people coming out of a supermarket who are willing to participate). However, both convenience sampling and quota sampling are potentially biased because not everyone in the target population has a chance of selection. Quota sampling may be the best we can do if we are limited on time or money, or if a sampling frame is not available.

Sample Size

Valid statistical inference requires that the study is sufficiently powered. There are various approaches for calculating sample size, which depend on the type of data involved and whether the study design is descriptive or analytic. In general, the required sample size increases when a greater confidence level is desired, when there is more variability in the population, and when the desired precision increases (width of the confidence interval decreases). In this section, some basic sample size techniques will be presented for descriptive and analytic epidemiologic studies.

DESCRIPTIVE STUDIES

In this section we will present the sample size formula for conducting different descriptive evaluations, each followed by an example.

Sample Size Equation for Estimating the Mean, σ Known

$$n = \frac{4 \times Z^2_{\alpha/2}\sigma^2}{\text{width}^2}$$

To illustrate, we know that the standard deviation of IQ among a group of college freshmen is 10 points. The investigator wants to estimate the mean IQ to within ± 3 points, with 95% confidence and $Z_{0.05/2} = 1.96$. Thus,

$$n = \frac{4 \times 1.96^2 \times 10^2}{6^2} = 42.7$$

Rounding up a sample size of n = 43 will give us an interval that allows us to estimate the population mean IQ to within 3 points with 95% confidence.

Sample Size Equation for Estimating the Mean, σ Not Known

$$n = \frac{4 \times t^2_{\alpha/2,n-1}s^2}{\text{width}^2}$$

To illustrate, a hospital administrator wants to know the mean length of time it takes physicians to see emergency room patients during the evening shift. She wishes to estimate μ to within ± 4 minutes with 95% confidence. She does not know the value of σ, the population standard deviation, so she takes a preliminary sample of $n = 10$ emergency room patients and finds the standard deviation of $s = 13$ minutes. How large does the sample size need to be in order to obtain the desired confidence interval?

A confidence level of 95% and a sample size of 10 give $t_{0.025,9} = 2.26$. Then

$$n = \frac{4 \times (2.26)^2 13^2}{8^2} = 53.95$$

Rounding up a sample size of $n = 54$ will give us an interval that allows us to estimate the population mean time of seeing a physician while attending the emergency room to within 4 points with 95% confidence. If we include the original 10 patients, then $54 - 10 = 44$ additional patients are needed to complete the sample. This process is known as *two-stage sampling*.

Although we used $t_{0.05/2,9} = 2.26$, if we had based the t-value on the total number of patients needed for this study, then there are $54 - 1 = 53$ degrees of freedom. Since $t_{0.05/2,53} = 2.00 < t_{0.05/2,9} = 2.26$, the actual confidence interval obtained will be narrower than ± 4 specified in the problem. Therefore, the sample size is conservatively large.

A similar approach is used with a proportion for a single group. It is comparable to estimating the proportion of successes in a binomial population π.

Sample Size Equation for Estimating a Proportion

$$n = \frac{4 \times Z^2_{\alpha/2}\pi(1-\pi)}{\text{width}^2}$$

To illustrate, an investigator wants to determine the sensitivity of a new diagnostic test for lung cancer. Based on a preliminary study involving 30 patients, she finds that 25 patients (83.3%) test positive. How many patients are needed to estimate a 95% confidence interval for the test's sensitivity of ± 0.05?

From the statement of the problem, a confidence level of 95% gives $Z_{0.05/2} = 1.96$, a confidence interval width of 0.1, and the standard deviation of 0.1391 (i.e., 0.833 × (1-0.833)). Thus,

$$n = \frac{4 \times 1.96^2 \times 0.1391}{(0.1)^2} = 213.7$$

Consequently the researcher needs to test $214 - 30 = 184$ more patients. Had a pilot study not been used and the value for π was not known, then a conservative approach would be to use $\pi = 0.5$, which gives

$$n = \frac{4 \times 1.96^2 \times 0.5(0.5)}{(0.1)^2} = 384.2$$

Thus the sample size based on the preliminary sample results required $385 - 214 = 171$ fewer patients. We therefore see the advantage of conducting a pilot study to determine the proportion used in the sample size calculation.

ANALYTIC STUDIES

To estimate the sample size for an analytic study we formulate our hypotheses, specify whether it is a one- or two-sided test, select a statistical test based on whether the data for the exposure and outcome variables are dichotomous or continuous, estimate the effect size and variability (if necessary), and specify the values of α and β based on a tolerable level of committing a type I or type II error.

Equation for Estimating the Sample Size for One Mean

$$n = \left[\frac{(Z_\alpha - Z_\beta)\sigma}{\mu_1 - \mu_0} \right]^2$$

To illustrate, a study evaluated whether adherence to a 6-month dietary program could cause body mass index (BMI) to significantly decrease. Suppose the investigators wanted to know prior to the intervention whether mean BMI is different than 28 by either plus or minus 2. Assume the standard deviation is 5, and let $\alpha = 0.05$ and $\beta = 0.20$. Therefore,

$$n = \left[\frac{(1.96 - [-0.84])5}{2} \right]^2 = 49$$

Thus, to conclude that mean BMI differs from 28 by 2 or more with standard deviation of 5 and a 95% confidence level requires a sample size of 49.

Equation for Estimating the Sample Size for One Proportion

$$n = \left[\frac{Z_\alpha \sqrt{\pi_0(1-\pi_0)} - Z_\beta \sqrt{\pi_1(1-\pi_1)}}{\pi_1 - \pi_0} \right]^2$$

To illustrate, suppose you are interested in identifying the prevalence of eating five or more servings of fruit and vegetables per day in a college student population. In the past, it has been assumed that about 25% of the students ate five or more servings of fruit and vegetables per day. However, you suspect that the true percentage is at least 30%. Let $\alpha = 0.05$ and $\beta = 0.10$. Therefore,

$$n = \left[\frac{1.645\sqrt{0.25(1-0.25)}-(-1.282)\sqrt{0.30(1-0.30)}}{0.30-0.25} \right]^2 = 675.8$$

Hence, the required sample size is 676.

Equation for Estimating the Sample Size for Two Means

$$n = 4\left[\frac{(z_\alpha - z_\beta)\sigma}{\mu_1 - \mu_2} \right]^2$$

n = Total number of participants required.

To illustrate, an exercise program has been developed for improving breathing. Researchers want to test whether it is better than the status quo. A randomized trial is planned to assess whether the forced expiratory volume in 1 second differs between those in the exercise program and those who continue with their regular activities. Forced expiratory volume is typically 1.5 liters, with a standard deviation of 1.0 liters. We want to know how many participants are needed in each group to detect a 20% difference, with $\alpha = 0.05$ and $\beta = 0.20$. The difference in means is 0.30 (1.5 × 0.20). Therefore,

$$n = 4\left[\frac{(1.96-[-0.84])1}{0.3} \right]^2 = 348.4$$

The required sample size is 175 per group.

If the standard deviation is not known such that s is used rather than σ in the equation, the sample size will be slightly underestimated if n is less than 30.

Equation for Estimating the Sample Size for Two Proportions

The total sample size required is

$$n = \left[\frac{z_\alpha\sqrt{4\pi(1-\pi)} - z_\beta\sqrt{2\pi_1(1-\pi_1)+2\pi_2(1-\pi_2)}}{\pi_1 - \pi_2} \right]^2$$

where the symbol $\pi = (\pi_1 + \pi_2)/2$, π_1 is the proportion in one group and π_2 is the proportion in the other group, z_α is the two-tailed z value related to the null hypothesis, and z_β is the lower one-tailed z value related to the alternative hypothesis. The required sample size per group is

$$n = \left[\frac{z_\alpha \sqrt{2\pi(1-\pi)} - z_\beta \sqrt{\pi_1(1-\pi_1) + \pi_2(1-\pi_2)}}{\pi_1 - \pi_2} \right]^2$$

To illustrate, suppose you are interested in investigating whether adults who lift weights for exercise have a lower risk of developing back pain than adults who jog for exercise. A review of the literature indicates that the risk of back pain is about 0.25 in adults who jog for exercise. You hope to show that lifting weights lowers the risk by at least 0.10. The number of subjects needed to determine if the incidence of developing back pain is 0.15 or less in those who lift weights, assuming $\alpha = 0.05$ and $\beta = 0.20$, is

$$n = \left[\frac{1.96\sqrt{2 \times 0.2(1-0.2)} - [-0.84]\sqrt{0.25(1-0.25) + 0.15(1-0.15)}}{0.25 - 0.15} \right]^2 = 249.7$$

Thus, the required sample size is 250 per group.

Sample Size Formula for the Correlation Coefficient

$$n = \left([z_\alpha - z_\beta]/C \right)^2 + 3$$

where
$C = 0.5 \times ln([1 + r]/[1 - r])$ and r is the correlation coefficient.

To illustrate, suppose you are interested in determining whether an association exists between BMI and the Beck Depression Inventory (BDI) score among a group of adults. A small preliminary study found a modest correlation ($r = 0.25$). The number of participants needed to be enrolled in the study, with α (one-tailed) $= 0.05$, $\beta = 0.2$, and $C = 0.5 \times ln\left(\frac{[1+0.25]}{[1-0.25]}\right) = 0.2554$, is

$$n = ([1.645 - (-0.84)]/0.2554)^2 + 3 = 97.7$$

Therefore, 98 participants are required for this study.

Because some subjects in a study are likely to drop out, the estimated required sample size should account for loss to follow-up.

Sample Size Adjustment Factor for Dropouts

$$\frac{1}{1-X}$$

where X is the expected proportion that drops out of the study.

Suppose 20% of participants in the previous example are expected to drop out of the study. The sample size adjustment factor is

$$\frac{1}{1-0.20} = 1.25$$

Therefore, the sample size should be 123 (98 ×1.25).

Equation for Estimating the Effect Size for Fixed Sample Size

$$\mu_1 - \mu_2 = \frac{2(z_\alpha - z_\beta)\sigma}{\sqrt{n}}$$

To illustrate, researchers find that 150 subjects with mild to moderate depression are willing to participate in a study of whether a 6-week dietary program affects their BDI score. Subjects are randomly assigned to the dietary program or their normal diet. If the standard deviation of the change in the BDI score is expected to be 10 points in both the intervention and control groups, the size difference the investigator will be able to detect between the two groups, at α (two-sided) = 0.05 and β = 0.20, is

$$\mu_1 - \mu_2 = \frac{2(1.96 - [-0.84])10}{\sqrt{150}} = 4.57$$

In other words, 75 subjects per group will be able to detect a difference of about 5 points between the two groups.

Questionnaires, Interviews, and Online Surveys

For many behavior epidemiologic studies, the quality of the results is dependent on the quality and appropriateness of the questionnaire, interview, or online survey. The primary methods of administration, and strengths and weaknesses of questionnaires and interviews, are presented in **Table 8-1**. Regardless of the approach taken for obtaining data, it needs to be valid and reliable.

Table 8-1			
Questionnaires versus Interviews			
	Method of administration	Strengths	Weaknesses
Questionnaires	• Mail • Email • Websites • Handheld electronic devices (to produce cleaner data)	• More efficient and uniform way to administer simple questions • Less expensive • More easily standardized	• Susceptible to imperfect memory • Affected by respondent giving socially acceptable responses
Interviews	• In person • Computer-assisted telephone interviewing (CATI) • Interactive voice response (computer-generated questions that collect subject responses over the telephone via keypad or voice recognition)	• Better for getting answers to more complicated questions • Can assure the answers are complete • Can be the only option when respondents have poor eyesight or cannot read • Can have a higher response rate	• More expensive • More time consuming • May be influenced by the relationship between the interviewer and the interviewee • More difficult to standardize (e.g., inconsistent probing) • May introduce bias by word choice, facial expressions, or tone of voice • Susceptible to imperfect memory • Affected by respondent giving socially acceptable responses

OPEN-ENDED VERSUS CLOSED-ENDED QUESTIONS

Questions may be open-ended or closed-ended. Open-ended questions do not restrict the subject's response. Closed-ended questions require the subject to choose from a list of possible responses. Closed-ended questions should allow for a set of mutually exclusive and exhaustive responses. Including the option "All that apply" is not recommended because it does not force people to consider the individual options and, if left blank, it does not tell us whether none applied or if the question was overlooked. While open-ended questions are often useful in focus groups and for narrowing possible responses that can be incorporated into a closed-ended question, closed-ended questions have the advantage in that they are easier to answer and the answer is easier to analyze.

FORMAT

At the beginning of a questionnaire or an interview, there should be a brief description of the purpose of the study and how the data will be used. Instructions on how to complete the instrument (along with a possible example) can improve the accuracy and standardization of the responses. Questions should be grouped according to topic areas with a heading. It is better to start with emotionally neutral questions and finish with more sensitive questions. The visual design should be simple, neat, and have plenty of space. Sometimes certain responses will lead to follow-up questions, which is best handled using branching questions, such as in the following box.

Have you ever smoked marijuana?
  ] *Yes → How old were you when you first smoked marijuana?*____
  ] *No → Go to question 13.*

Branching questions cause the respondent to focus only on the relevant questions and, therefore, save time.

An advantage of online surveys is that they are often easier to complete because they can incorporate skip logic. For example, a male respondent would not see specific questions about uterine bleeding, fibrosis, or menopausal status, and a nonsmoker would not see questions about current level of use. However, skip logic requires careful design and validation.

WORD CHOICE

The wording of a question can influence its reproducibility and validity. To encourage accurate and honest responses, it is important that the questions be clear, simple, and neutral. Questions should be as clear as possible. For example, asking a group of current smokers, "How much do you smoke?" is less clear than asking, "During a typical day, how many cigarettes do you smoke?" Questions should use simple, clear wording. For example, it is clearer to ask, "Do you take any cholesterol-lowering medications?" than to ask, "Do you take statins?" Questions should avoid using loaded words and phrases that have strong emotional overtones or connotations that can evoke a reaction beyond its literal meaning (e.g., weed versus marijuana, elitist versus expert, child murder versus abortion, or put up with versus tolerate). For example, rather than asking, "During the past week, did you talk too much?" it is better to ask, "During the past week, how often did you talk to the point that your speech felt strained and required effort?"

Respondents may feel more comfortable answering a sensitive question on a questionnaire rather than in an interview setting. However, the presence of the interviewer can help a person be more honest in his or her response to sensitive questions. For example, an interviewer asking about income may elicit more accurate responses if he or she is not dressed to intimidate. Similarly, asking women about their weight may be more effective if the interviewer is overweight rather than a slim, very fit-looking individual. Another strategy is to preface a question by saying something like, "Many people experience anxiety. In the past week, did you ever have excessive feelings of fear, unease, or worry?"

TIME FRAME

Questions about a behavior should be relative to some time period, such as per day, within the past 30 days, or within the past year. For example, selected questions from the 2013 Behavioral Risk Factor Surveillance System (BRFSS) asked, "During the past 30 days, for about how many days did pain make it hard for you to do your usual activities, such as self-care, work, or recreation?" "How many times have you been to a doctor, nurse, or other health professional in the past 12 months?" "During the past month, not counting juice, how many times per day, week, or month did you eat fruit?" and "On average, how many hours of sleep do you get in a 24-hour period?" (Centers for Disease Control and Prevention, 2012). The first three questions try to identify the frequency of a behavior during a specified time period. The last question tries to get at what is usual or typical behavior.

Questions should ask about the shortest recent segment of time that best represents the characteristic over the period of interest (Cummings, Kohn, & Hulley, 2013). The appropriate segment of time depends on the characteristic. For example, how many times a person sees a doctor, nurse, or other health professional can vary considerably from month to month, but the past year may adequately represent such patterns. Juice consumption may vary considerably from day to day, but the past week may adequately represent this behavior.

Diary records may be a useful way to collect information regarding a behavior. By looking at diary records, researchers can find information regarding the time and place of the behavior and possibly factors immediately preceding the behavior. In general, diary studies allow us to collect longitudinal and temporal information; report events and experiences in context; and determine the antecedents, correlates, and consequences of daily experiences (Lallemand, 2012). The use of diaries in research assumes that the time period assessed is typical and that self-awareness from using a diary does not alter the behavior being recorded (Cummings et al., 2013).

PITFALLS

Three potential pitfalls in designing a good instrument have been iden-tified: double-barreled questions, hidden assumptions, and when the question and answer options do not match (Cummings et al., 2013). A double-barreled question contains more than one issue. For example, "Is running good for your health and fun?" While many people may run because they think it is good for their health, it does not neces-sarily mean they think it is fun. When questions include two issues, it is better to divide the issues into two questions: "Is running good for your health?" "Do you consider running to be a fun activity?"

It may be that some questions contain assumptions that do not apply to all people in the study. For example, a question might ask, "How often in the past week did you exercise because your spouse/partner wanted to exercise with you?" This assumes that the respon-dents have a spouse/partner. Or, "How often do you play video games with friends?" This assumes that you play video games and that you have friends. A hidden assumption can make it confusing for some individuals to know how to respond to the question.

Questions in which the answer choices do not match the questions can also make it difficult for individuals to know how to respond. For example, the question, "Have you done anaerobic exercise in the past week?" should not be matched with the possible responses "never," "seldom," "often," and "very often." The question should instead ask, "How often did you do anaerobic exercise in the past week?" or the response should be changed to "yes" or "no." Questions that involve intensity of a behavior can also be problematic. For example, sup-pose the question "I sometimes argue with other people" has possible responses of "agree" or "disagree." A person may disagree because they never argue with other people or because they often argue with other people. It would be clearer to ask, "Do you argue with other people?" with possible responses of "often," "sometimes," and "never."

MEASURING ABSTRACT VARIABLES

In behavioral research, abstract concepts are often being studied, such as awareness, knowledge, beliefs and perceptions (e.g., perceived susceptibility, perceived severity, perceived benefits, and perceived barriers), attitudes and values, readiness to change, motivation, self-efficacy, confidence, skills, capacity, personality traits, or behavioral intentions. Because it is difficult to quantitatively assess such variables, it is common practice to measure these abstract concepts using scores based on a series of questions that are organized into a scale (McDow-ell, 2006; Streiner & Norman, 2009).

Likert scales are psychometric scales commonly used in research that employ abstract variables. They assume that the strength or intensity of experience is on a continuum from strongly agree to strongly disagree. Respondents are given a list of questions or comments with corresponding responses that have a number assigned to each possible response. For example, the Center for Epidemiologic Studies Depression (CES-D) Scale presents a list of ways a person might have felt or behaved (Radloff, 1977). Respondents are asked how often they felt this way during the past week (**Table 8-2**).

Table 8-2

Center for Epidemiologic Studies Depression Scale				
	Rarely or none of the time (less than 1 day)	Some or a little of the time (1–2 days)	Occasionally or a moderate amount of time (3–4 days)	Most or all of the time (5–7 days)
1. I was bothered by things that usually don't bother me.	1	2	3	4
2. I did not feel like eating; my appetite was poor.	1	2	3	4
3. I felt that I could not shake off the blues, even with help from my family or friends.	1	2	3	4
4. I felt I was just as good as other people.	1	2	3	4
5. I had trouble keeping my mind on what I was doing.	1	2	3	4
6. I felt depressed.	1	2	3	4
7. I felt that everything I did was with effort.	1	2	3	4
8. I felt hopeful about the future.	1	2	3	4
9. I thought my life had been a failure.	1	2	3	4
10. I felt fearful.	1	2	3	4
11. My sleep was restless.	1	2	3	4
12. I was happy.	1	2	3	4
13. I talked less than usual.	1	2	3	4
14. I felt lonely.	1	2	3	4
15. People were unfriendly.	1	2	3	4
16. I enjoyed life.	1	2	3	4
17. I had crying spells.	1	2	3	4
18. I felt sad.	1	2	3	4
19. I felt that people dislike me.	1	2	3	4
20. I could not get going.	1	2	3	4

Data from Radloff, LS (1977). The CES-D Scale: A Self-Report Depression Scale for Research in the General Population. Applied Psychological Measurement, 1(3), 385-401.

For many scales, an overall score for each respondent's answers may simply be the sum of all scores or the average of the scores, which gives equal weight to each item. The scoring rule for the CES-D Scale is 0 for answers in the first column, 1 for answers in the second column, 2 for answers in the third column, and 3 for answers in the fourth column. The scoring of positive items is reversed. The possible range of scores is 0 to 60, with the higher scores indicating a higher presence of depression.

Cronbach's *alpha* is a reliability coefficient used to measure internal consistency of a scale (Cronbach, 1951). This statistic ranges between 0 and 1 and is an accepted rule of thumb for describing internal consistency (**Table 8-3**). The rating of internal consistency should be viewed as a guide, with the goal to include items that are internally consistent and also provide unique information about what is being measured.

To illustrate, suppose we want to measure how well three questions on the Oxford Happiness Questionnaire correlate (Hills & Argyle, 2002). We select three questions from the survey that we believe will help us understand who is happy and who is not, according to our own definition of happiness. Individuals are asked to rate how strongly they agree or disagree with the following three statements:

1. I am intensely interested in other people.

   a. Strongly agree
   b. Moderately agree
   c. Slightly agree
   d. Slightly disagree
   e. Moderately disagree
   f. Strongly disagree

2. I feel that life is very rewarding.

   a. Strongly agree
   b. Moderately agree
   c. Slightly agree
   d. Slightly disagree
   e. Moderately disagree
   f. Strongly disagree

3. I laugh a lot.

   a. Strongly agree
   b. Moderately agree
   c. Slightly agree
   d. Slightly disagree
   e. Moderately disagree
   f. Strongly disagree

To know whether or not these questions are internally consistent (i.e., they all get at the same idea), we can use Cronbach's alpha, which

Table 8-3		
Cronbach's Alpha for Evaluating Internal Consistency		
Cronbach's alpha	**Internal consistency**	
$\alpha \geq 0.9$	Excellent	
$0.9 > \alpha \geq 0.8$	Good	
$0.8 > \alpha \geq 0.7$	Acceptable	
$0.7 > \alpha \geq 0.6$	Questionable	
$0.6 > \alpha \geq 0.5$	Poor	
$0.5 > \alpha$	Unacceptable	

Data from George, D, and Mallery, P (2003). *SPSS for windows step by step: A simple guide and reference*, 4th ed. Boston, MA: Allyn & Bacon.

is calculated by correlating ratings between questions for each individual then taking the mean of these correlations. Assume we find that Cronbach's alpha for these three questions is 0.80. This means that respondents who agreed with question 1 generally also agreed with questions 2 and 3, which shows that the questions seem to be getting at the same concept. However, if we find that Cronbach's alpha is low, such as 0.30, it could mean that respondents who agreed with one question frequently disagreed with the others, showing that the test questions are not well correlated.

If we used SAS procedure code to estimate Cronbach's coefficient alpha, we would use the ALPHA option with the CORR procedure. The output provides both the estimated alpha and an estimated standardized alpha. If the variances of some of the variables vary widely, we should use the standardized score to estimate reliability. The standardized alpha coefficient tells us how each variable reflects the reliability of the scale with standardized variables.

CREATING A NEW SCALE

Many instruments are available that have been shown to be reliable and valid. It is good practice to first see if an existing scale is available to measure a characteristic of interest before trying to create your own. Developing a reliable and valid instrument can take considerable time and resources, and it should involve consideration of reliability and validity (i.e., face validity, content validity, construct validity, and criterion-related validity). If possible, a new instrument may be compared with a gold standard to assess validity. Oftentimes these issues are explored using focus groups, which are small groups of participants (e.g., 8–12) who are willing to spend an hour or so to discuss the topic because they are relevant to the research question.

Initial and subsequent focus groups can be helpful in identifying relevant variables, reviewing questions, and reviewing and modifying an instrument. Pretesting the instrument in a larger pilot study can provide valuable information about reliability, validity, and whether the questions provide a sufficient range of responses.

Interviewer Training

Interviewer training may involve both classroom and field training. It should occur with members of the actual sample. It is also important to provide interviewers with a reference manual that contains instructions for fieldwork. Interviewers should also be supplied with cards or pictures that accompany the questionnaire, a letter of appointment or ID card, and maps or instructions on how to locate the respondents. Herold (2008) presented selected items that should be included in training interviewers:

1. How to locate the correct households or sample points.
2. How to approach respondents to assure they agree to be interviewed.
3. How to inform respondents that their identity is anonymous and confidential.
4. How to introduce the consent form, if applicable.
5. How to administer the questionnaire so the words are not changed or emphasized inconsistently, skip patterns are adhered to, and other issues related to filling out the questionnaire properly are carried out.
6. How to define terms used in the questionnaire so all respondents have the same understanding of terms.
7. How to contact a supervisor in the event a new or unexpected situation arises in the field.
8. How to dress for interviewing so the respondent feels most comfortable with the interviewer.
9. How to review the completed questionnaire for accuracy, consistency, and completeness while there is still an opportunity to return to the respondent for corrections.
10. How to adhere to the overall sample design, find respondents, and minimize refusal.

The time spent in training interviewers with respect to these items is critical to the success of the study. It is also helpful for the interviewer to understand the purpose of the study, the effort that has gone into creating a valid and reliable instrument, the value of the representativeness of the study, and the need to minimize bias.

Data Management

Data management involves creating data tables, developing the data entry system, extracting data (queries) for monitoring and analysis, and assuring confidentiality and security of the data (Kohn, Newman, & Hulley, 2013). All epidemiologic researchers should be familiar with these data management issues. In this section, we will provide a brief overview of data management.

The information we obtain through direct and indirect measures of subjects and variables will be stored in a computer database. The database can then be updated, monitored, and formatted for data analysis. The study database will consist of one or more line listings where the rows correspond to the study subjects and the columns correspond to attributes of the subjects. A unique subject identification number that does not have meaning beyond the study database should be used for linking purposes and for maintaining confidentiality. Databases with personal identifying information must be securely stored (i.e., restricted access, password protected computer, and secure server).

Data entry is the means for populating the data tables. Double data entry is often used with survey data; the entered data are compared for accuracy, and discrepancies are corrected. However, electronic data captured through online surveys are becoming more common. There are many advantages to using online data entry: the data are keyed directly into the data tables without the need for a second transcription step and the corresponding potential for error; the computer can include validation checks to give immediate feedback if there is a data entry error (e.g., entered value is out of range); the computer can incorporate skip logic; and data may be viewed and entered using portable, wireless devices (e.g., iPad, iPhone, or notebook computer) (Kohn et al., 2013).

A spreadsheet is adequate for many study databases. However, complex databases may require database management software. Database queries are used to sort and filter the data. They are useful for monitoring data entry, providing reports about the study's progress, and formatting the results for analysis.

The data dictionary provides a list of the variables in the database, along with their data type, description, and range of allowed values. The variables should not contain spaces because most statistical packages will incorrectly treat a variable name with a space as two variables. An example of a data dictionary from a SAS dataset is shown in **Figure 8-1**.

The study database should be backed up on a regular basis, and the backup copy should be located at an alternate site. It is also

#	Variable	Type	Len	Format	Informat	Label
1	NAME	Char	80	$80.	$80.	School Name
2	SURVEY	Char	8	$SURVEY.	$8.	Survey type
3	Q43	Num	8	Q43A.		30 day Alcohol use frequency
4	Q44	Num	8	Q44A.		30 day Marijuana use frequency
5	Q45	Num	8	Q45A.		30 day Hallucinogen use frequency
6	Q46	Num	8	Q46A.		30 day Cocaine use frequency
7	Q47	Num	8	Q47A.		30 day Inhalant use frequency
8	Q48	Num	8	Q48A.		30 day Phenoxydine use frequency
9	Q49	Num	8	Q49A.		30 day Methamphetamine use frequency
10	Q50	Num	8	Q50A.		30 day Prescription stimulant use frequency
11	Q51	Num	8	Q51A.		30 day Prescription sedative use frequency
12	Q52	Num	8	Q52A.		30 day Prescription tranquilizer use frequency
13	Q53	Num	8	Q53A.		30 day Narcotic prescription drug use frequency
14	Q54	Num	8	Q54A.		30 day Heroin use frequency
15	Q55	Num	8	Q55A.		30 day Steroid use frequency
16	Q56	Num	8	Q56A.		30 day Ecstasy use frequency
17	Q57	Num	8	Q57A.		30 day Synthetic marijuana use frequency

Figure 8-1 Alphabetical list of variables and attributes

important to have multiple backups to avoid having an error in the database (e.g., inadvertent deletion of some data) be backed up to your only copy. After the study is completed, the final data set and its data dictionary should be archived for possible future use.

Sources of Error

At the heart of the matter, subjective collection of behavior data is fraught with potential for error. Although it is unrealistic to eliminate all error, we can recognize and attempt to minimize certain sources of error. A number of areas for potential error should be considered when designing and planning a survey:

- ■ *Coverage error* occurs when the sample is not equivalent to the target population. An outdated or poorly constructed sampling frame may be the cause of coverage error. It is important to know the quality of the sampling frame and its representation of the target population before drawing a sample. If coverage error is discovered after the data are collected, the resulting potential for bias should be reported with the results of the study.

- ▨ *Sampling error* is determined by the study design and the sample size. Sampling error is less problematic in that it is quantifiable and unbiased.
- ▨ *Measurement error* occurs from various sources in the data collection process and is the error that makes one respondent's answers incomparable with another's. Measurement error may be the most difficult to avoid and often goes undetected. Measurement error may occur because a study subject chooses to incorrectly respond or not respond to an item because the question is of a sensitive nature, threatening, or difficult to understand. Complicated skip patterns can contribute to measurement error. Recall or interviewer biases are types of errors that occur in certain types of studies.
- ▨ Error attributed to *nonresponse*. If the response rate is low, the representative properties of the sample are lost. Nonresponse may occur because the interviewer fails to locate the respondent or the respondent does not consent to participate in the study. Both of these factors can be controlled by appropriate study selection and interviewer training. It should not be concluded that a person could not be located unless several attempts were made to contact him or her. Often five or six attempts are recommended. The response rate will likely be higher for face-to-face surveys than for telephone or mail surveys.
- ▨ *Data processing errors* are becoming less of a problem with electronic data capture. However, manual data entry is always susceptible to error, especially if the questions are open ended and the responses are being coded (Herold, 2008).

Misclassification of subjects in case-control and cohort studies is a measurement error that can occur in either the exposure or the outcome variables. Imagine that an adult who smoked regularly as a teenager and is now a nonsmoker answers no to the question "Have you ever smoked 100 cigarettes?" This error in reporting could have occurred for several reasons, including misinterpretation or misreading of the question (e.g., the respondent thought the question was asking about recent smoking) or intentional misreporting (e.g., because smoking is viewed negatively, the respondent did not want to admit to having ever smoked). Although the underlying reason for the error may be important in the interpretation of study results, it is unlikely that a researcher will be able to determine which responses are errors, much less the underlying reason for the error.

In case-control studies, misclassification occurs when either the exposure or outcome status is incorrectly assigned. For example, suppose we are interested in assessing the association between hypertension and stroke. If classification of a history of hypertension is accurate in 90% of cases and 90% of controls, misclassification occurs at the same level in cases and controls. Because the level of misclassification is the same in cases and controls, we refer to this as nondifferential (also called random) misclassification. Alternatively, suppose that classification of a history of hypertension is accurate in 90% of cases and 70% of controls. This situation is referred to as differential (also called nonrandom) misclassification. Nondifferential misclassification will always lead to an underestimation of the odds ratio, and differential misclassification can lead to either an overestimation or underestimation of the odds ratio.

Misclassifying exposure or outcome status in a cohort study also yields biased results. When misclassification of the outcome is related to the exposure in a cohort study, differential (nonrandom) misclassification occurs. Consequently, the estimated rate ratio or risk ratio is distorted. If misclassification of the outcome is not related to the exposure, it is nondifferential (random). For example, consider a group of women who were classified as sexually active or not sexually active, then they were followed into the future to compare their respective risk of cervical cancer. If the sexually active women were more likely to pursue medical attention than those who were not, cervical cancer was likely to be more frequently and accurately diagnosed. Thus, the measured association between being sexually active and cervical cancer will be overestimated.

On the other hand, random misclassification in a cohort study can occur because of inaccuracies in classifying the outcome status of subjects, but these misclassifications occur similarly between exposed and unexposed groups. For example, suppose we are interested in measuring the association between physical demands on the job and risk of heart disease. However, some job switching and time working can result in misclassification of some employees. Nevertheless, this misclassification is likely to be unrelated to myocardial infarction. The effect of random misclassification is to make the groups more similar, thereby underestimating the association between exposure and outcome variables.

Differential misclassification is perhaps more common in case-control studies because being a case may affect a person's recall of exposure status differently than controls. For example, a woman who has a child with a neurological disorder is likely to recall exposures during pregnancy better than a woman who has a normal child. Being a case may also make a person more hesitant to identify a certain exposure. For example, a woman who has a child with a neurological problem may be less likely to admit drinking alcohol during pregnancy than a woman who has a normal child.

Consider a hypothetical case-control study of birth defects and alcohol consumption during pregnancy for 100 cases and 100 controls (**Table 8-4**).

Table 8-4		
Hypothetical Case-Control Data of Alcohol Drinking during Pregnancy and Birth Defects		
	Birth defect	
Alcohol drinking during pregnancy	Yes	No
Yes	80	20
No	20	80

The odds ratio is 16 (95% CI: 8.00–31.99). Since drinking alcohol during pregnancy is viewed negatively in society, mothers of infants who have birth defects may be more reluctant to report alcohol consumption. If 40% of mothers in cases who consumed alcohol during pregnancy indicated that they had not drunk alcohol, the data would appear as shown in **Table 8-5**. The odds ratio is 2.67 (95% CI: 1.42–5.02). There remains a significant relationship between alcohol drinking during pregnancy and having a child with a birth defect, but the association is much smaller than the true level of association. If half the women who drank alcohol during pregnancy and who had a child with a birth defect simply did not respond, the odds ratio would be 8.00 (95% CI: 3.87–16.55). Thus we see how differential recall or missing data can have a large impact on the resulting measure of association.

Now consider a hypothetical cohort study assessing unprotected sex and sexually transmitted infections (STI). The subject responses are shown in **Table 8-6**. The risk ratio is 2.33 (95% CI: 1.59–3.42). If some of the data in the table were misclassified because of mistakes in identifying the status of sexually transmitted infection, bias would occur. Consider the level of misclassification in **Table 8-7**. The risk ratio is 2.62 (95% CI: 1.82–3.79).

Now let's consider the effect of missing information due to loss to follow-up. Suppose 10% of all subjects were lost to follow-up. The

Table 8-5		
Hypothetical Case-Control Data with Misclassification		
	Birth defect	
Alcohol drinking during pregnancy	Yes	No
Yes	40	20
No	60	80

Table 8-6		
Hypothetical Cohort Assessing Unprotected Sex and Sexually Transmitted Infections		
	Sexually transmitted infection	
Unprotected sex	Yes	No
Yes	40	80
No	40	240

Table 8-7		
Hypothetical Cohort with Misclassification		
	Sexually transmitted infection	
Unprotected sex	Yes	No
Yes	45	75
No	40	240

risk ratio remains unchanged at 2.33, but the 95% confidence interval becomes a little wider: 1.56–3.49. If loss to follow-up is 10% of those with unprotected sex only, the risk ratio remains unchanged at 2.33 (95% CI: 1.58–3.45). If loss to follow-up is 10% of those with protected sex only, the risk ratio remains unchanged at 2.33 (95% CI: 1.57–3.46). However, if 10% loss to follow-up occurred in just those who would have had a sexually transmitted infection in the future, the risk ratio becomes 2.38 (95% CI: 1.58–3.58); 2.17 (95% CI: 1.46–3.22) for 10% loss in just the unprotected group who would have gone on to have a sexually transmitted infection; or 2.56 (95% CI: 1.72–3.80) for 10% loss in just the protected group who would have gone on to have a sexually transmitted infection. Thus we see that the risk ratio is biased only if the loss to follow-up differs according to outcome status.

Missing Data

We discussed certain precautions that can be taken to improve response rates and, therefore, the representativeness of a sample. If the response rate is too low, analysis and reporting of the data should only be done if it can be argued that those who responded to the study are representative of the target population. Making such a case can be very challenging.

A well-designed instrument is the best approach to avoid missing data. In clinical trials, having a tolerable intervention and treatment, excluding those less likely to comply, and offering incentives are proven ways to reduce loss to follow-up. In some situations it may be appropriate to replace missing data with substitute values (imputation). There are several excellent sources that cover this topic (Enders, 2010; Little, 1988; Little & Rubin, 2002; Rahman & Davis, 2012; Rubin, 1976; Rubin, 1987). If missing data or loss to follow-up is too high, then analyses may produce biased and misleading results. There may also be an insufficient number to address the study hypotheses. A rule of thumb for what would be considered a large number of missing observations is 10%.

Summary

1. Original direct measures of behavior include personal monitoring (quantitative measurements of personal behavior) and biologic markers. Original indirect measures of behavior include questionnaires, interviews, and online surveys. The reliability and validity of these instruments should be determined prior to administration.

2. Reasons for sampling include being able to study sample data more quickly and more economically; it may be the only feasible approach, especially in studies with long follow-up; greater effort can be devoted to accurately measuring a fewer number of subjects; probability methods can be used to estimate error in the statistics; and a sample can be selected to reduce variability in the group.

3. A sufficient sample size is needed for there to be sufficient power to evaluate our hypotheses. Several sample size equations covering different situations are given in this chapter.

4. Probability samples (i.e., samples with a random process such as simple random sampling, systematic sampling, stratified sampling, and cluster sampling) are the best approach to ensure reliable and valid inferences.

5. Two types of nonprobability sampling methods are convenience samples or quota samples. A convenience sample is a type of nonprobability sampling in which a sample population is selected because it is readily available and convenient. Quota sampling is the nonprobability equivalent of stratified sampling. Both convenience sampling and quota sampling are potentially biased because not everyone in the target population has a chance of selection.

6. Methods, strengths, and weaknesses of questionnaires and interviews were presented, along with several aspects relevant to these indirect sources of data (i.e., open versus closed-ended questions, format, word choice, time frame, pitfalls, measuring abstract variables, and creating a new scale).

7. Interviewer training may involve both classroom and field training and involve members of the actual sample. Interviewers should have a reference manual that contains instructions for fieldwork. As part of the training, interviewers should learn about the purpose of the study, the effort that has gone into creating a valid and reliable instrument, the value of the representativeness of the study, and the need to minimize bias. Spending sufficient time to train interviewers is critical to the success of the study.

8. Data management involves creating data tables, developing the data entry system, extracting data (queries) for monitoring and analysis, and assuring confidentiality and security of the data.

9. Five areas of potential error that should be considered when developing a survey instrument are coverage error, sampling error, measurement error, error because of nonresponse, and data processing error.

10. A well-thought-out study and carefully designed instrument are the best approaches to improve response rates and avoid missing data.

References

Centers for Disease Control and Prevention. (2012). *Behavioral risk factor surveillance system questionnaire—2013*. Retrieved from http://www.cdc.gov/brfss/questionnaires /pdf-ques/2013%20BRFSS_English.pdf

Cronbach, L. J. (1951). Coefficient alpha and the internal structure of tests. *Psychometrika, 16*(3), 297–334.

Cummings, S. R., Kohn, M. A., & Hulley, S. B. (2013). Designing questionnaires, interviews, and online surveys. In S. B. Hulley, S. F. Cummings, W. S. Browner, D. G. Grady, & T. B. Newman (Eds.), *Designing clinical research* (4th ed., pp. 223–236). Baltimore, MD: Williams & Wilkins.

Enders, C. K. (2010). *Applied missing data analysis*. New York, NY: Guilford Press.

George, D., & Mallery, P. (2003). *SPSS for Windows step by step: A simple guide and reference* (4th ed.). Boston, MA: Allyn & Bacon.

Herold, J. M. (2008). Surveys and sampling. In M. Gregg (Ed.), *Field epidemiology* (3rd ed., pp. 97–117). New York, NY: Oxford University Press.

Hills, P., & Argyle, M. (2002). The Oxford Happiness Questionnaire: A compact scale for the measurement of psychological well-being. *Personality and Individual Differences, 33*(7), 1073–1082.

Kohn, M. A., Newman, T. B., & Hulley, S. B. (2013). Data management. In S. B. Hulley, S. F. Cummings, W. S. Browner, D. G. Grady, & T. B. Newman (Eds.), *Designing clinical research* (4th ed., pp. 237–249). Baltimore, MD: Williams & Wilkins.

Lallemand, C. (2012). Dear diary: Using diaries to study user experience. Retrieved from http://uxpamagazine.org/dear-diary-using-diaries-to-study-user-experience/

Little, R. J. A. (1988). Missing-data adjustments in large surveys. *Journal of Business and Economic Statistics, 6*(3), 287–296.

Little, R. J. A., & Rubin, D. B. (2002). *Statistical analysis with missing data* (2nd ed.). New York, NY: Wiley & Sons.

McDowell, I. (2006). *Measuring health: A guide to rating scales and questionnaires* (3rd ed.). New York, NY: Oxford University Press.

National Cancer Institute. (2013). Biomarkers. Retrieved from http://appliedresearch .cancer.gov/areas/biomarkers/

Radloff, L. S. (1977). The CES-D scale: A self-report depression scale for research in the general population. *Applied Psychological Measurement, 1*(3), 385–401.

Rahman, M. M., & Davis, D. N. (2012). Fuzzy unordered rules induction algorithm used as missing value imputation methods for K-mean clustering on real cardiovascular data. *Proceedings of The World Congress on Engineering, 1*(1), 391–394.

Rubin, D. B. (1976). Inference and missing data. *Biometrika, 63,* 581–592.

Rubin, D. B. (1987). *Multiple imputation for nonresponse in surveys.* New York, NY: Wiley & Sons.

Streiner, D. L., & Norman, G. R. (2009). *Health measurement scales: A practical guide to their development and use* (4th ed.). New York, NY: Oxford University Press.

Vasan, R. S. (2006). Biomarkers of cardiovascular disease: Molecular basis and practical considerations. *Circulation, 113,* 2335–2362.

© Dmytro Hurnytskiy/ShutterStock, Inc.

Chapter 9

Statistical Application to Behavior Data

Many disciplines are involved in public health research, but it primarily rests upon epidemiology for monitoring, diagnosing, and investigating disease and health-related events. Biostatistics also plays an important role in public health and, in particular, is fundamental to carrying out descriptive and analytic epidemiologic studies. *Biostatistics* is the science of statistics applied to biologic or medical data; it is a contraction of biology and statistics. It differs from epidemiology in two important ways. First, biostatistics is not restricted to studies involving human populations; it can investigate all living organisms. Second, biostatistics does not explore causal factors and causal mechanisms, whereas this is a primary function of epidemiology.

The word *statistics* has multiple meanings, such as data or numbers, the process of collecting and analyzing data for patterns and relationships, and description of a field of study. Working with numbers can involve applying statistical methods to summarize and describe person, place, and time variables, as well as using statistical methods to draw certain conclusions that can be applied to public health. There are four areas of statistics: descriptive, probability, inferential, and statistical techniques. *Descriptive statistics* involves organizing, summarizing, and describing numerical data. Descriptive statistics are used in epidemiology to study the distribution (frequency and pattern) of health-related states or events and to provide a description of who, what, when, and where aspects of health-related states or events in selected populations. *Probability* is used extensively in epidemiology to assess the likelihood of experiencing an outcome, based on exposure information. Probability also provides a basis for assessing the reliability of the conclusions we reach and the inferences we make. *Inferential statistics* involves drawing conclusions about a population's characteristics from information obtained from sample data. Epidemiologic studies often rely on sample data. Finally, *statistical techniques* are analytic approaches that utilize statistical methods to investigate a range of problems. Epidemiology relies on a number of statistical techniques in its overall study of health-related states or events and in evaluating public health interventions.

The purpose of this chapter is to provide a brief introduction to each of the four areas of statistics.

Descriptive Statistics

There are many approaches for evaluating and describing data. Nominal and ordinal data are often described using counts and proportions. Discrete and continuous data are often summarized and described using measures of central tendency (e.g., arithmetic mean, geometric mean, median, and mode) and measures of dispersion (e.g., range, interquartile range, variance, standard deviation, and coefficient of variation). Data are often presented in tables. Graphs are used to help clarify exposure and outcome information. Descriptions of several types of graphs commonly used in describing epidemiologic data are presented in **Table 9-1**. Tables and graphs are useful for showing patterns, trends, aberrations, similarities, and differences in the data

Table 9-1	
Graphs for Describing Epidemiologic Data	
Type of graph	**Description**
Arithmetic-scale line graph	Line graphs are used mostly for data plotted against time. An arithmetic graph has equal quantities along the *y*-axis. An arithmetic graph shows actual changes in magnitude of the number or rate of a health-related state or event across time.
Logarithmic-scale line graph	The *y*-axis is changed to a logarithmic scale. In other words, the axis is divided into cycles, with each being 10 times greater than the previous cycle. The focus is on the rate of change. A straight line reflects a constant rate of change.

Table 9-1 (Continued)

Graphs for Describing Epidemiologic Data

Type of graph	Description
Simple bar chart	This chart is a visual display of the magnitude of the different categories of a single variable, with each category or value of the variable represented by a bar.
Grouped bar chart	Multiple sets of data are displayed as side-by-side bars.
Stacked bar chart	This chart is similar to a grouped bar chart, except each of the segments in which the bar or column is divided belongs to a different data series. It shows how a total entity is subdivided into parts.
Deviation bar chart	This chart illustrates differences, both positive and negative, from the baseline.
100% component bar chart	The bar is divided into proportions that are the same as the proportions of each category of the variable; it compares how components contribute to the whole in different groups.
Pie chart	This chart shows components of a whole.
Population pyramid	This is a graphical illustration that shows the distribution of age groups in a population for males and females.
Histogram	This is a graphic representation of the frequency distribution of a variable. Rectangles are drawn in such a way that their bases lie on a linear scale representing different intervals, and their heights are proportional to the frequencies of the values within each of the intervals.
Frequency polygon	This is a graphical display of a frequency table. The intervals are shown on the x-axis, and the frequency in each interval is represented by the height of a point located above the middle of the interval. The points are connected so that together with the x-axis they form a polygon.
Cumulative frequency	This is a running total of frequencies. A cumulative frequency polygon is used to graphically represent it.
Spot map	This map indicates the location of each case of a rare health-related state or event by a place that is potentially relevant to the health event being investigated, such as where each case lived or worked.
Area map	This map indicates the number or rate of a health-related state or event by place, using different colors or shadings to represent the various levels of the disease, event, behavior, or condition.
Stem-and-leaf plot	This is a method of organizing numerical data in order of place value. The stem of the number includes all but the last digit. The leaf of the number is always one digit.
Box plot	Also called a box-and-whisker plot, this is a graphical depiction of numerical data through six-number summaries: the mean, the smallest observation, the first quartile, the median, the third quartile, and the largest observation. The box portion of the graph represents the middle 50% of the data. The plot is useful for describing the distribution of the data, whether it is skewed, and if outliers are present.
Scatter plot	This graph is a useful summary of the association between two numerical variables. It is usually drawn before calculating a linear correlation coefficient or fitting a regression line because these statistics assume a linear relationship in the data. It provides a good visual picture of the relationship between the two variables and aids in the interpretation of the correlation coefficient or regression model.

Data from Merrill, RM (2013). *Fundamentals of Epidemiology and Biostatistics: Combining the Basics* (pp. 69-71). Burlington, MA: Jones & Bartlett Learning.

(numbers, ratios, proportions, or rates). Tables and graphs are useful for communicating epidemiologic data according to person, place, and time factors.

Probability

Most of us understand the word *probability*, which we apply to our lives when we consider the chance or likelihood that a given event will occur. For example, a person undergoes a medical procedure with consideration of the chance it will make him or her feel better. Probability provides a basis for assessing the reliability of the conclusions we make under conditions of uncertainty. Probability theory is applied extensively in epidemiology. We are often interested in the prevalence of a health-related state or event in a specified population. Conditional probability is also commonly employed. For example, consider the following calculations for an odds ratio or a risk ratio:

$$\text{Odds Ratio} = \frac{P(\text{Exposed} \mid \text{Disease})/P(\text{Unexposed} \mid \text{Disease})}{P(\text{Exposed} \mid \text{No Disease})/P(\text{Unexposed} \mid \text{No Disease})}$$

or

$$\text{Risk Ratio} = \frac{P(\text{Disease} \mid \text{Exposed})}{P(\text{Disease} \mid \text{Unexposed})}$$

Here, $P(\text{Event}_2 \mid \text{Event}_1)$ represents the probability of some event, given " $\mid$ " another event has occurred. In diagnostic testing, we may be interested in the probability of a positive test given having the disease (sensitivity); the probability of a negative test given not having a disease (specificity); the probability of having a disease given a positive test (predictive value positive); or the probability of not having a disease given a negative test (predictive value negative).

Epidemiologic studies often rely on sampled data. Probability sampling is a sampling approach in which each individual in the target population has a known chance of being sampled. In random sampling, for example, each person has an equal chance of being selected. This approach is used to obtain a representative group from the population of interest. We also use random assignment in experimental studies so each person has an equal chance of being in any given arm of the study. This approach helps balance out the effect of confounding factors.

In statistical hypothesis testing in epidemiologic studies, we use probability. Probability is employed in statistical inference to capture the chance of error. For example, hypothesis testing may result in committing a type I error or a type II error. We also compare our calculated test statistics with critical values obtained from probability distribution tables to determine statistical significance.

Statistical Inference

Statistical inference is the process of drawing conclusions about the population based on a representative sample of the population. We often use data from samples or experiments to estimate the values of unknown parameters or in testing hypotheses concerning these values. In sampling from a population, our goal is to construct a sample quantity (estimator) that estimates an unknown parameter. The actual numerical value obtained for an estimator is called an estimate or point estimate. For example, the sample mean $\overline{X}$ is an estimator of the population parameter μ.

A hypothesis test is a way of generalizing the population based on sample information. A hypothesis test makes an assumption about the population, and probability is used to estimate the likelihood that the results obtained from the sample meet the assumption about the population. Hypotheses are expressed in terms of population parameters, such as $\mu = 50$, $\mu \geq 50$ (population mean at least 50), or $\mu \leq 50$ (population mean is no greater than 50). A hypothesis test is a statistical procedure used to make a decision about the value of a population parameter. Hypotheses may involve a single variable or a relation between or among variables. Hypotheses are shown to be consistent or inconsistent with the facts. If established information or facts are lacking to support a hypothesis, more information should be obtained, or we fail to reject the null hypothesis. After the null and alternative hypotheses are formulated in statistical terms in the first two steps, the level of significance for the statistical test and the sample size are given in the third step. An appropriate test statistic, degrees of freedom, and the critical value are given in the fourth step. Then we calculate the statistic in the fifth step and state our conclusion in the sixth step.

Our choice of a test statistic to evaluate our hypotheses is influenced by the type of data involved. In the remainder of this section we will present the Z statistic, t statistic, F statistic, and χ^2 (chi-square) statistic for testing certain hypotheses. Each of the tests described assumes that random samples have been taken. When two samples are taken for the same test, they are assumed to be independent.

THE Z STATISTIC

The standard normal distribution is a normal distribution that has mean 0 and variance 1. The Z distribution is a theoretical probability distribution that is symmetric, bell shaped, and has a mean of 0 and a variance of 1. The Z statistic is equal to the estimator $(\hat{\theta})$ minus the hypothesized parameter value $(E(\theta))$ divided by the standard error of the estimate (σ_θ), written as

$$Z = \frac{\hat{\theta} - E(\theta)}{\sigma_\theta}$$

If $\hat{\theta}$ is normally distributed, Z is a standard normal distribution. The Z can be used to evaluate a single normally distributed variable, as follows:

$$Z = \frac{X - \mu_0}{\sigma}$$

If n is large (> 30), then

$$Z = \frac{\overline{X} - \mu_0}{\sigma/\sqrt{n}}$$

$\overline{X}$ has approximately a normal distribution with mean μ_0 and standard error $\sigma/\sqrt{n}$. Hypotheses can be formulated about the mean as follows, depending on whether a lower, upper, or two-tailed test is involved, respectively:

$$H_0 : \mu \geq \mu_0 \ H_1 : \mu < \mu_0$$
$$H_0 : \mu \leq \mu_0 \ H_1 : \mu > \mu_0$$
$$H_0 : \mu = \mu_0 \ H_1 : \mu \neq \mu_0$$

If $|Z| > Z_\alpha$ (one-tailed test), reject H_0 and conclude H_1.
If $|Z| > Z_{\alpha/2}$ (two-tailed test), reject H_0 and conclude H_1.

Suppose it is assumed that a given group of adults consume on average no more than 2,300 milligrams of sodium per day. However, you think it is higher than this. In a sample of 100 individuals, you estimate that the average sodium intake over a week is 2,500 milligrams. The standard deviation is 800. Applying the steps of hypothesis testing gives the following:

1. $H_0 : \mu \leq 2,300$
2. $H_1 : \mu > 2,300$
3. $\alpha = 0.05$, n = 100
4. Z statistic
5. $Z = 2.5$
6. From a Z table, we obtain a critical value of 1.645. Since 2.5 > 1.645, we reject the null hypothesis and conclude that the

average sodium intake for this population of adults is significantly greater than 2,300 milligrams per day.

For one binomial population, hypotheses may be formulated as follows:

$$H_0: \pi \geq \pi_0 \; H_1: \pi < \pi_0$$

$$H_0: \pi \leq \pi_0 \; H_1: \pi > \pi_0$$

$$H_0: \pi = \pi_0 \; H_1: \pi \neq \pi_0$$

The test statistic for evaluating the number of successes is

$$Z = \frac{X - \pi_0}{\sqrt{n\pi_0(1 - \pi_0)}}$$

The test statistic for evaluating the proportion or fraction (f) of successes is

$$Z = \frac{f - \pi_0}{\sqrt{\pi_0(1 - \pi_0)/n}}$$

These tests require large samples where $n\pi_0(1 - \pi_0) \geq 5$.

Suppose that the percentage of individuals aged 45–54 years who have been told that they have arthritis is 42.1%, according to the Behavior Risk Factor Surveillance System (BRFSS) (Centers for Disease Control and Prevention [CDC], 2009b). Since this statistic is based on personal reporting, you would like to test whether a survey of 1,000 randomly chosen physician records of adults gives a similar result. The survey of medical records resulted in 43.6%. Is there a statistically significant difference? Applying the steps of hypothesis testing gives the following:

1. $H_0: \mu = 0.421$
2. $H_1: \mu \neq 0.421$
3. $\alpha = 0.05$, n = 1,000
4. Z statistic
5. Z = 0.961
6. From a Z table, we obtain a critical value of 1.96. Since 0.961 < 1.96, we fail to reject the null hypothesis and conclude that there is no difference in the proportion of arthritis cases in the adult population between the two sampling approaches.

THE t STATISTIC

The t distribution is a theoretical probability distribution that is symmetric, bell shaped, and has a mean of 0. The variability of the t distribution depends on the sample size n and has n − 1 degrees of freedom. *Degrees of freedom* are independent pieces of data being used to make a calculation. The smaller the number of degrees of freedom associated with the t statistic, the more variable will be its sampling distribution.

The t statistic is equal to the estimator $(\hat{\theta})$ minus the hypothesized parameter value $(E(\theta))$ divided by the standard error of the estimate (s_θ); that is, the t statistic has the form

$$t = \frac{\hat{\theta} - E(\theta)}{s_\theta}$$

If n < 30, the population should be approximately normally distributed. If the standard error of the estimate is known (σ_θ), rather than s_θ, then the ratio is a Z value. When n > 30, then t ≈ Z, even if the population is not normally distributed, according to the central limit theorem.

For a single numerical population value, hypotheses are formulated as shown under the Z statistic section, that is,

$$H_0 : \mu \geq \mu_0 \ H_1 : \mu < \mu_0$$
$$H_0 : \mu \leq \mu_0 \ H_1 : \mu > \mu_0$$
$$H_0 : \mu = \mu_0 \ H_1 : \mu \neq \mu_0$$

The test statistic is computed and compared with the critical value from the t table based on n−1 degrees of freedom, that is,

$$t = \frac{\overline{X} - \mu_0}{s/\sqrt{n}}$$

If $|t| > t_{\alpha, n-1}$ (one-tailed test), reject H_0 and conclude H_1.
If $|t| > t_{\alpha/2, n-1}$ (two-tailed test), reject H_0 and conclude H_1.

To illustrate, consider a random sample of 10 states from 50 U.S. states from which aggregated data are available on the percentage of adults aged 65 years and older who have had a flu shot within the past year (CDC, 2012b). You are interested in whether the mean of these 10 states is significantly different than the projected goal of 65% in this age group being vaccinated. The 10 randomly selected states (and their vaccination rates for flu) are Wisconsin (50.5%), Michigan (55.4%), Oklahoma (67.8%), Idaho (52.0%), New York (55.1%), Florida (54.7%), Hawaii (62.7%), Wyoming (53.3%), Maryland (63.2%), and Texas (59.4%). Applying the steps of hypothesis testing gives the following:

1. $H_0 : \mu = 0.65$
2. $H_1 : \mu \neq 0.65$
3. $\alpha = 0.05$, n = 10

4. t statistic
5. $t = -4.27$
6. From a t table, we obtain a critical value of 2.262. Since $|-4.27| > 2.262$, we reject the null hypothesis and conclude that there is a difference in the proportion of individuals aged 65 years and older who received a flu shot in the past year. The negative t test indicates that the actual sample mean of the proportions is significantly lower than 0.65.

In some situations, the mean of the same group is measured at baseline and at a follow-up period. We use the t test to evaluate whether a significant change occurred in the mean values. The difference score is assumed to be normally distributed with the population variance (σ^2) unknown. Examples of statistical hypotheses for paired data are

$$H_0 : \delta \geq 0 \text{ versus } H_a : \delta < 0$$

$$H_0 : \delta \leq 0 \text{ versus } H_a : \delta > 0$$

$$H_0 : \delta = 0 \text{ versus } H_a : \delta \neq 0$$

The t statistic can be used with the following modification:

$$t = \frac{\bar{d} - 0}{s_d / \sqrt{n}}$$

The denominator is the standard error of the mean differences with

$$s_d = \sqrt{\frac{\sum (d - \bar{d})^2}{n - 1}}$$

There are $n - 1$ degrees of freedom.

A sample of 10 adults each had their daily exercise time measured in minutes, averaged over 5 work days in June. They then attended a 2-hour health education class that stressed the importance of exercise and other healthy behaviors. They then had their daily exercise time measured again, averaged over 5 work days in the same month. Data in the first/second session were 23/38, 40/38, 33/40, 25/26, 18/41, 38/25, 5/31, 50/40, 22/35, and 36/40. We believe the health education class will cause exercise time to increase. Applying the steps of hypothesis testing gives the following:

1. $H_0 : \delta \leq 0$
2. $H_1 : \delta > 0$
3. $\alpha = 0.05, n = 10$

4. t statistic
5. t = 1.55
6. From a t table, we obtain a critical value of 1.833. Since 1.55 < 1.833, we fail to reject the null hypothesis and conclude that there is not an increase in minutes exercised from before to after the health education intervention.

When assessing a research question about means in two separate groups, the t statistic can be used if certain assumptions hold. First, the samples need to be independent random samples, such that knowing the values of the observations in one group does not tell us anything about the observations in the other group. Second, the populations both need to be normally distributed. However, this is less a concern when the sample size is at least 30, according to the central limit theorem. For smaller sample sizes where the two separate groups are not normally distributed, a nonparametric procedure called the Wilcoxon rank sum test is preferred. Third, the population variances for both groups are equal. However, the t test is robust to deviation in the variances.

If the variances are approximately equal, as determined by an F test, then we can compute a pooled standard deviation, as follows:

$$S_p = \sqrt{\frac{\left(n_1 - 1\right)s_1^2 + \left(n_2 - 1\right)s_2^2}{n_1 + n_2 - 2}}$$

We then use the pooled standard deviation to calculate the standard error of the difference in means, as follows:

$$SE_{(\bar{X}_1 - \bar{X}_2)} = s_P \sqrt{\frac{1}{n_1} + \frac{1}{n_2}}$$

The standard error of the difference is used in the denominator of the t statistic when evaluating the difference between means from two independent groups.

Three forms of hypotheses are as follows:

$$H_0 : \mu_1 \geq \mu_2 \ H_a : \mu_1 < \mu_2$$

$$H_0 : \mu_1 \leq \mu_2 \ H_a : \mu_1 > \mu_2$$

$$H_0 : \mu_1 = \mu_2 \ H_a : \mu_1 \neq \mu_2$$

The t statistic is then computed as follows:

$$t_{n_1 + n_2 - 2} = \frac{\left(\bar{X}_1 - \bar{X}_2\right) - 0}{s_P \sqrt{\left(\frac{1}{n_1} + \frac{1}{n_2}\right)}}$$

The pooled standard error will be underestimated if the variances are not equal. When the variances are not equal, the following form of the t statistic should be used:

$$t_v = \frac{\left(\overline{X}_1 - \overline{X}_2\right) - 0}{\sqrt{\left(\dfrac{s_1^2}{n_1} + \dfrac{s_2^2}{n_2}\right)}}$$

The next step is to calculate the approximate degrees of freedom as

$$v = \frac{\left[\left(\dfrac{s_1^2}{n_1}\right) + \left(\dfrac{s_2^2}{n_2}\right)\right]^2}{\left[\left(\dfrac{s_1^2}{n_1}\right)^2 / (n_1 - 1) + \left(\dfrac{s_2^2}{n_2}\right)^2 / (n_2 - 1)\right]}$$

In the Coronary Health Improvement Project (CHIP), there were 337 participants aged 43–81 years (Aldana et al., 2005). We were interested in whether our random assignment balanced out the age distribution between intervention and control groups of the study. The mean age in the intervention was 50.39 (SD = 10.97, n_1 = 167), and in the control group it was 50.83 (SD = 11.13, n_2 = 170). Applying the steps of hypothesis testing to these data gave the following:

1. $H_0 : \mu_1 = \mu_2$
2. $H_1 : \mu_1 \neq \mu_2$
3. $\alpha = 0.05$, n_1 = 167, n_2 = 170
4. t statistic
5. t = −0.37. This is based on a pooled standard deviation of 11.05. We pooled because the variances were not significantly different, based on the F test, as will be illustrated in the next section.
6. From a t table, we obtain a critical value of 1.96. Since $|-0.37| < 1.96$, we fail to reject the null hypothesis and conclude that the mean age was similar between the two groups; our randomization appeared to successfully balance out the age distribution between the intervention and control groups.

THE F TEST

The F distribution is an asymmetric probability distribution that ranges from 0 to infinity. It has two degrees of freedom: v_1 for the numerator, and v_2 for the denominator. For each combination of these degrees of freedom, there is a different F distribution. The distribution has the greatest spread when the degrees of freedom are small. The hypothesis of equality of variances that is evaluated when considering whether it is appropriate to pool the variances in a t test is evaluated using an F test, that is,

$$H_0 : \sigma_1^2 = \sigma_2^2 \quad H_1 : \sigma_1^2 \neq \sigma_2^2$$

If $F > F_{\alpha/2, \, v_1, \, v_2}$, then reject H_0, where $F = \frac{s_1^2}{s_2^2}$ and the degrees of freedom are $v_1 = n_1 - 1$ and $v_2 = n_2 - 1$. Note that the largest sample variance is always placed in the numerator of the ratio.

On the basis of the data in the previous example, $F = \frac{123.88}{120.34} = 1.03$. Since $1.03 < 1.35$, we fail to reject the null hypothesis of equality of means.

THE CHI-SQUARE TEST

The chi-square distribution is a continuous distribution derived as a sampling distribution of a sum of squares of independent standard normal variables. It is a skewed distribution where only nonnegative values of the variable are possible. Its shape depends on the degrees of freedom. To test the hypothesis that the criteria of classification in the rows R_i and columns C_j of a contingency table (**Table 9-2**) are independent, we compute an expected number of sample elements for each cell, m_{ij}, and employ a χ^2 that approximately follows a chi-square distribution. The symbol χ^2 refers to the chi-square statistic.

$$\chi^2 = \sum_i \sum_j \frac{(n_{ij} - m_{ij})^2}{m_{ij}}$$

where $m_{ij} = \frac{R_i C_j}{n}$.

For example, consider the following 2 × 2 contingency table:

Passive smoking	Preterm birth (< 32 weeks of gestation)	Term births	Row totals
Yes	60	1,680	1,740
No	126	7,405	7,531
Column total	186	9,085	9,271

Data from Qiu, J, He, X, Cui, H, Zhang, C, Zhang, H, Dang, Y, …, Zhang, Y (2014). Passive smoking and preterm birth in urban China. *American Journal of Epidemiology. 180*(1), 94–102.

A table of expected values for the cells is shown as follows:

Passive smoking	Preterm birth (< 32 weeks of gestation)	Term births
Yes	34.91	1,705.09
No	151.09	7,379.91

Table 9-2		
	$r \times c$ Contingency Table	
Rows	**1 2 3 ... c**	**Row totals**
1	$Y_{11}Y_{12}Y_{13}...Y_{1c}$	R_1
2	$Y_{21} Y_{22} Y_{23}...Y_{2c}$	R_2
3	$Y_{31} Y_{32} Y_{33}...Y_{3c}$	R_3
.	... .	.
.	... .	.
.	... .	.
r	$Y_{r1} Y_{r2} Y_{r3}... Y_{rc}$	R_r
Column totals	$C_1 C_2 C_3... C_c$	n

$$\chi^2 = \frac{(60 - 34.91)^2}{34.91} + \frac{(1,680 - 1,705.09)^2}{1,705.09}$$
$$+ \frac{(126 - 151.09)^2}{151.09} + \frac{(7,405 - 7,379.91)^2}{7,379.91} = 22.65$$

Computational formulas that are easier to derive for the chi-square will be given later (Table 9-4).

Statistical Techniques

A number of statistical techniques are used in epidemiology to investigate a range of public health issues. For example, statistical techniques commonly used for assessing proportions, rates, and time to failure are as follows: regression methods have been used extensively for assessing proportions, rates, matched studies, and much more; and power and sample size estimation techniques are basic to epidemiologic studies.

The number of statistical techniques currently available to epidemiologists is extensive, some requiring a fairly sophisticated understanding of statistics. Some of these techniques can be applied using a spreadsheet, but others require the use of computer software. Statistical techniques are tools for addressing questions of scientific interest. Therefore, the process begins with the research question, which corresponds to a public health problem.

For nominal and ordinal scaled variables, data are entered into a contingency table, and the frequency distribution of one variable is compared across the levels of the other variable. If the data are discrete or continuous, some common measures of association are the correlation coefficient, Spearman's rank correlation coefficient, the coefficient of determination, and the slope coefficient in regression analysis.

The *correlation coefficient* (denoted by r) measures the strength of the association between two variables (also called the Pearson correlation). The method assumes both variables are normally distributed and that a linear association exists between the variables. When normality does not hold, Spearman's rank correlation coefficient can be used, which is not sensitive to outliers that skew the data distribution. When the latter assumption is violated, the investigator may choose to apply the correlation measure over a subsection of the data where linearity holds. The correlation coefficient ranges between -1 and $+1$.

Let x be the exposure variable and y be the outcome variable. The lowercase letter indicates that sample data are involved. The mean of x is $\bar{x}$ and the mean of y is $\bar{y}$. The correlation coefficient for these two variables is

$$r = \frac{\sum (x - \bar{x})(y - \bar{y})}{\sqrt{\sum (x - \bar{x})^2 \sum (y - \bar{y})^2}}$$

When the population parameter (ρ) is hypothesized to be zero, the following mathematical expression involving the correlation coefficient, often called the t ratio, has a t distribution with $n - 2$ degrees of freedom, that is,

$$t = \frac{r\sqrt{n - 2}}{\sqrt{1 - r^2}}$$

We then compare the calculated t value with the critical value obtained from a t table with $n - 2$ degrees of freedom. For example, suppose the correlation coefficient between exercise (minutes per week) and a depression score (from 1 to 100) for a sample of 25 adults is -0.4. Applying the steps of hypothesis testing gives the following:

1. $H_0: \rho = 0$
2. $H_1: \rho \neq 0$
3. t test, sample size $= 25$, and the level of significance is 0.05
4. Degrees of freedom $= 25 - 2 = 23$
5. $t = \frac{-0.4\sqrt{25-2}}{\sqrt{1-0.4^2}} = 2.09$
6. The critical t value obtained from a t table using a two-sided test, level of significance of 0.05, and 23 degrees of freedom is 2.07. Since the calculated t is greater than the critical t, we reject the null hypothesis of no association and conclude that exercise is significantly associated with a lower depression score.

The correlation coefficient is very sensitive to outliers in the data, especially when a small number of observations are involved. The alternative to the correlation coefficient when the data are not normally distributed is the Spearman's rank correlation coefficient. It is calculated as follows:

$$r_s = \frac{\sum \left(R_x - \overline{R}_x\right)\left(R_y - \overline{R}_y\right)}{\sqrt{\sum \left(R_x - \overline{R}_x\right)^2 \sum \left(R_y - \overline{R}_y\right)^2}}$$

where the ranked x data are depicted as R_x and the ranked y data are depicted as R_y.

To illustrate, in the 2012 BRFSS, questions were asked whether you were "ever told you had a heart attack (myocardial infarction)?" or "ever told you had skin cancer?" (CDC, 2012a). Based on these data, the correlation coefficient is r = 0.570. Spearman's rank correlation coefficient is r_s = 0.490 If you were to plot the data, the distribution of heart attack is slightly skewed to the right, whereas the distribution of skin cancer is close to being symmetric. Because there are not large departures from normality, the correlation coefficient is preferred. Applying the steps of hypothesis testing gives the following:

1. $H_0: \rho = 0$
2. $H_1: \rho \neq 0$
3. t test, sample size = 51, and the level of significance is 0.05
4. Degrees of freedom = 51 − 2 = 49
5. $t = \frac{0.57\sqrt{51-2}}{\sqrt{1-0.57^2}} = 4.86$
6. The critical t value obtained from a t table using a two-sided test, level of significance of 0.05, and 49 degrees of freedom is 2.01. Since the calculated t is greater than the critical t, we reject the null hypothesis of no association and conclude that there is a significant linear association between heart attack and skin cancer. Of course, this does not mean there is a causal association, which can only be concluded after consideration of other factors.

The *coefficient of determination* (denoted by r^2) is the square of the correlation coefficient, and it represents the proportion of the total variation in the outcome variable that is determined by the exposure variable. If a perfect positive or negative association exists, then all of the variation in the outcome variable would be explained by the exposure variable. Generally, however, only part of the variation in the outcome variable can be explained by a single exposure variable. For example, suppose that systolic blood pressure and exercise are correlated with r = 0.50 and the coefficient of determination r^2 = 0.25. If we believe that exercise influences systolic blood pressure, we can say that 25% of the variation in systolic blood pressure is explained by variation in exercise. The remaining 75% is attributed to other factors.

Regression analysis provides an equation that estimates the change in the outcome variable (*y*) per unit change in the exposure variable (*x*). This method assumes that for each value of *x*, *y* is normally distributed, that the standard deviation of the outcomes *y* do not change over *x*, that the outcomes *y* are independent, and that a linear relationship exists between *x* and *y*. Regression methods have been used extensively for assessing proportions, rates, proportional hazards, and matched studies.

REGRESSION FUNCTION

A regression function describes the association between the dependent variable and one or more independent variables. In epidemiology, we often refer to the dependent variable as the outcome or response variable and the independent variable as the explanatory, predictor, or exposure variable. Confounding or interacting variables are also of primary interest. The frequentist view of regression describes how the outcome variable Y changes by the level of the predictor variable X. The regression function can be expressed as $E(Y|X = x)$, which is the expected average (population mean) of the response variable Y when the predictor variable X takes on a specific value *x*.

The researcher selects the relevant explanatory variable(s) and decides on the functional form of the model. The selected form of the relationship between Y and X should be based on judgment and experience. In addition, the following error term is included in the model:

$$E(Y|X = x) = f(x) + \epsilon$$

Note that $f(x)$ is some function, such as $\beta_0 + \beta_1 x$, which expresses the relation between the two variables. The error term is included to capture the effects of variables we did not consider in the model. Unlike a functional relation, a statistical relation is not a perfect one.

SIMPLE LINEAR REGRESSION

Simple linear regression is statistical technique used to explore the relationship between a continuous outcome variable and a continuous, ordinal, or categorical predictor variable. It allows us to identify how an outcome variable changes, given variation in an exposure variable. In regression analysis, we are interested in estimating the value of the outcome variable that is related to a fixed exposure variable. The standard assumptions for simple linear regression are as follows: (1) for each value of X, the distribution of Y is normally distributed; (2) the standard deviation of the outcomes Y do not change over X; (3) the outcomes Y are independent; and (4) a linear relationship exists between X and Y. The equation for simple linear regression may be written as

$$Y_i = \beta_0 + \beta_1 X_i + \epsilon_i$$

where $\epsilon_i \sim N(0, \sigma^2)$ and independent. The relationship between X and Y is linear in the parameter β_1. If X is fixed, then $Y_i \sim N(\mu_i, \sigma^2)$. The mean or expected value of Y is

$$E(Y_i) = E(\beta_0 + \beta_1 X_i + \epsilon_i)$$
$$= \beta_0 + \beta_1 X_i + E(\epsilon_i)$$
$$= \beta_0 + \beta_1 X_i$$

If y_i is the observed outcome of Y_i for a particular value x_i, and $\hat{y}_i$ is the corresponding predicted value, then

$$e_i = y_i - \hat{y}_i$$

The distance e_i is known as the *residual*, which estimates the random population error.

The intercept and the slope of the regression line passing through a set of points are estimated using a method called *least-squares*. The sum of squares of the deviations of the observed minus the estimated values is the fitted line that makes this sum of squares a minimum, or least. The best-fitting line is the one that minimizes the sum of squares of the deviations. It is calculated as

$$b_1 = \frac{\sum \left(x_i - \bar{x} \right)\left(y_i - \bar{y} \right)}{\sum \left(x_i - \bar{x} \right)^2}$$

$$b_0 = \bar{y} - b_1 \bar{x}$$

The estimated regression line is

$$\hat{y}_i = b_0 + b_1 x_i$$

The parameter estimate b_0 represents the y-intercept of the linear fitted line, and b_1 represents the slope. The slope is a measure of association that indicates how y changes when x changes by one unit. The hat ^ means the outcome is estimated.

In regression analysis, we can use the t test to evaluate hypotheses related to the slope coefficients. We usually test whether the slope is significantly different than zero and formulate the hypotheses as follows:

$$H_0 : \beta_1 \geq 0 \quad H_1 : \beta_1 < 0$$

$$H_0: \beta_1 \leq 0 \; H_1: \beta_1 > 0$$

$$H_0: \beta_1 = 0 \; H_1: \beta_1 \neq 0$$

The t test can be used to evaluate the hypotheses, as follows:

$$t = \frac{b_1 - \beta_1}{se_{b_1}}$$

The 95% confidence interval for the slope is computed as $b_1 \pm 1.96 \times se_{b_1}$.

The error sum of squares is the sum of the squared deviations of each observation y_i around its estimated expected value; that is,

$$SSE = \sum [y_i - (b_0 + b_1 x_i)]^2 = \sum (y_i - \hat{y}_i)^2$$

In other words, SSE measures the variability of y_i observations in relation to the fitted regression line. The sum of squares is

$$SST = \sum (y_i - \overline{y})^2$$

The test statistic for evaluating the significance of the model is

$$F^* = \frac{SST - SSE}{df_T - df_E} \div \frac{SSE}{df_E} = \frac{SST - SSE}{(n-1) - (n-2)} \div \frac{SSE}{(n-2)}$$

$$= \frac{SSR}{1} \div \frac{SSE}{(n-2)} = \frac{MSR}{MSE}$$

which is an F distribution when H_0 holds. In addition, this is the same as the test statistic for the analysis of variance test statistic, which will be shown. In simple regression, $t^2 = F^*$.

The F statistic can be used to evaluate the overall significance of both a simple and multiple regression model, with the following decision rule: If $F^* \leq F(1 - \alpha, v_1, v_2)$, fail to reject H_0. If $F^* > F(1 - \alpha, v_1, v_2)$, reject H_0.

In the previous example, the linear association between heart attack and skin cancer was assessed using ecologic data. We will now use that data in a simple regression model, with heart attack regressed on skin cancer. Applying the steps of hypothesis testing gives the following:

1. $H_0: \beta_1 = 0$
2. $H_1: \beta_1 \neq 0$
3. t test, sample size = 51, and the level of significance is 0.05

4. Degrees of freedom $= 51-2 = 49$
5. $t = \frac{0.45294-0}{0.09337} = 4.85$
6. The critical t value obtained from a t table using a two-sided test, level of significance of 0.05, and 49 degrees of freedom is 2.01. Since the calculated t is greater than the critical t, we reject the null hypothesis of no association and conclude that there is a significant linear association between heart attack and skin cancer, that is,

$$F^* = \frac{14.975}{1} \div \frac{31.182}{49} = \frac{14.975}{0.636} = 23.53$$

$$t^2 = 4.85^2 = F^*$$

LOGISTIC REGRESSION

Logistic regression is a type of statistical model that is often used to assess the relationship between a categorical response variable and categorical and/or continuous independent variables. Suppose the outcome responses are binary 0/1 observations, then

$$Y_i = \beta_0 + \beta_1 X_i + \epsilon_i \quad Y_i = 0, 1$$

Let π_i be the probability $Y_i = 1$ and $1 - \pi_i$ be the probability that $Y_i = 0$. However, special problems exist when the outcome variable is binary. First, the assumption that the ϵ_i are normally distributed is not appropriate. Second, the error terms ϵ_i do not have constant variance. Third, the mean response is constrained to

$$0 \le E(Y) = \pi \le 1$$

This last problem is the most serious, making linear regression inappropriate.

The simple logistic regression function can be written as

$$E(Y) = \pi = \frac{\exp(\beta_0 + \beta_1 X)}{1 + \exp(\beta_0 + \beta_1 X)}$$

The mean response, denoted by π, is a probability when the dependent variable is a 0, 1 indicator variable. The logistic response function can be expressed as a linear model, making the transformation

$$\pi' = \log_e \left(\frac{\pi}{1 - \pi} \right)$$

This is called the *logit transformation* of the probability π. The ratio $\frac{\pi}{1-\pi}$ in the logit transformation is called the odds. With some algebra, it can be shown that

$$\pi' = \log_e\left(\frac{\pi}{1-\pi}\right) = \beta_0 + \beta_1 X$$

where π' ranges from $-\infty$ to $+\infty$ as X ranges from $-\infty$ to $+\infty$.

When the independent variable is an exposure $(1 = \text{Yes}, 0 = \text{No})$, then

$$\log_e(\text{odds})_{\text{Exposed}} = b_0 + b_1 \times 1 = b_0 + b_1$$

$$\log_e(\text{odds})_{\text{Unexposed}} = b_0 + b_1 \times 0 = b_0$$

$$b_1 = \log_e(\text{odds})_{\text{Exposed}} - \log_e(\text{odds})_{\text{Unexposed}} = \log_e(\text{Odds Ratio})$$

$$\text{Odds Ratio} = e^{b_1}$$

The 95% confidence interval for the odds ratio is computed as $e^{b_1 \pm 1.96 \times se_{b_1}}$.

In a case-control study, researchers explored whether acoustic neuroma (a benign tumor that develops on the hearing and balance nerves near the inner ear) was associated with exposure to loud noise (Fisher et al., 2014). Several loud noise activities were assessed. One involved working out with loud music. Of those with the disease, 31 worked out with loud music and 188 did not. Of those without the disease, 18 worked out with loud music and 315 did not. Applying the steps of hypothesis testing gives the following:

1. $H_0: \beta_1 = 1$
2. $H_1: \beta_1 \neq 1$
3. $\alpha = 0.05, n = 552$
4. Wald chi-square (using SAS) with 1 degree of freedom
5. The logistic regression (using SAS) is $b_1 = 1.0597$. Then, *Odds Ratio* $= e^{1.0597} = 2.885$. The 95% confidence interval is $1.571 - 5.301$. The Wald chi-square $= 11.6598$.

   The SAS code is as follows:

   ```
   DATA NOISE;
   INPUT X Y COUNT;
   DATALINES;
   1 1 62
   1 2 60
   2 1 188
   2 2 315
   ;
   PROC LOGISTIC DATA=NOISE DESC;
   ```

```
MODEL Y=X;
WEIGHT COUNT;
RUN;
```

6. At the 0.05 level of significance, the critical value from the chi-square table at 1 degree of freedom is 3.84. Since 11.66 > 3.84, we reject the null hypothesis and conclude that there is a positive association between workouts with loud music and acoustic neuroma. Note that the 95% confidence interval will not overlap 1 as long as the test statistic is significant at the 0.05 level.

POISSON REGRESSION

Poisson regression is appropriate when the dependent events occur infrequently, the events occur independently, and the events occur over some continuous medium such as time or area. Counts or rates of rare diseases are well suited for modeling with Poisson regression (Frome & Checkoway, 1985). When counts or rates are not rare, then logistic regression is more appropriate for assessing the data. We will now describe the meaning of the slope coefficient in a Poisson model when the independent variable is an exposure ($1 = $ Yes, $0 = $ No):

$$\log_e(\text{Rate})_{\text{Exposed}} = b_0 + b_1 \times 1 = b_0 + b_1$$

$$\log_e(\text{Rate})_{\text{Unexposed}} = b_0 + b_1 \times 0 = b_0$$

$$b_1 = \log_e(\text{Rate})_{\text{Exposed}} - \log_e(\text{Rate})_{\text{Unexposed}} = \log_e(\text{Rate Ratio})$$

$$\text{Rate Ratio} = e^{b_1}$$

The 95% confidence interval for the rate ratio is computed as $e^{b_1 \pm 1.96 \times se_{b_1}}$.

In a cohort study, Iso and colleagues (2005) assessed the association between current tobacco smoking and cardiovascular disease. The study identified 882 cases (220,965 person years) with the disease who smoked. It also identified 673 cases (189,254 person years) with the disease who did not smoke. Applying the steps of hypothesis testing gives the following:

1. $H_0 : \beta_1 = 1$
2. $H_1 : \beta_1 \neq 1$
3. $\alpha = 0.05$, $n = 1,555$
4. Wald chi-square (using SAS) with 1 degree of freedom
5. The Poisson regression (using SAS) is $b_1 = 0.1156$. Then, Rate Ratio $= e^{0.1156} = 1.1225$. The 95% confidence interval is $1.015 - 1.241$. The Wald chi-square $= 5.10$.

The SAS code is as follows:
```
DATA SMOKING;
INPUT EXPOSED $ CASES PYEARS;
LPYEARS=LOG(PYEARS);
DATALINES;
1 882 220965
2 673 189254
;

PROC GENMOD DATA=SMOKING;
CLASS EXPOSED;
MODEL CASES=EXPOSED/DIST=POISSON LINK=LOG
OFFSET=LPYEARS;
ESTIMATE 'SMOKER' EXPOSED 1 -1/EXP;
RUN;
```
6. Since 5.10 > 3.84, we reject the null hypothesis and conclude that there is a positive association between current smoking and cardiovascular disease. We also see that the 95% confidence interval does not overlap 1.

Multiple Regression

In this section, we will extend the simple regression models to more than one independent variable. The linear (in the parameters) model for a continuous outcome variable (Y) and continuous, ordinal, or nominal predictor variables (Xs) is

$$Y_i = \beta_0 + \beta_1 X_{1i} + \ldots + \beta_n X_{ni} + \epsilon_i$$

where $\epsilon_i \sim N(0, \sigma^2)$ and independent.

The estimated models presented in the **Table 9-3** each have multiple independent variables. Hence, they are called multiple regression models as opposed to simple regression models, where a single independent variable is employed. Multiple regression models are

Table 9-3		
Multiple Regression Models and Interpretation of the Slope Coefficient b_1		
	Multiple regression model	Interpretation of b_1
Linear	$y_i = b_0 + b_1 x_{1i} + \ldots + b_n x_{ni}$	Change in y mean value per unit change in x_1, adjusted for the other variables in the model
Logistic	$\log_e (odds) = b_0 + b_1 x_{1i} + \ldots + b_n x_{ni}$	Change in the log odds of the outcome per unit change in x_1, adjusted for the other variables in the model
Poisson	$\log_e (rate) = b_0 + b_1 x_{1i} + \ldots + b_n x_{ni}$	Change in the log rate of the outcome per unit change in x_1, adjusted for the other variables in the model

useful for adjusting for potential confounding effects of an exposure–outcome relation and are generally more efficient than stratified simple regression models when data in the stratified combinations are sparse.

To illustrate linear multiple regression, body mass index (BMI) was regressed on diabetes, age (years), sex (1 = Male, 0 = Female), and race (1 = Caucasian, 0 = other) for 1,102 adults. The estimated model using SAS is as follows:

SAS code:

PROC REG:
MODEL BMI=DIABETIC AGE SEX RACE;
RUN;

Partial SAS output:

Parameter Estimates					
Variable	DF	Parameter Estimate	Standard Error	t Value	Pr > |t|
Intercept	1	24.73268	0.94700	26.12	<.0001
DIABETIC	1	3.83907	0.74689	5.14	<.0001
AGE	1	0.01787	0.01325	1.35	0.1778
SEX	1	1.53499	0.28246	5.43	<.0001
RACE	1	0.67495	0.62837	1.07	0.2830

The estimated model indicates that BMI is 3.84 greater among diabetics than nondiabetics, on average, after adjusting for age, sex, and race. Only diabetic and sex are significant variables in the model.

To illustrate logistic multiple regression, suppose we are interested in assessing whether hypertension predicts diabetes among the 1,102 adults. Individuals were classified as having diabetes (yes/no) and having hypertension (yes/no). Age, sex, and race were scaled as indicated in the previous example. The estimated model using SAS is as follows:

SAS code:

PROC LOGISTIC DESC;
MODEL DIABETIC=HYPERTENSION AGE SEX1 RACE;
RUN;

Partial SAS output:

Analysis of Maximum Likelihood Estimates					
Parameter	DF	Estimate	Standard Error	Wald Chi-Square	Pr > ChiSq
Intercept	1	−6.0504	1.3298	20.7008	<.0001
Hypertension	1	1.3813	0.3360	16.9049	<.0001
Age	1	0.0295	0.0151	3.8541	0.0496
SEX1	1	0.1596	0.3378	0.2232	0.6366
race	1	0.6458	1.0293	0.3937	0.5304

The adjusted odds ratio $= e^{1.3813} = 3.98$. The 95% confidence interval is $0.3813 - 7.689$.

To illustrate Poisson multiple regression, based on 18 tumor registries in the Surveillance, Epidemiology, and End Results (SEER) Program (2014) for the years 2009–2011, we were interested in whether lip cancer incidence for whites was significantly associated with age (0–49, 50–59, 60–69, and 70 and older), sex, and Hispanic status. We used PROC GENMOD in SAS to evaluate the data.

SAS code:

```
PROC GENMOD DATA=SMOKING;
CLASS AGE1 HISP SEX;
MODEL COUNT=AGE1 HISP SEX/DIST=POISSON LINK=LOG
OFFSET=LPYEARS;
ESTIMATE 'SEX' SEX 1 -1/EXP;
ESTIMATE 'HISP' HISP 1 -1/EXP;
ESTIMATE 'AGE' AGE1 -1 1 0 0/EXP;
ESTIMATE 'AGE' AGE1 -1 0 1 0/EXP;
ESTIMATE 'AGE' AGE1 -1 0 0 1/EXP;
RUN;
```

Partial SAS Output:

Contrast Estimate Results								
Label	Mean Estimate	Mean		L'Beta Estimate	Standard Error	Alpha	L'Beta		Chi-Square	Pr > ChiSq
		Confidence Limits					Confidence Limits			
SEX	3.2003	2.8664	3.5731	1.1632	0.0562	0.05	1.0530	1.2734	428.04	<.0001
Exp(SEX)				3.2003	0.1799	0.05	2.8664	3.5731		
HISP	2.4606	2.0475	2.9572	0.9004	0.0938	0.05	0.7166	1.0842	92.18	<.0001
Exp(HISP)				2.4606	0.2308	0.05	2.0475	2.9572		
AGE	8.2545	6.8645	9.9260	2.1108	0.0941	0.05	1.9264	2.2952	503.33	<.0001
Exp(AGE)				8.2545	0.7766	0.05	6.8645	9.9260		
AGE	12.3818	10.3108	14.8687	2.5162	0.0934	0.05	2.3332	2.6993	726.02	<.0001
Exp(AGE)				12.3818	1.1563	0.05	10.3108	14.8687		
AGE	27.2003	23.0559	32.0896	3.3032	0.0843	0.05	3.1379	3.4685	1533.9	<.0001
Exp(AGE)				27.2003	2.2941	0.05	23.0559	32.0896		

The mean estimates indicate that the rate of malignant lip cancer in whites is 3.2 times (220%) greater in males than in females; 2.46 times (146%) greater in non-Hispanics compared with Hispanics; 8.25 (725%) times greater in ages 50–59 compared with ages 0–49; 12.38 (1,238%) times greater in ages 60–69 compared with ages 0–49; and 27.20 (2,620%) times greater in ages 70 and older compared with ages 0–49.

Analysis of Variance

When certain assumptions are met, testing the equality of several means requires the use of a procedure called analysis of variance (ANOVA). The assumptions of ANOVA are that the error terms are normally distributed, the error variances for different groups are equal, the slopes for different group regression lines are equal, and linearity holds. When the sample size is large, the normality assumption is less important than the other assumptions.

To conduct an ANOVA wherein we test the null hypothesis of equality of several means, independent samples are taken from j independent groups, that is,

$$H_0 : \mu_1 = \mu_2 = \ldots = \mu_k$$
$$H_1 : \text{Otherwise}$$

Let

X_{ij} be the ith observation in the jth group.

$\overline{X}_j$ be the mean of all observations in the jth group.

$\overline{\overline{X}}$ be the grand mean of the observations.

The total sum of squares (SS_T) the sum of squares among groups (SS_A) plus the error sum of squares (SS_E); that is,

$$\sum \left(X_{ij} - \overline{\overline{X}} \right)^2 = \sum \left(\overline{X}_j - \overline{\overline{X}} \right)^2 + \sum \left(X_{ij} - \overline{X}_j \right)^2$$

Computational formulas for the equations are as follows:

$$SS_T = \sum \left(X_{ij} - \overline{\overline{X}} \right)^2 = \sum X_{ij}^2 - \frac{\left(\sum X_{ij} \right)^2}{n}$$

$$SS_A = \sum \left(\overline{X}_j - \overline{\overline{X}} \right)^2 = \sum n_j \overline{X}_j^2 - \frac{\left(\sum X_{ij} \right)^2}{n}$$

$$SS_E = SS_T - SS_A$$

$$MS_A = \frac{SS_A}{j - 1}$$

$$MS_E = \frac{SS_E}{n - j}$$

The final step in ANOVA is to obtain the F ratio, which is $F = \frac{MS_A}{MS_E}$. If F is greater than the critical $F_{\alpha, v_1, v_{12}}$ value obtained from an F table with $v_1 = j - 1$ and $v_2 = n - j$, then reject the null hypothesis of equality of means.

To illustrate, suppose we were interested in whether the number of times bullied at age 8 (i.e., 0, 1, 2, 3, or more) was related to the family wealth index. Applying the steps of hypothesis testing gives the following:

1. $H_0: \mu_1 = \mu_2 = \mu_3 = \mu_4$
2. $H_1:$ Otherwise
3. $\alpha = 0.05$, n = 714
4. F statistic with 3 numerator degrees of freedom and 710 denominator degrees of freedom
5. $F = \frac{0.436/3}{23.983/710} = \frac{0.1453}{0.0338} = 4.30$, p = 0.0051
6. Reject the null hypothesis.

When the F test is significant, which indicates that the population means are not all equal, we can now perform the following number of two-sample t tests:

$$\binom{k}{2} = \frac{k!}{2!(k-2)!}$$

If k = 4, then $\binom{4}{2} = \frac{4!}{2!(4-2)!} = \frac{4 \times 3 \times 2 \times 1}{2 \times 1(2 \times 1)} = 6$. However, multiple tests increase the probability of committing a type 1 error. The Bonferroni correction of our individual α level should be used to evaluate statistical significance, that is,

$$\alpha^* = \frac{\alpha}{\binom{k}{2}}$$

If $\alpha = 0.05$ and 6 pair-wise mean comparisons are being evaluated, we would use $\alpha^* = \frac{0.05}{6} = 0.0083$ as our level of significance.

Chi-Square for Evaluating Ratios and Proportions

The hypotheses and test statistics associated with ratios, proportions, rates, and measures of association (odds ratio, rate ratio, risk ratio, and prevalence proportion) between dichotomous scaled exposure and outcome variables are shown in **Table 9-4**.

In the Fisher and colleagues (2014) case-control study that was previously referred to, the authors also investigated the association between acoustic neuroma and motorcycle racing or riding. Of those with acoustic neuroma, 28 raced or rode motorcycles and 188 did not.

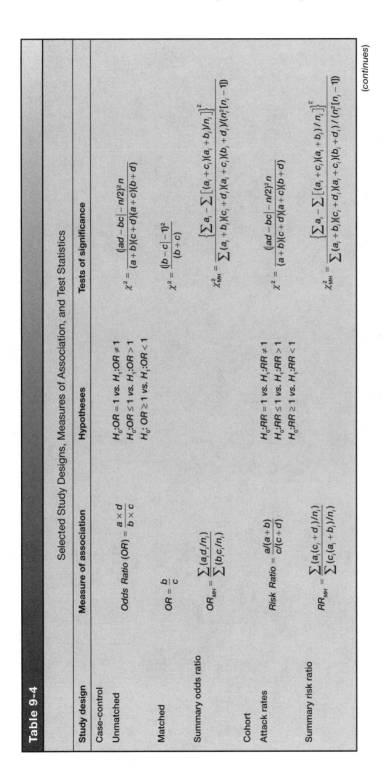

Table 9-4

Selected Study Designs, Measures of Association, and Test Statistics

Study design	Measure of association	Hypotheses	Tests of significance
Case-control			
Unmatched	$Odds\ Ratio\ (OR) = \dfrac{a \times d}{b \times c}$	$H_0{:}OR = 1$ vs. $H_1{:}OR \neq 1$ $H_0{:}OR \leq 1$ vs. $H_1{:}OR > 1$ $H_0{:}OR \geq 1$ vs. $H_1{:}OR < 1$	$\chi^2 = \dfrac{(|ad - bc| - n/2)^2 n}{(a+b)(c+d)(a+c)(b+d)}$
Matched	$OR = \dfrac{b}{c}$		$\chi^2 = \dfrac{(|b-c|-1)^2}{(b+c)}$
Summary odds ratio	$OR_{MH} = \dfrac{\sum(a_i d_i / n_i)}{\sum(b_i c_i / n_i)}$		$\chi^2_{MH} = \dfrac{\left\{\sum a_i - \sum\left[(a_i + c_i)(a_i + b_i)/n_i\right]\right\}^2}{\sum(a_i + b_i)(c_i + d_i)(a_i + c_i)(b_i + d_i)/(n_i^2[n_i - 1])}$
Cohort			
Attack rates	$Risk\ Ratio = \dfrac{a/(a+b)}{c/(c+d)}$	$H_0{:}RR = 1$ vs. $H_1{:}RR \neq 1$ $H_0{:}RR \leq 1$ vs. $H_1{:}RR > 1$ $H_0{:}RR \geq 1$ vs. $H_1{:}RR < 1$	$\chi^2 = \dfrac{(|ad - bc| - n/2)^2 n}{(a+b)(c+d)(a+c)(b+d)}$
Summary risk ratio	$RR_{MH} = \dfrac{\sum(a_i(c_i + d_i)/n_i)}{\sum(c_i(a_i + b_i)/n_i)}$		$\chi^2_{MH} = \dfrac{\left\{\sum a_i - \sum\left[(a_i + c_i)(a_i + b_i)/n_i\right]\right\}^2}{\sum(a_i + b_i)(c_i + d_i)(a_i + c_i)(b_i + d_i)/(n_i^2[n_i - 1])}$

(continues)

Table 9-4 (Continued)

Selected Study Designs, Measures of Association, and Test Statistics

Study design	Measure of association	Hypotheses	Tests of significance
Person-time rates	Rate Ratio $= \dfrac{a/T_e}{c/T_o}$		$\chi^2 = \dfrac{\{a - [T_e(a+c)]/T\}^2}{T_e[T_o(a+c)]/T^2}$
Summary rate ratio	$RR_{MH} = \dfrac{\sum(a_i T_o/T)}{\sum(c_i T_e/T)}$		$\chi^2 = \dfrac{\left\{\sum a_i - \sum[T_e(a_i+c_i)]/T\right\}^2}{\sum T_e[T_o(a_i+c_i)]/T^2}$
Cross-sectional	Prevalence Ratio $= \dfrac{a/(a+b)}{c/(c+d)}$	$H_0:PR = 1$ vs. $H_1:PR \neq 1$ $H_0:PR \leq 1$ vs. $H_1:PR > 1$ $H_0:PR \geq 1$ vs. $H_1:PR < 1$	$\chi^2 = \dfrac{(|ad - bc| - n/2)^2 n}{(a+b)(c+d)(a+c)(b+d)}$

Note: MH = Mantel-Haenszel
a = Number of exposed individuals with the outcome
b = Number of exposed individuals without the outcome
c = Number of unexposed individuals with the outcome
d = Number of unexposed individuals without the outcome
n = Total number of individuals in the sample
i = Level of stratification
T = Total time a cohort of exposed (e) and unexposed (o) people are followed

Of those without the disease, 20 raced or rode motorcycles and 315 did not. Applying the steps of hypothesis testing gives the following:

1. H_0:Odds Ratio $= 1$
2. H_1:Odds Ratio $\neq 1$
3. $\alpha = 0.05$, n $= 551$
4. A chi-square statistic will be used with 1 degree of freedom:

$$\chi_1^2 = \frac{\left(|ad - bc| - n/2\right)^2 n}{(a+b)(c+d)(a+c)(b+d)}$$

5. OR $= 2.35$, $\chi^2 = 7.22$
6. At the 0.05 level of significance, the critical value from the chi-square table at 1 degree of freedom is 3.84. Since $7.22 > 3.84$, we reject the null hypothesis and conclude that there is a positive association between motorcycle racing or riding and acoustic neuroma.

In a cohort study, researchers were interested in the relationship between antibiotic use during the first year of life and celiac disease (Canova et al., 2014). Among the cases, 129 (160,573 person years of follow-up) used cephalosporins during the first year of life, and 592 (970,712 person years of follow-up) did not. Applying the steps of hypothesis testing gives the following:

1. H_0:Rate Ratio $= 1$
2. H_1: Rate Ratio $\neq 1$
3. $\alpha = 0.05$, n $= 721$ cases and 1,131,285 person years
4. A chi-square statistic will be used with 1 degree of freedom:

$$\chi_1^2 = \frac{\{a - [T_e(a+c)]/T\}^2}{T_e[T_o(a+c)/T^2}$$

5. RR $= 1.32$, $\chi^2 = 8.10$
6. Since $8.10 > 3.84$, we reject the null hypothesis and conclude that there is a positive association between cephalosporin use during the first year of life and celiac disease. Those who used cephalosporins were 1.32 times (32%) more likely to develop celiac disease.

Summary of Statistical Techniques and Tests by Variable Type

A description of selected types of analyses for measuring the association between variables, depending on the type of data involved and if the assumption of normality holds, is shown in **Table 9-5**. Graphs are

---

Table 9-5

Classifications of Selected Statistical Techniques (and Tests) by Types of Variables

	Outcome variable			
Exposure variable	Nominal with 2 categories (dichotomous)	Nominal with > 2 categories (multichotomous)	Continuous, not normally distributed, or ordinal with > 2 categories	Continuous, normally distributed
Continuous, normally distributed	Logistic regression (likelihood ratio test)	Analysis of variance (*F* test)	*Spearman rank correlation*	Correlation coefficient (*t* test) Linear regression (*t* test, *F* test)
Continuous, not normally distributed, or ordinal with > 2 categories	*Wilcoxon rank sum*	*Kruskal-Wallis*	*Spearman rank correlation*	*Spearman rank correlation*
Nominal with > 2 categories	Logistic regression (likelihood ratio test) Contingency table (chi-square)	Contingency table (chi-square)	*Kruskal-Wallis*	Analysis of variance (*F* test)
Nominal with 2 categories	Logistic regression (likelihood ratio test) Poisson regression (chi-square) Contingency table (chi-square)	Contingency table (chi-square)	*Wilcoxon rank sum*	Comparison of means (*t* test)

Note: Nonparametric tests (shown in italics) are distribution free tests because they do not follow a specific distribution. The Kruskal-Wallis test evaluates whether the population medians on a dependent variable are the same across all levels of an independent variable. The Wilcoxon rank sum test is a nonparametric alternative to the two sample *t* test that is based solely on the order in which the observations from the two samples fall.

Data from Feigal, D., Black, D., Grady, D., & et al. (1988). Planning for data management and analysis. In S. B. Hulley, & S. F. Cummings (Eds.), *Designing clinical research: An epidemiologic approach* (pp. 159–171). Baltimore, MD: Williams & Wilkins.

---

useful for checking the assumptions of normality and linear association among variables. There are also formal tests available, such as the Kolmogorov-Smirnov test, which is a goodness-of-fit test that assesses whether a distribution is normally distributed. Data transformations and other methods are used to respond to violations of these assumptions. In some situations when outliers exist, the model is estimated without the outliers. In situations when a linear relationship between variables does not hold, piecewise linear regression or polynomial regression may be employed. Several nonparametric tests, which do not assume a distribution for the variables, are also available (e.g., Spearman's rank correlation coefficient).

Group Behavior Clusters

A cluster is an unusual number, real or perceived, of health events grouped together in time and location (CDC, 2009a). In epidemiology, a cluster is a grouping of cases of disease. A cluster can also refer to a co-occurrence of unhealthy behaviors among population subgroups at increased risk of disease. Certain social determinants (e.g., poverty, low educational level, lack of work skills, and adverse environment) are associated with clusters of unhealthy behaviors in the population (Marmot, Friel, Bell, Houweling, & Taylor, 2008; Rose, 1985). Given that the social environment has been associated with risk behavior clustering (Schneider, Huy, Schuessler, Diehl, & Schwarz, 2009; Singh, Rouxel, Watt, & Tsakos, 2013), it has been supposed that the provision of resources (e.g., information, education, and environmental improvements) will improve health behaviors in a parallel fashion (Spring, Moller, & Coons, 2012). An advantage of identifying subgroups of people with similar behavioral characteristics associated with health-related states or events is that interventions might then be developed that can more efficiently target these groups. The tailored interventions might be more effective at influencing group behavior and impacting enabling and reinforcing factors.

Group health behavioral cluster investigations require accurate grouping according to the behavior; case information according to person, place, and time; length of time cases lived in the area in question; potential changes in the given behavior; and migration patterns. In addition, a sufficient number of people with the behavior is needed to rule out chance as an explanation for the cluster finding. The primary statistical challenge with cluster investigations involves the fact that most cluster analyses involve posteriori rather than a priori hypotheses.

Posteriori refers to a formulation of the hypotheses after observation of an event such as putative excess in a given health-risk behavior. Hypotheses of this type are problematic because the conventional P value is only interpretable with *a priori* hypotheses—that is, those hypotheses established without prior knowledge of the level of the health events in a specified population. Selectively choosing a suspected cluster for statistical testing is equivalent to multiple testing. This is because the probability of finding a significant result increases as we become highly selective in testing only a given area out of many.

A second challenge is that rates have the danger of being overestimated because of *boundary shrinkage* of the population where the cluster is presumed to exist. That is, in calculating the rate of a putative cluster, the at-risk population that should go into the denominator of the rate calculation may be underrepresented. This situation has been compared by Rothman to the Texas sharpshooter who first fires his gun and then draws a target around the bullet hole (Rothman, 1990). With post hoc hypotheses, where significance tests are inappropriate, alternative methods of assessment include the following:

- Performing the study in a different location with a similar exposure (e.g., similar social environment)
- Excluding the cases in the original cluster and using new cases in the test of significance, assuming further case ascertainment occurred
- Looking for factors that distinguish the cases from others in the cluster, other than their residence
- Evaluating a dose–response relationship between the exposure and health event (Wilkinson, 2006)

Summary

1. There are four areas of statistics: descriptive, probability, inferential, and statistical techniques. Each of these areas of statistics is commonly employed in epidemiology.

2. Descriptive statistics are used in epidemiology to study the distribution (frequency and pattern) of health-related states or events and to provide a description of who, what, when, and where aspects of health-related states or events in selected populations.

3. Probability is used extensively in epidemiology to assess the likelihood of experiencing an outcome, based on exposure information. Probability also provides a basis for assessing the reliability of the conclusions we reach and the inferences we make.

4. Inferential statistics involves drawing conclusions about a population's characteristics from information obtained from sample data. Epidemiologic studies often rely on sample data. The following statistical hypothesis tests were presented: Z test, t test, F test, and chi-square test.

5. A number of statistical techniques are used in epidemiology to investigate a range of public health issues, such as proportions, rates, and time to failure; regression methods for assessing proportions, rates, matched studies, and much more; and power and sample size estimation techniques, which are basic to epidemiologic studies.

6. The correlation coefficient measures the strength of the linear association between two variables. The nonparametric equivalent to this measure is Spearman's rank correlation coefficient.

7. The coefficient of determination is the square of the correlation coefficient, and it represents the proportion of the total variation in the outcome variable that is determined by the exposure variable.

8. Regression is a method of estimating the functional relationship between an outcome (y or dependent variable) and one or more postulated risk factors (or independent variables). Simple regression involves one independent variable.

Logistic regression is a type of regression in which the dependent variable is a categorical variable (usually dichotomous). Poisson regression is a type of regression in which the dependent variable is a count or a rate.

9. Multiple regression is an extension of simple regression analysis in which there are two or more independent variables. In multiple regression, the effects of multiple independent variables on the dependent variable can be simultaneously assessed. This type of model is useful for adjusting for potential confounders.

10. A behavior cluster may be thought of as a co-occurrence of unhealthy behaviors among population subgroups at increased risk of disease. The social environment has been associated with clustering of unhealthy behaviors in the population. Tailored interventions (e.g., information, education, and environmental improvements) might be more effective at influencing group behavior and impacting enabling and reinforcing factors.

References

Aldana, S. G., Greenlaw, R. L., Diehl, H. A., Salberg, A., Merrill, R. M., Ohmine, S., & Thomas, C. (2005). Effects of an intensive diet and physical activity modification program on the health risks of adults. *Journal of the American Dietetic Association, 105*(3), 371–381.

Canova, C., Zabeo, V., Pitter, G., Romor, P., Baldovin, T., Zanotti, R., & Simonato, L. (2014). Association of maternal education, early infections, and antibiotic use with celiac disease: A population-based birth cohort study in Northeastern Italy. *American Journal of Epidemiology, 180*(1), 76–85.

Centers for Disease Control and Prevention. (2009a). Glossary of terms. Retrieved from http://www.atsdr.cdc.gov/glossary.html#G-A-

Centers for Disease Control and Prevention. (2009b). Prevalence and trends data: Nationwide (states and DC)–2009 arthritis. Retrieved from http://apps.nccd.cdc.gov/brfss/age.asp?cat=AR&yr=2009&qkey=4498&state=UB

Centers for Disease Control and Prevention. (2012a). Prevalence and trends data: Nationwide (states and DC)–2012 chronic health indicators. Retrieved from http://apps.nccd.cdc.gov/brfss/list.asp?cat=CH&yr=2012&qkey=8091&state

Centers for Disease Control and Prevention. (2012b). Prevalence and trends data: Nationwide (states and DC)–2012 immunization. Retrieved http://apps.nccd.cdc.gov/brfss/list.asp?cat=IM&yr=2012&qkey=8341&state=All

Feigal, D., Black, D., Grady, D., Hearst, N., Fox, C., Newman, T. B., & Hulley, S. B. (1988). Planning for data management and analysis. In S. B. Hulley & S. F. Cummings (Eds.), *Designing clinical research: An epidemiologic approach* (pp. 159–171). Baltimore, MD: Williams & Wilkins.

Fisher, J. L., Petterson, D., Palmisano, S., Schwartzbaum, J. A., Edwards, C. G., Mathiesen, T., ... Feychting, M. (2014). Loud noise exposure and acoustic neuroma. *American Journal of Epidemiology, 180*(1), 58–67.

Frome, E. L., & Checkoway, H. (1985). Use of Poisson regression models in estimating incidence rates and ratios. *American Journal of Epidemiology, 212*, 309–323.

Iso, H., Date, C., Yamamoto, A., Toyoshima, H., Watanabe, Y., Kikuchi, S., ... Tamakoshi, A. (2005). Smoking cessation and mortality from cardiovascular disease among Japanese men and women: The JACC study. *American Journal of Epidemiology*, 161(2), 170–179.

Marmot, M., Friel, S., Bell, R., Houweling, T. A. J., & Taylor, S. (2008). Closing the gap in a generation: Health equity through action on the social determinants of health. *The Lancet*, 372, 1661–1669.

Merrill, R. M. (2013). *Fundamentals of epidemiology and biostatistics: Combining the basics*. Burlington, MA: Jones & Bartlett Learning.

Qiu, J., He, X., Cui, H., Zhang, C., Zhang, H., Dang, Y., ... Zhang, Y. (2014). Passive smoking and preterm birth in urban China. *American Journal of Epidemiology*, 180(1), 94–102.

Rose, G. (1985). Sick individuals and sick populations. *International Journal of Epidemiology*, 14(1), 32–38.

Rothman, K. J. (1990). A sobering start for the cluster busters' conference. *American Journal of Epidemiology*, 132(Suppl.), S6–S13.

Schneider, S., Huy, C., Schuessler, M., Diehl, K., & Schwarz, S. (2009). Optimising lifestyle interventions: Identification of health behaviour patterns by cluster analysis in a German 50+ survey. *European Journal of Public Health*, 19(3), 271–277.

Singh, A., Rouxel, P., Watt, R. G., & Tsakos, G. (2013). Social inequalities in clustering of oral health related behaviors in a national sample of British adults. *Preventive Medicine*, 57(2), 102–106.

Spring, B., Moller, A. C., & Coons, M. J. (2012). Multiple health behaviours: Overview and implications. *Journal of Public Health* (Oxf.), 24(Suppl. 1), i3–i10.

Surveillance, Epidemiology, and End Results Program. (2014). Incidence—SEER 18 Regs Research Data + Hurricane Katrina Impacted Louisiana Cases, Nov 2013 Sub (2000–2011) <Katrina/Rita Population Adjustment>. Retrieved from http://seer.cancer.gov/data/seerstat/nov2013/

Wilkinson, P. (Ed.). (2006). *Environmental epidemiology*. New York, NY: Open University Press.

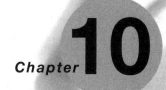

Epidemiological Input for Selecting Behavioral Intervention Targets

The phases of research in behavioral epidemiology to promote health and prevent disease consist of the following: (1) developing measures of behavior, (2) identifying influences on behavior, (3) establishing a link between behaviors and health, (4) evaluating interventions to change behavior, and (5) translating research into practice (Sallis, Owen, & Fotheringham, 2000). Public health literature contains many examples of studies devoted to these different areas. In this text we have presented several measures of behavior, influences on behavior, and ways to study associations between behaviors and health. Tools for monitoring and evaluating interventions to change behavior have also been discussed, and ways to disseminate research findings to encourage translating research into practice have been presented. Targeting each of these areas and studying them in combination is fundamental to effective health promotion and disease prevention.

In studying behavior, we are interested in the causal factors that influence them and the causal link between the behavior and health-related states or events. An understanding of the cause and routes of transmission for health-related states or events allows us to remove, eliminate, modify, or contain the cause, disrupt and block the chain of disease transmission, and protect the susceptible population against further health problems. For example, for thousands of years diseases like malaria, yellow fever, encephalitis, and, more recently, West Nile virus have been associated with marshes, swamps, and other wetlands. However, the mosquito was not identified as a vector for such diseases until 1900; the discovery was made by Walter Reed, a U.S. Army physician (Pierce & Writer, 2005). With this knowledge, interventions against these diseases have often involved spraying watery breeding places (environments) to kill this vector.

In 1964, the surgeon general of the United States concluded that, based on results from 29 case-control studies and 7 cohort studies, smoking was causally linked with lung cancer (U.S. Department of Health and Human Services, 1964). It has also been shown that exposure to carcinogens from tobacco use (e.g., aminostilbene; arsenic; benzene; cadmium; chrysene; N-dibutylnitrosamine; 2,3-dimethylchrysene; nickel compound; polonium-210; and many more) increases the risk of several other types of cancer (e.g., bladder, mouth, lip, throat, voice box, and esophagus). Many tobacco-related prevention and control programs have since been effective at lowering the prevalence of tobacco use in many populations. Plague is another major cause of death in which the flea vector was not identified until Paul-Louis Simond made the discovery of transmission by rat fleas in 1898 (Simond, Godley, & Mouriquand, 1998).

Understanding the cause and causal mechanisms is the highest form of scientific knowledge and is a central aim of epidemiology. Epidemiology contributes to our understanding of cause-and-effect relationships by identifying associations between postulated causal factors and health-related states or events. Causal models have been developed in epidemiology that provide a framework for interpreting and applying evidence. Causal models broaden causal perspectives. Epidemiologic study designs can be applied to provide evidence, along with reasoning and judgment, for drawing conclusions about causal relationships. For a behavioral intervention to be successful, the targeted behavior must be a cause of the health-related state or event.

The purpose of this chapter is to review basic principles of causal theory and discuss how causal inference and modeling can play an important role in behavioral intervention.

Cause and Causal Inference

A *cause* produces an effect, result, or consequence. It is an event, condition, characteristic, or behavior that precedes the outcome. A cause can also be thought of as an explanation or answer as to why something happened. In epidemiology, a cause is something that alters the frequency of a health-related state or event. Causality is supported by demonstrating a mechanism (i.e., the means by which an effect is obtained; a description of the chain of events in a particular process). When talking about causal relationships, we use words like *cause, influence, change, increase, decrease,* and *promote* (Pearl, 2002). *Etiology* is the study of causation; that is, etiology is the study of why and how things occur.

Trying to understand why and how things occur is part of human nature. Our actions are largely influenced by conclusions we make about causal connections. Causality is based on judgment through hypothesis generation and testing, data interpretation, and other evidence, and it is open to change with new evidence. All judgments about cause-and-effect relationships are tentative.

Causal inference in epidemiology is a conclusion about the presence of a health-related state or event and the reasons for its existence. Statements about the relationship between human health and physical, chemical, biological, social, and psychosocial factors are based on causal inference. Epidemiologic studies generally approach causal inference using statistical data. While identifying a valid statistical association does not necessarily mean there is a causal association, it does provide support, along with other evidence, for drawing conclusions about cause–effect relationships.

Understanding causal mechanisms is complex and involves the interplay of several factors. Attempting to make sense of this interplay of factors is the purpose of causal modeling, which we will discuss shortly. The factors that contribute to a health problem are referred to as risk factors. Any given risk factor (i.e., a characteristic, condition, or behavior that increases the possibility of disease or injury; something that contributes to the production of an adverse health outcome) may or may not be sufficient to cause the health problem, but generally, combinations of risk factors are required before health problems occur.

Epidemiologic research has identified risk factors for the eight leading causes of death in the United States (**Table 10-1**). Many of the risk factors are associated with more than one leading cause of death. The risk factors are also interrelated and, in combination, explain these diseases. For example, a sufficient cause of heart disease may include social, behavioral, and genetic risk factors, with interactions among these factors. Risk factors can also be thought of as predisposing factors, reinforcing factors, enabling factors, and precipitating factors. In the table, predisposing factors are represented by genetic factors. Other predisposing factors include age and immune status. Reinforcing and enabling factors are represented in the table as environmental factors. The precipitating factors are represented in the table as behaviors.

In the late 1800s and early 1900s, researchers began to identify several vitamin and nutritional deficiencies that were statistically

Table 10-1

Top Eight Leading Causes of Death in the United States According to Selected Risk Factors

Risk factors	Heart disease	Cancer	Stroke	Accidents	Diabetes	Cirrhosis	Suicide	Homicide
Physical, chemical and biological environments								
Worksite risks/ exposures		X		X				
Environmental hazards		X		X				
Vehicular hazards				X				
Household hazards				X				
Medical care risks		X	X	X	X	X	X	
Radiation exposures		X		X				
Infectious pathogens	X	X						
Engineering/ design hazards				X				
Social environment								
Poverty	X	X	X	X	X	X	X	X
Low educational level	X	X	X	X	X	X	X	X
Lack of work skills	X	X	X	X	X	X	X	X
Disrupted families	X	X	X	X	X	X	X	X
Behaviorally related								
Smoking/ tobacco use	X	X	X	X				
Alcohol use/ abuse	X	X	X	X		X	X	X
Nutrition/diet	X	X	X		X	X		
Lack of exercise/ fitness	X	X	X		X			
High blood pressure	X		X					
LDL cholesterol levels	X		X					
Overweight/ obesity	X	X			X			

Table 10-1 (Continued)								
Top Eight Leading Causes of Death in the United States According to Selected Risk Factors								
Risk factors	Heart disease	Cancer	Stroke	Accidents	Diabetes	Cirrhosis	Suicide	Homicide
Stress	X		X	X			X	X
Drug use/ abuse	X		X	X			X	X
Lack of seat belt use				X				
Genetic related								
Chromo- some/ genetic defects	X	X	X		X	X	X	
Congenital anomalies	X	X	X		X	X	X	
Developmen- tal defects	X	X	X		X	X	X	

Data from Centers for Disease Control and Prevention. (1992). Chronic Disease and Health Promotion reprints from MMWR, 1985–1989. Hyattsville, MD: Public Health Services, U.S. Department of Health and Human Services; National Centers for Health Statistics. (1991). Health in the United States—1990. Hyattsville, MD: Public Health Services, U.S. Department of Health and Human Services; National Cancer Institute. (1992). Strategies to control tobacco use in the United States. Hyattsville, MD: U.S. Dept. of Health and Human Services, Public Health Services; Green, L.W., & Kreuter, M.W. (1991). Health promotion planning: An educational and ecological approach. Mountain View, CA: Mayfield Publishing. Hardman, J.G., Limbird, L.E., & Gilman, G.G. (2001). Goodman and Gilman's Pharmacological Basis of Therapeutics (10th ed., p. 992).

associated with disease (Keusch, 2003). The statistical evidence and other evidence led researchers to conclude that selected adverse health effects are caused by vitamin deficiency and overdose (**Table 10-2**). The environments presented in Table 10-1 play an important role in the susceptibility of people to these vitamin- and nutrient-related diseases.

Historical Thinking about Causality

In ancient history, disease was believed to be caused by God. Hippocrates (460–377 BC), on the other hand, used observation and reason to try to identify natural explanations for disease (Garrison, 1926). He ascribed to what we now call *atomic theory*, wherein every-thing is made of tiny particles (i.e., earth, air, fire, and water) and the body consists of four humors: phlegm (earth and water atoms), yellow bile (fire and air atoms), blood (fire and water atoms), and black bile (earth and air atoms). Sickness was believed to be caused by an imbalance of these humors, and fever was thought to be caused by too much blood. He also considered diet to be a cause and a cure for disease. Aristotle (384–322 BC) also believed disorders of the human

Table 10-2		
Diseases Caused by Vitamin Deficiency and Overdose		
Vitamin	**Deficiency disease**	**Overdose disease**
Vitamin A	Night blindness or inability to see in dim light, keratomalacia, xerophthalmia	Hypervitaminosis A
Vitamin B$_1$ (thiamin)	Beriberi, Wernicke-Korsakoff syndrome	Rare hypersensitive reactions resembling anaphylactic shock—injection only, drowsiness
Vitamin B$_2$	Ariboflavinosis	?
Vitamin B$_3$	Pellagra	Liver damage (doses > 2 g/day) and other problems
Vitamin B$_5$	Paresthesia	?
Vitamin B$_6$	Anemia peripheral neuropathy	Impairment of proprioception, nerve damage (doses > 100 mg/day)
Vitamin B$_7$	Dermatitis, enteritis	?
Vitamin B$_9$	Deficiency during pregnancy associated with birth defects, such as neural tube defects	Possible decrease in seizure threshold
Vitamin B$_{12}$	Megaloblastic anemia	No known toxicity
Vitamin C	Scurvy	Vitamin C megadosage
Vitamin D	Rickets and osteomalacia	Hypervitaminosis D
Vitamin E	Deficiency is very rare, mild hemolytic anemia in newborn infants	Increased congestive heart failure seen in one large randomized study
Vitamin K	Bleeding diathesis	Increases coagulation in patients taking warfarin

Data from Kutsky, R (1973). *Handbook of vitamins and hormones*. New York: Van Nostrand Reinhold; Hardman, JG, Limbird, LE, Gilman, GG (2001). *Goodman and Gilman's Pharmacological Basis of Therapeutics* (10th ed., p. 992); Vitamin A— Health Professional Fact Sheet. (n.d.). Retrieved December 17, 2009, from http://dietary-supplements.info.nih.gov/factsheets/vitamina.asp; Vitamin and Mineral Supplement Fact Sheets: Vitamin B6. Retrieved December 17, 2009, from http://ods.od.nih.gov/factsheets/VitaminB6-HealthProfessional/; Vitamin and Mineral Supplement Fact Sheets: Vitamin B12. Retrieved December 17, 2009, from http://ods.od.nih.gov/factsheets/VitaminB12-HealthProfessional/; The Merck Manual. Disorders of Nutrition and Metabolism. Retrieved December 17, 2009, from http://www.merck.com/mmhe/sec12/ch154/ch154a .html; Rohde, LE, de Assis, MC, Rabelo, ER (1997). Dietary vitamin K intake and anticoagulation in elderly patients. *Current Opinion in Internal Medicine, 10*(1), 1–5.

body were caused by an upset in the balance of humors (Singer, 1928). In 1856, John Stuart Mill presented the following three ways to consider disease etiology (Mill, 1862):

■ *Method of difference* says if the frequency of a health problem is different between two places, times, or circumstances, the health problem is caused by a factor that differs between them. For example, if colon cancer rates are high in the United States but are low in Japan, and the rates among Japanese immigrants begin to approach those in the United States, it might mean that different dietary behaviors are causing the difference.

- *Method of agreement* refers to a single factor in common to places, times, and circumstances in which the health problem exists. For example, higher levels of tobacco smoking are directly associated with increasing trends in lung cancer rates in many different places throughout the world.
- *Method of concomitant variation* is where the frequency of a factor varies in direct proportion to the health problem. For example, low immunization rates are inversely associated with higher vaccine-preventable disease rates.

Ignaz Semmelweis (1818–1865), a Hungarian physician, discovered that the incidence of puerperal fever could be drastically cut by the use of hand-washing standards in obstetrical clinics (Semmelweis, 1988). This may have influenced the idea of microorganisms that was presented in the Henle-Koch postulates in 1877. Four criteria were given that must be met before an association between an infectious agent and disease could be considered a causal association (Koch, 1893):

1. The microorganism must be found in abundance in all organisms suffering from the disease, but it should not be found in healthy organisms.
2. The microorganism must be isolated from a diseased organism and grown in pure culture.
3. The cultured microorganism should cause disease when introduced into a healthy organism.
4. The microorganism must be re-isolated from the inoculated, diseased experimental host and identified as being identical to the original specific causative agent.

Koch later abandoned the first postulate because asymptomatic carriers of cholera were identified (Mill, 1874). These postulates are also insufficient for diseases that have multiple potential causes and for noninfectious diseases because they assume that causal agents are both necessary and sufficient. Nevertheless, these postulates enabled the germ theory of disease to gain acceptance in medicine. Robert Koch (1843–1910), a German physician, took the first photographs of microbes in the early 1900s and showed the world that microorganisms exist and can cause various diseases (Cumston, 1926; Garrison, 1926; Rosen 1993).

In 1965, Sir Austin Bradford Hill built on Mill's postulates and presented nine criteria of causation (Hill, 1965):

1. Strength of association: The larger the relative effect, the more likely the causal influence of the factor.
2. Consistency: If similar associations are found in different studies using different methods and involving different populations, the more likely the causal influence of the factor.

Look for literature reviews or meta-analyses if you want to determine consistency and strength of association in a study.

3. Dose–response: If the risk is positively associated with an increased dose of the risk factor, the more likely the causal influence of the factor. This effect is particularly common for environmental contaminants, such as lead or arsenic poisoning.

4. Temporal relationship: The risk factor exposure must precede the outcome. Temporality is not always easy to establish. For example, in cross-sectional studies, depression might show an association with obesity, but does obesity lead to depression or does depression lead to obesity? Cohort studies that can establish temporality are usually needed to establish this criterion.

5. Biological plausibility: The association is biologically supported through assessment based on experiments in controlled laboratory environments. Biologic plausibility is where biology and epidemiology merge. To determine whether an observed association is causal, you naturally need to see if it is biologically feasible for that to occur. Biologists provide invaluable information on physiological processes that allow us to determine potential pathways for disease occurrence.

6. Specificity: The risk factor exposure is associated with one outcome, and a given outcome is associated with one risk factor.

7. Coherence: Associations between the risk factor and the outcome must be consistent with existing epidemiologic knowledge.

8. Experiment: It is not clear what Hill meant by this criterion. He may have meant that experimental study designs are better for supporting statements about causality because of their greater control over measurements, subjects, confounding, and bias.

9. Analogy: Analogous situations with previously demonstrated causal associations provide support for there being a causal association.

In a paper published by Sir Richard Doll, he referred to Hill's use of the word *criteria* as a misnomer. He thought these nine items should be considered "guides to causality" (Doll, 2002, p. 501) since many of them are not necessary for causality to exist. However, some of these criteria are essential, such as strength of association. They can be evaluated using statistics and a temporal relationship, which can best be established using cohort/experimental study designs.

Some of the statistical measures used to assess associations include regression coefficients, correlation coefficients, risk ratios, rate ratios, and odds ratios. Although an association does not imply causation, statistically valid associations of quantitative data do provide information about causal relationships; that is, a statistical association may be judged to be causally associated based on the statistical evaluation of association and other evidence, as presented by Sir Bradford Hill (Hill, 1965).

A recommended systematic approach to causal inference is shown in **Figure 10-1**.

Causal Models

The epidemiologic notion of cause–effect is that health-related states or events almost always involve an interplay of the environment, the genetic and physical makeup of the individual, and the behavior or agent of disease. When a disease is attributed to a single cause, it is invariably by definition; that is, to say that tuberculosis is caused by the tubercle bacillus is according to definition. In reality, the epidemiologic perspective of the cause of tuberculosis is that it is not just the tubercle bacillus, but also factors like malnutrition and overcrowding that contribute to the disease. We attempt to capture this idea by various disease causation models. All of the models presented in this section are simplifications of the truth. The models provide a schema of the levels of prevention to devise a comprehensive framework for thinking about possible action.

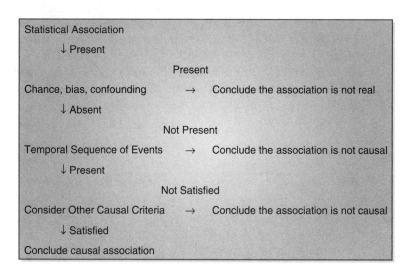

Figure 10-1 Systematic approach to causal inference

THE LINE MODEL

The line model explores whether the disease is predominantly genetic or environmental (**Figure 10-2**). Genetic-related diseases tend to have stable incidence rates over time, and they cluster in families. For example, certain cancers have been shown to cluster in families such as hereditary retinoblastoma; xeroderma pigmentosum for skin cancer; Wilms' tumor for kidney cancer; Li-Fraumeni syndrome for sarcomas, brain cancer, breast cancer, and leukemia; family adenomatous polyposis for colon and rectal cancers; Paget's disease of the bone for bone cancer; and Fanconi's aplastic anemia for leukemia, liver, and skin cancer. Nevertheless, heredity is thought to affect less than 10% of all cancer cases (American Cancer Society, 2014).

In cancer research, the environment is defined as everything outside the body that can enter and interact with the body. This interaction is referred to as exposure, such as sunlight, radiation, viruses, bacteria, chemicals, and behaviors (e.g., tobacco smoking, excessive alcohol drinking, poor diet, low physical activity, or sexual behavior that influences exposure). Behaviors, in turn, have been associated with diarrheal diseases, cardiovascular diseases, lung cancer, acquired immunodeficiency syndrome (AIDS), and other sexually transmitted diseases. Most cancer is attributed to some type of environmental factor, which is largely modifiable through lifestyle choices. Doll (1998) reported the proportion of cancer deaths linked to avoidable risk factors as follows: 29–31% tobacco; 20–50% diet; 10–20% infections (bacteria, viruses); 5–7% ionizing and ultraviolet light; 2–4% occupation; and 1–5% pollution (air, water, food). Consistent with Mill's (1862) method of difference, U.S.-born Japanese men and women have colon cancer rates about 40% higher than their counterparts born in Japan (142.5 for males and 90.1 for females in the United States, compared with 69.3 for males and 63.5 for females in Japan; rates per 100,000 person years) (Flood et al., 2000).

While environmental exposures can cause gene changes that cause cancer, there may also be randomly occurring gene changes

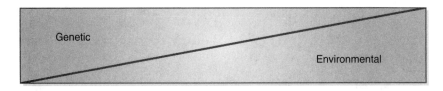

Figure 10-2 Line model for genetic and environmental influences

that accumulate in our body's cells over a lifetime. The unique patterns that result may put some people at increased risk after exposure to a given agent or because of a certain behavior. Other factors that may influence cancer risk include the immune systems, variations in detoxifying enzymes or repair genes, and hormones (Ankathil, 2011; Fulop et al., 2013; Hankinson & Eliassen, 2010).

THE WHEEL MODEL

The wheel model emphasizes the unity of the gene and host within an interactive environmental envelope (Mausner & Bahn, 1985). It also emphasizes the interplay of physical, biological, and social environments, with genetic factors in the core of the wheel (**Figure 10-3**). The size of the host and the environmental components depend on their influence for a given disease process (Krieger, 1994). The total environment surrounding the host is divided into biological, physical, and social environments. Interactions exist among these different types of environments. Many environmental factors may be considered for a given health-related state or event, including behaviors. Many environmental factors for inflammatory bowel disease have been investigated, including infectious agents, diet, drugs, stress, and social status, and they probably involve an interaction between genetic and environmental factors (Sicilia et al., 2001; Uzoigwe, Khaitsa, & Gibbs, 2007). For example, at the genetic core, a family may have an inherited mutation that increases their risk of developing cancer of the colon and rectum. In addition to this genetic predisposition for the disease, there may need to be

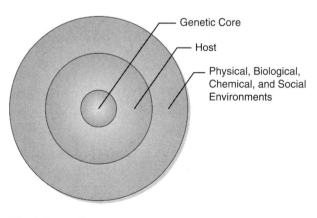

Figure 10-3 Wheel of causation

certain environmental influences, such as available dietary content and social influence on diet.

Understanding the source and nature of environmental conditions, ways people are exposed, and dose effects often requires the combined efforts of epidemiologists, biologists, toxicologists, respiratory physiologists, and public health officials. Effective prevention may require determining the source and nature of each environmental contaminant or stress, assessing how and in what form it comes into contact with people, measuring the health effect, and applying controls when and where appropriate (Moeller, 1992).

THE TRIANGLE MODEL

The epidemiology triangle is an infectious disease model that consists of a host that harbors the disease, an agent that causes the disease, an environment that includes those surroundings and conditions external to the host that causes or allows disease transmission, and time that accounts for the incubation period (**Figure 10-4**). Epidemiologists study the interactions that may occur among the host, agent, and environment. The host offers subsistence and lodging for a pathogen. The agent of infectious disease includes bacteria, viruses, parasites, fungi, and molds. The environment is the favorable surroundings and conditions external to the host that allow disease transmission (e.g., temperature, moisture, families and households, socioeconomic conditions, social networks, social support, neighborhoods and communities, institutions, and public policy). Finally, time includes severity of illness in relation to how long a person is infected or until the condition causes death or passes the threshold of danger toward recovery. Interventions on the host level may include protective measures (isolate and treat cases), nutrition, and immunization; on the agent level they may include thoroughly cooking meat and using antibiotics sensibly; and on the environment level they may include housing, income, and education.

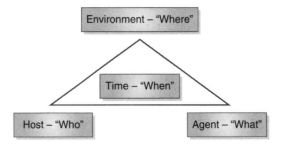

Figure 10-4 Epidemiology triangle of infectious disease

The epidemiology triangle is basic and foundational to epidemiology. We can apply the model to more than just infectious diseases. The agent can be a behavior, such as physical inactivity. The environment can be those factors that influence the behavior such as labor-saving devices, built/physical conditions, social/cultural conditions, economic circumstances, and policy. This model allows us to consider a health problem in a broader view, which presents more options for interventions. Swinburn and Egger (2002) used the epidemiologic triangle to identify prevention strategies against weight gain and obesity. In their model, the agent represented chronic positive energy balance (overeating) with specific behaviors consisting of eating energy-dense foods and large portion sizes, labor-saving devices, and physical inactivity. The model clarifies the interrelationship among the behaviors, the environment, and the affected individual.

ROTHMAN'S PIES

The interaction among the host, agent, and environment can be complex, especially when the agent represents behaviors and the outcome is a chronic disease. A simple way of looking at different factors that explain the health-related state or event was presented in a paper by Kenneth Rothman, published in 1976. Factors contributing to a given health-related state or event were represented by pieces of a pie, with the entire pie making up the sufficient cause for the health outcome (Rothman, 1976). The health-related state or event may have more than one sufficient cause, with each sufficient cause consisting of multiple contributing factors that are called component causes (i.e., represented by the pieces of the pie). To illustrate, component causes A, B, and C may be sufficient to cause a disease, but component causes A, D, and E may also be sufficient to cause the disease (**Figure 10-5**). In this case, A is necessary because it is required in each of the sufficient causes.

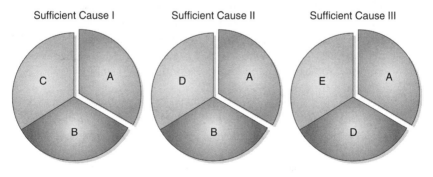

Figure 10-5 Three sufficient causes of an adverse health outcome

Suppose that A represents a necessary cause such as exposure to Rubivirus for rubella-related birth defects to occur. Exposure to this virus is not sufficient for birth defects to occur, but component causes may be required to make a sufficient cause, such as illness and a lack of immunity during the first few months of pregnancy. A component cause of lung cancer is tobacco smoking. Smoking alone may not be sufficient to cause lung cancer; it must be combined with component causes such as age and genetic susceptibility. Another example involves classic Kaposi's sarcoma, which is a soft tissue cancer found primarily in the lower limbs of older men, mainly of Mediterranean, eastern European, or Middle Eastern descent. Kaposi's sarcoma-associated herpes virus (KSHV) is necessary but not sufficient to cause classic Kaposi's sarcoma. Other component causes that, when combined with KSHV, may be sufficient to cause classic Kaposi's sarcoma include cigarette smoking, diabetes, asthma, allergies in males, corticosteroid use, infrequent bathing, education, and residential chronic Luvisol exposure (Anderson et al., 2008; Goedert et al., 2002; Pelser et al., 2009).

The component causes may be thought of as risk factors. A risk factor is a condition or behavior variable associated with the increased probability of a human health problem. It may be thought of as a component cause because it must be combined with other factors before an adverse health outcome occurs. Risk factors are identified through analytic epidemiologic studies. Behavioral risk factors are common and often involved in the combination of component causes that are sufficient for disease. In other words, although a behavioral risk factor may not be necessary or sufficient in and of itself, it is often a critical component that, when combined with other component causes, is sufficient to produce adverse health outcomes.

CAUSAL DIAGRAMS

A causal diagram is similar to a causal pie in that it illustrates how risk factors contribute to the onset of disease. A causal diagram can put many different causal pies in one image by using a series of boxes and arrows (Joffe, Gambhir, Chadeau-Hyam, & Vineis, 2012). An effective feature of this method is that it enables us to visualize multiple routes of disease transmission in a population instead of one specific cause at a time.

Directed acyclic graphs (DAGs) are a simple way to show the relationship of variables (**Figure 10-6**). The causal interpretation in DAGs depends on the direction of the arrows. For example, low education (X) may lead to poor nutrition (Y) that leads to heart disease (Z).

Diagrams used in behavioral epidemiology may attempt to explain a system consisting of a human population within its environment.

1. $X \to Y \to Z$	Y is a mediator for X and Z
2. $X \gets Y \gets Z$	Y is a mediator for Z and X
3. $X \to Y \gets Z$	Both X and Z cause Y; the path between X and Z is blocked
4. $X \gets Y \to Z$	Y is a cause of X and of Z

Figure 10-6 DAGs showing the relationship of X, Y, and Z variables

Models concerned with only a single causal pathway include compartmental models like the Susceptible–Infected–Recovered (SIR) model, which divides the population according to the state in the disease process.

WEB OF CAUSATION

A *web of causation* is a graphic, pictorial, or paradigm representation of complex sets of events or conditions caused by an array of activities connected to a common core, common experience, or event. In webs of causation, the final outcome is the disease or condition. Webs have many arms, branches, sources, inputs, and causes that are somehow interconnected or interrelated to the outcome. Webs can also have a chain of events in which some events must occur before others. Some behavior-related diseases or conditions develop from multiple exposures (physical, chemical, social, and biological environments; inherent conditions).

A web of causation for heart disease shows several heart disease promoters and inhibitors that involve behavior (**Figure 10-7**). The web of causation could be further expanded by including environmental and genetic factors that may lead to these behaviors.

There are two approaches available to enhance webs of causation: decision trees and fish bone diagrams. A *decision tree* is a flowchart that uses lines and symbols to visually present the process in which understanding takes place and proper decisions are made about the role of certain risk factors in webs of causation. Whereas a web of causation is a flowchart that identifies risk factors that eventually lead to the disease or condition, a decision tree is established and worked through to assure that the correct decision is being made and leads to the causation of the outcome. A decision tree asks questions that are answered with yes or no, leading the investigator down the correct path toward discovery. This assumes the questions are answered correctly. By convention, rectangular boxes are used to depict activities, and diamond-shaped boxes are decision points. For example, a diamond-shaped box may say "positive reaction." If yes, a rectangular box may say "chest radiograph." This is illustrated in **Figure 10-8**.

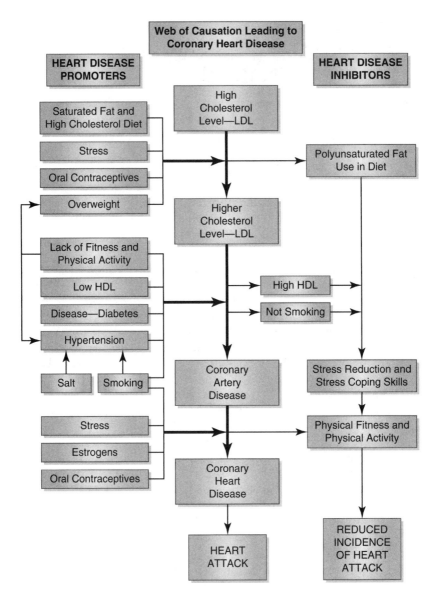

Figure 10-7 Web of causation for coronary heart disease

Data from Sherwin, R. (1985). In Mausner, J.S., & Kramer, S. *Epidmeiology: An Introductory Text.* Philadelphia, PA: WB Saunders.

The following steps may be useful to consider when constructing webs of causation and decision trees:

1. Identify the problem, affirm the condition, and obtain an accurate diagnosis of the disease.
2. Place the diagnosis at the center or bottom of the web.

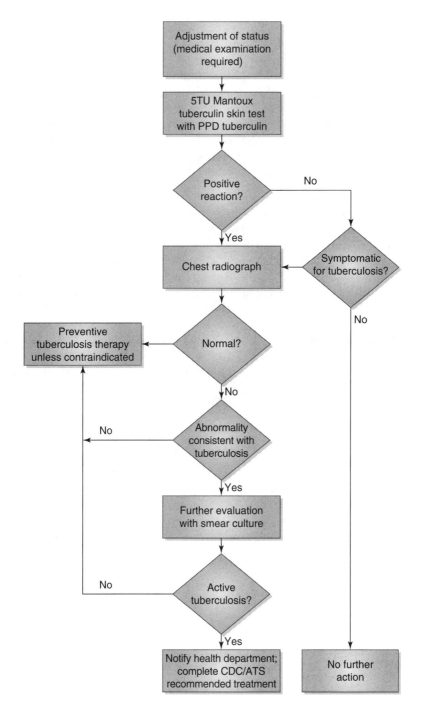

Figure 10-8 Decision tree for decision making showing decision making activities for tuberculosis screening in the United States for individuals seeking permanent residence

Data from CDC. Tuberculosis among foreign-born persons entering the United States – Recommendations of the advisory committee for elimination of tuberculosis. *MMWR*. 1990/39(RR 18);1–13, 18–21.

3. Brainstorm and list all possible sources of the disease.
4. Brainstorm and list all risk factors and predisposing factors of the disease.
5. Develop subwebs and tertiary-level subwebs for the various branches of webs if needed.
6. Organize lists of sources and risk factors for the disease. Arrange them in steps from general and most distant to more specific and focused as they move closer to the diagnosis.
7. Develop and work through causation decision trees for each element under consideration on the way toward the diagnosed disease.

Fish bone diagrams are cause–effect diagrams that provide visual presentations of all possible factors that may contribute to the health outcome (**Figure 10-9**). They are useful to help epidemiologists define, determine, uncover, or eliminate possible causes.

To construct a fish bone diagram, brainstorm lists of all potential causes or contributing risk factors. Place the categories of causes on the bones of the diagram, making it a visual display for easy study and analysis. Then develop subcategories of all specific causes for each of the major category areas. Label each branch of the fish bone. It is also possible to add a third (tertiary) level of cause to the bones of the diagram. The effect or outcome box at the head of the diagram is the

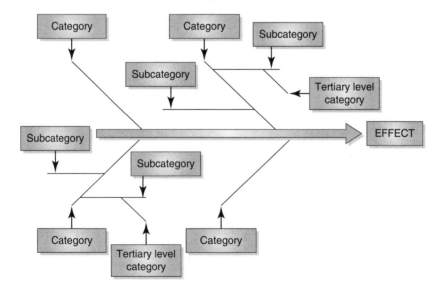

Figure 10-9 Approach for constructing a fish bone diagram

outcome of interest. The diagram is complete when all possible risk factors or causes have been properly placed within the categories and subcategories of the diagram on the lines that create the fish bone effect.

Causal Assumption in Epidemiologic Measures

Selected measures are referred to as attributable risk, attributable risk percentage, population attributable risk, and population attributable risk percentage. A related measure is the prevented fraction in the exposed group. Briefly, attributable risk is the excess risk of the health-related state or event among the exposed group that is attributed to the exposure; the attributable risk percentage for cases that are exposed is the percentage of disease cases attributed to their exposure; the population attributable risk is the excess risk of the health-related state or event in the population that is attributed to the exposure; and the population attributable risk percentage is the percent of the health-related state or event in the population that can be attributed to the exposure. If the risk ratio (or rate ratio) is less than 1.0, the prevented fraction in the exposed group can be used, which is the proportion of potential new cases that would have occurred in the absence of the exposure. That is, the prevented fraction is the proportion of potential cases prevented by some beneficial exposure, such as a vaccination; that is,

$$\frac{\text{Prevented}}{\text{Fraction}} = \frac{\text{Incidence Rate (unexposed)} - \text{Incidence Rate (exposed)}}{\text{Incidence Rate (unexposed)}} = 1 - \text{RR}$$

The prevented fraction has perhaps been most commonly used to evaluate the protective effect of vaccination. For example, Kostova and colleagues (2013) used this statistic to evaluate influenza illness and hospitalizations averted by influenza vaccination in the United States from 2005 to 2011. They found that the six-season total prevented fraction was 15.7% (95% CI = 14.8–16.3%) for ages 0–4; 7.3% (6.7–7.8%) for ages 5–19; 7.4% (6.9–7.7%) for ages 20–64; and 18.4% (15.3–20.7%) for ages 65 and older. For all ages, the prevented fraction was 10.2% (9.2–10.9%). Therefore, overall the vaccination prevented roughly 10.2% of the cases that would have otherwise occurred among vaccinated individuals had they not been vaccinated (also called vaccine efficacy).

Statistical tests of significance can be used to determine if the observed results could have resulted by chance alone if exposure was not actually associated with the disease. Both the null and alternative hypotheses should be stated in advance. If little is known about the association being tested, the null hypothesis should be specified as

H_0:RR = 1. An alternative hypothesis of H_1:RR $\neq$ 1 indicates the possibilities that the exposure may increase or decrease the risk of disease. If we are studying a vaccine where we expect there to be a protective relation, the alternative hypothesis should be formulated as H_1:RR < 1. The chi-square test or the Fisher exact test (if the expected value in any cell is less than 5) is then used to evaluate the hypotheses. Confidence intervals can also be constructed to indicate statistical significance. If the confidence overlaps 1, then we fail to reject the null hypothesis. In the preceding example, all the estimated prevented fractions were statistically significant at the 0.05 level.

The terms *attributable* and *prevented* imply more than just statistical association. They convey a causal association between the exposure and outcome variables. Therefore, these measures should be used only after thoughtful consideration has been given to causality.

Developing Interventions

When a public health problem is identified, there is a societal expectation for public health officials to intervene as quickly as possible to solve the problem. Interventions designed to prevent and control health problems should be scientifically based according to facts and data from epidemiologic research and from knowledge about previous interventions and studies. The nature of the intervention will depend on the type of problem involved, its cause, and the causal mechanisms involved. In addition, two-way communication between government agencies and the public is expected and may be required for the intervention to be successful (Goodman, Fontaine, Hadler, & Vugia, 2008).

Determinants for the timing and choice of public health interventions include three key components: severity of the problem, epidemiologic information, and causal inference (Goodman et al., 2008). The greater the perceived severity of a problem, the greater the expectation is for public health intervention. Severity may be reflected by incidence, disability, mortality, or survival rates. The economic impact of the health problem may also be a measure of severity. For example, fatal accidents may be a useful measure of severity. In the United States, highway deaths claim more than 30,000 lives each year (National Highway Traffic Safety Administration [NHTSA], 2012). In the same year, seat belts in passenger vehicles saved an estimated 12,174 lives (among those aged 5 years and older) (NHTSA, 2013). An estimated 3,031 additional lives would have been saved at 100% seat belt use (NHTSA, 2013).

When a public health problem is identified, the level of certainty about the cause and causal mechanism may cover a range from known to unknown. Where there is better knowledge about the cause and causal mechanisms, policy and practice guidelines can be put in place to minimize the public health problem. For example, in 2012, laws involving car seats, motorcycle helmets, and minimum drinking age helped save an estimated 284 children younger than 5 years of age, 1,699 motorcyclists, and 525 young people, respectively (NHTSA, 2013). When little is known about the cause or causal mechanisms of a health problem, epidemiologic investigation is needed before interventions are developed and implemented. However, preliminary control measures are often in order (e.g., quarantine), based on limited initial information, then they are modified as the epidemiologic investigation proceeds. In his article on criteria for assessing causal association, Hill (1965) concluded that public health action should weigh the strength of the epidemiologic evidence against the consequences of delayed or premature action. Criteria presented by Hill (previously discussed) may increase confidence to initiate action. Data are needed to satisfy as many of the criteria as possible before drawing conclusions about causality. Satisfying a combination of these criteria, thereby providing evidence about cause and causal mechanisms, can facilitate support and confidence for directed interventions.

Interventions for preventing and controlling public health problems that are related to behavior can be approached by targeting specific aspects of the host, behavior, and environment. As discussed, there are primary, secondary, and tertiary prevention options. After those aspects have been targeted, research-based interventions can be implemented. Long-term prevention and control measures require community support. Failure to gain the community's trust and support can disable or constrain the intervention. This may be particularly true of public health problems that affect certain groups disproportionately. Those groups may be marginalized or reluctant to work with public health officials. Failure to gain community trust can also impact the effectiveness of health education and promotion efforts. The fact that car restraint and motorcycle helmet laws have not gained 100% acceptance may be partially explained by a lack of trust in the importance of restraints and helmet use as conveyed by community leaders.

An evaluation of interventions is important to determine whether to continue, modify, or stop intervention measures. After the public health intervention is implemented, data should be generated by epidemiologic methods to assess the effectiveness of the intervention. Such information should also guide the decision to modify or terminate an existing intervention. Keeping an intervention for the long run may be reasonable when the public health risk cannot be eliminated and thus continues to be an ongoing threat, such as many vaccine-preventable diseases, required seat belt use, or bans on texting while driving.

Research steps in the development and evaluation of public health interventions have been described by de Zoysa, Habicht, Pelto, & Martines (1998). The authors presented a flow diagram that shows the conceptual framework for nine steps to develop and evaluate public health interventions (**Figure 10-10**).

The main points of the nine steps are as follows (de Zoysa et al., 1998):

1. Monitoring trends in incidence rates, mortality rates, or prevalence proportions can often reveal a public health problem beyond what we would normally expect. Describing the problem according to person, place, and time factors can give us a sense as to who is at greatest risk, where the problem is greatest, and the time frame when the problem is greatest.

2. Research is carried out to identify whether selected exposures (e.g., behavior) are a risk factor for disease. This process can provide clues about causal mechanisms and further help specify those at greatest risk. This level of research is based on carefully conducted analytic epidemiologic studies. Most behavioral risk factors are

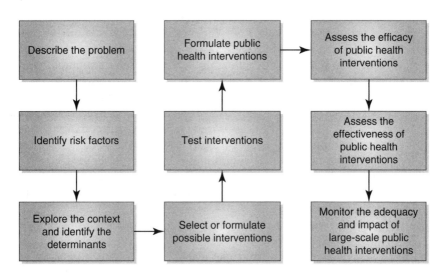

Figure 10-10 Flow diagram of the conceptual framework for research steps in developing and evaluating public health interventions

Data from De Zoysa, I, Habicht, JP, Pelto, G, Martines, J (1998). Research steps in the development and evaluation of public health interventions. *Bulletin of the World Health Organization, 76*(2), 127–133.

based on observational studies, although experimental studies are also used to identify risk factors. For example, tobacco smoking has been shown to increase the risk of many types of cancer, heart disease, and other health problems through case-control and cohort study designs. Five randomized controlled trials have shown that aspirin reduces the risk of myocardial infarction by about 28% (U.S. Preventive Services Task Force, 2002, 2009).

3. When the exposure is a behavior, it is very important to try to identify why people behave the way they do. It may be that successful behavior interventions must take into account social, physical, chemical, and biological environments that can facilitate or constrain behavior change. This research step can be qualitative and quantitative. It should refer to theoretical models of behavior.

4. In this step we develop a solution to the problem such as a vaccine, a medical or surgical procedure, or a physical aid such as a condom. Behavioral solutions are also required, given that all public health interventions have a behavioral component. For example, condoms are of little value if they are not properly and consistently used. The approaches to change behavior should build on previous knowledge about factors influencing behavior, such as predisposing and precipitating factors, then build on the reinforcing and enabling factors that sustain the behavior. Such models of behavior change can be used to design and plan interventions such as for the prevention of sexually transmitted diseases (Hornik, 1991).

5. This step involves tests that examine safety, feasibility, acceptability, and efficacy of the intervention. Clinical trials and community trials may be employed at this stage. Clinical trials may involve testing preventive measures or testing new treatment methods. Tests of community interventions are often designed for the purpose of evaluating educational and behavioral changes at the population level. Incorporating randomization and blinding are best for determining the efficacy of interventions, but it is often not feasible to incorporate this level of rigor into studies. Behavioral interventions in particular are often not amenable to trials with such stringent rules.

6. After the intervention is tested, the task is to take the appropriate steps to make it available to those who may benefit from it. This step is formative, involving decisions about alternative interventions based on the intervention's suitability in a particular setting.

7. This step involves assessing the efficacy of the intervention in terms of changes in behavior or health outcomes that could be achieved as a result of the intervention in the assigned setting.

8. This step involves assessing the effectiveness of the intervention; that is, the impact of the intervention delivered under normal program conditions is assessed. Public health studies focused on the effectiveness of an intervention are helpful to policy makers and program planners who want to know whether the program is having its intended effect. Cost-effectiveness studies may also be conducted at this step of research.

9. At this step, it is most important to ensure that the program goals are being met. It may also be necessary to modify the intervention as new information becomes available.

Irwig, Zwarenstein, Zwi, and Chalmers (1998) proposed a decision tree to facilitate selection of interventions for health care based on a systematic review (**Figure 10-11**). The flow diagram begins by asking whether there already exists an adequate systematic review showing the effects of all available alternative interventions that are designed to prevent or control the health problem. If not, it should be developed. Then, what conclusions can be drawn from the available review or newly prepared review? This leads to the crucial step of determining whether an intervention is likely to do more good than harm in some settings; the intervention is not likely to do more good than harm in any setting; or the intervention's ability to do more good than harm is uncertain. The intervention does more good than harm when, compared with the alternative (an existing intervention or nothing), the beneficial effects outweigh the harmful effects in selected settings (e.g., low-dose aspirin for reducing the risk of myocardial infarction). If it does more good than harm, we need to determine the applicability of the intervention in the particular setting of interest. Local populations or subgroups may differ in that they might benefit or be harmed by a given intervention. For example, cholesterol-lowering drugs would benefit only high-risk groups.

The cost-effectiveness of an intervention is influenced by the scale of provision and if it is to be provided alongside other interventions. In addition, it may be cost-effective in some areas but not others. For example, mammogram screening of women aged 50 years and older may be cost-effective in wealthy countries but not in poor countries, especially where the incidence rate of breast cancer is low. If the intervention is cost-effective, a pilot study may be used to determine whether it can be reasonably implemented. If so, it can be implemented with an ongoing audit of the process.

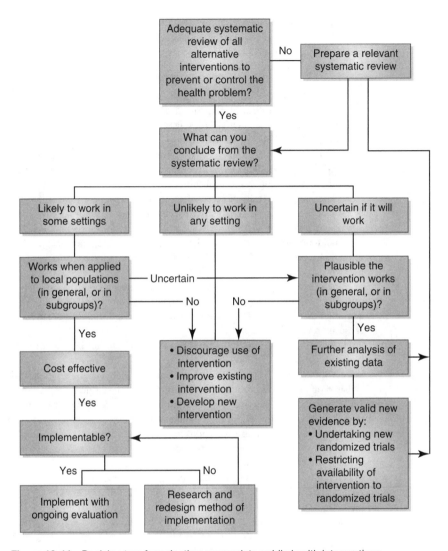

Figure 10-11 Decision tree for selecting appropriate public health interventions

Data from Irwig, L, Zwarenstein, M, Zwi, A, Chalmers, I (1998). A flow diagram to facilitate selection of interventions and research for health care. *Bulletin of the World Health Organization, 76*(1), 17-24.

Summary

1. Research in behavioral epidemiology consists of the following: (1) developing measures of behavior, (2) identifying influences on behavior, (3) establishing a link between behaviors and health, (4) evaluating interventions to change behavior, and (5) translating research into practice.

2. Understanding cause and causal mechanisms is the highest form of scientific knowledge and is a central aim of epidemiology. A cause produces an effect, result, or consequence. Causality is supported by demonstrating a mechanism, which is the chain of events by which an effect is obtained. Etiology is the study of causality, and causal inference is a conclusion about the presence of a health-related state or event and the reasons for its existence.

3. Guidelines or lists for drawing conclusions about causality have been provided by various researchers, such as Hill's list of nine criteria (1965): strength of association, consistency, dose–response, temporal relationship, biological plausibility, specificity, coherence, experiment, and analogy. Not all of these items need to be considered in causal inference, and some are more important than others (e.g., temporal relationship).

4. In epidemiology, the study of cause–effect relationships involves the interplay of how a given outcome is affected by environmental factors, the genetic and physical makeup of the individual, and the behavior or agent. Causation models attempt to capture the complex relationships among these factors. The models also provide a schema of the levels of prevention to devise a comprehensive framework for thinking about possible action.

5. In epidemiology, the terms *attributable* and *prevented* imply more than just statistical association; they suggest there is a causal association between the exposure and outcome variables. These measures require thoughtful consideration of cause and causal mechanisms.

6. Public health prevention and control interventions should be scientifically based according to facts and data from epidemiologic research and from knowledge of previous interventions and studies. Effective interventions will be based on the type of problem, its cause and the involved causal mechanisms, and whether there was two-way communication between the government agencies and the public with respect to the intervention.

7. Determinants for the timing and choice of public health interventions should include three key components: severity of the problem, epidemiologic information, and causal inference.

8. Interventions for preventing and controlling public health problems that are related to behavior can be approached by targeting specific aspects of the host, behavior, and environment.

9. Evaluations of interventions are important to determine whether to continue, modify, or stop intervention measures. After the public health intervention is implemented, data should be generated by epidemiologic methods to assess the effectiveness of the intervention. Such information should also guide the decision to modify or terminate an existing intervention.

10. Researchers have presented a useful flow diagram of the conceptual framework for research steps in developing and evaluating public health interventions: describe the problem, identify risk factors, explore the context and identify the determinants, select or formulate possible interventions, test the interventions, formulate public health interventions, assess the efficacy of public health interventions, assess the effectiveness of public health interventions, and monitor the adequacy and impact of the interventions.

References

American Cancer Society (2014). Family cancer syndromes. Retrieved from http://www.cancer.org/cancer/cancercauses/geneticsandcancer/heredity-and-cancer

Anderson, L. A., Lauria, C., Romano, N., Brown, E. E., Whitby, D., Graubard, B. I., ... Goedert, J. J. (2008). Risk factors for classical Kaposi sarcoma in a population-based case-control study in Sicily. Cancer Epidemiology Biomarkers and Prevention, 17(12), 3435–3443.

Ankathil, R. (2011). Low penetrance genetic variations in DNA repair genes and cancer susceptibility. In I. Kruman, DNA repair. ISBN: 978-953-307-697-3.

Centers for Disease Control and Prevention. (1990). Tuberculosis among foreign-born persons entering the United States. Morbidity and Mortality Weekly Report, 39(RR18), 1–13, 18–21.

Centers for Disease Control and Prevention. (1992). Chronic disease and health promotion reprints from MMWR, 1985–1989. Hyattsville, MD: Public Health Services, U.S. Department of Health and Human Services.

Cumston, C. G. (1926). An introduction to the history of medicine. New York, NY: Alfred A. Knopf.

de Zoysa, I., Habicht, J. P., Pelto, G., & Martines, J. (1998). Research steps in the development and evaluation of public health interventions. Bulletin of the World Health Organization, 76(2), 127–133.

Doll, R. (1998). Epidemiological evidence of the effects of behavior and the environment on the risk of human cancer. Recent Results in Cancer Research, 154, 3.

Doll, R. (2002). Proof of causality: Deduction from epidemiological observation. Perspectives in Biology and Medicine, 45(4), 499–515.

Flood, D. M., Weiss, N. S., Cook, L. S., Emerson, J. C., Schwartz, S. M., & Potter, J. D. Colorectal cancer incidence in Asian migrants to the United States and their descendants. Cancer Causes and Control, 11, 403–411.

Fulop, T., Larbi, A., Witkowski, J. M., Kotb, R., Hirokawa, K., Pawelec, G. (2013). Immunosenescence and cancer. Critical Reviews in Oncogenesis, 18(6), 489–513.

Garrison, F. H. (1926). History of medicine. Philadelphia, PA: Saunders.

Goedert, J. J., Vitale, F., Lauria, C., Serraino, D., Tamburini, M. Montella, M., ... Romano, N. (2002). Risk factors for classical Kaposi's sarcoma, 94(22), 1712–1718.

Goodman, R. A., Fontaine, R. E., Hadler, J. L., & Vugia, D. J. (2008). Developing interventions. In M. Gregg (Ed.), Field epidemiology (3rd ed., pp. 236–248). New York, NY: Oxford University Press.

Green, L. W., & Kreuter, M. W. (1991). Health promotion planning: An educational and ecological approach. Mountain View, CA: Mayfield.

Hankinson, S. E., & Eliassen, A. H. (2010). Circulating sex steroids and breast cancer risk in premenopausal women. Hormones and Cancer, 1(1), 2–10.

Hardman, J. G., Limbird, L. E., & Gilman, G. G. (2001). Goodman and Gilman's pharmacological basis of therapeutics (10th ed.). New York: McGraw-Hill.

Hill, A. B. (1965). The environment and disease: Association or causation? Proceedings of the Royal Society of Medicine, 58, 295–300.

Hornik, R. (1991). Alternative models of behavior change. In J. N. Wasserheit (Ed.), *Research issues in human behavior and sexually transmitted diseases in the AIDS era* (pp. 201–219). Washington, DC: American Society for Microbiology.

Irwig, L., Zwarenstein, M., Zwi, A., & Chalmers, I. (1998). A flow diagram to facilitate selection of interventions and research for health care. *Bulletin of the World Health Organization, 76*(1), 17–24.

Joffe, M., Gambhir, M., Chadeau-Hyam, M., & Vineis, P. (2012). Causal diagrams in systems epidemiology. *Emerging Themes in Epidemiology, 9*(1), 1. doi:10.1186/1742-7622-9-1

Keusch, G. T. (2003). The history of nutrition: Malnutrition, infection and immunity. *Journal of Nutrition, 133*(1), 336S–340S.

Koch, R. (1893). Über den augenblicklichen stand der bakteriologischen choleradiagnose. *Zeitschrift Für Hygiene Und Infectionskrankheiten, 14*(1), 319–338.

Kostova, D., Reed, C., Finelli, L., Cheng, P. Y., Gargiullo, P. M., Shay, D. K., ... Bresee, J. S. (2013). Influenza illness and hospitalizations averted by influenza vaccination in the United States, 2005–2011. *Public Library of Science, 8*(6), e66312.

Krieger, N. (1994). Epidemiology and the web of causation: Has anyone seen the spider? *Social Science & Medicine, 39*, 887–903.

Kutsky, R. (1981). *Handbook of vitamins, minerals, and hormones* (2nd ed.). New York, NY: Van Nostrand Reinhold.

Mausner, J. S., & Kramer, S. (1985). *Mausner & Bahn Epidemiology: An introductory text.* Philadelphia, PA: W. B. Saunders.

Merck Manual Home Edition. (2014). Overview of vitamins. Retrieved from http://www.merck.com/mmhe/sec12/ch154/ch154a.html

Mill, J. S. (1862). *A system of logic, ratiocinative and inductive* (5th ed.). London, UK: Parker, Son, and Bowin.

Mill, J. S. (1874). *A system of logic, ratiocinative and inductive; being a connected view of the principles of evidence, and the methods of scientific investigation.* New York, NY: Harper & Brothers.

Moeller, D. W. (1992). *Environmental health.* Cambridge, MA: Harvard University Press.

National Cancer Institute. (1992). *Strategies to control tobacco use in the United States.* Hyattsville, MD: U.S. Department of Health and Human Services, Public Health Services.

National Centers for Health Statistics. (1991). *Health in the United States—1990.* Hyattsville, MD: Public Health Services, U.S. Department of Health and Human Services.

National Highway Traffic Safety Administration. (2012). NHTSA data confirms traffic fatalities increased in 2012. Retrieved from http://www.nhtsa.gov/About NHTSA/Press Releases/NHTSA Data Confirms Traffic Fatalities Increased In 2012

National Highway Traffic Safety Administration. (2013). Lives saved in 2012 by restraint use and minimum drinking age laws. Retrieved from http://www-nrd.nhtsa.dot.gov/Pubs/811851.pdf

National Institutes of Health. (2011a). Vitamin B6: Dietary supplement fact sheet. Retrieved from http://ods.od.nih.gov/factsheets/VitaminB6-Health Professional/

National Institutes of Health. (2011b). Vitamin B12: Dietary supplement fact sheet. Retrieved from http://ods.od.nih.gov/factsheets/VitaminB12 -HealthProfessional/

National Institutes of Health. (2013). Vitamin A: Fact sheet for health professionals. Retrieved from http://dietary-supplements.info.nih.gov/factsheets /vitamina.asp

Pearl, J. (2002). Causal inference in the health sciences: A conceptual introduction. Health Services and Outcomes Research Methodology, 2(3–4), 189–220.

Pelser, C., Dazzi, C., Graubard, B. I., Lauria, C., Vitale, F., & Goedert, J. J. (2009). Annals of Epidemiology, 19(8), 597–601.

Pierce, J. R., & Writer, J. (2005). Yellow jack: How yellow fever ravaged America and Walter Reed discovered its deadly secrets. Hoboken, NJ: John Wiley and Sons.

Rohde, L. E., de Assis, M. C., & Rabelo, E. R. (1997). Dietary vitamin K intake and anticoagulation in elderly patients. Current Opinion in Internal Medicine, 10(1), 1–5.

Rosen, G. (1993). A history of public health (Rev. ed.). Baltimore, MD: Johns Hopkins University Press.

Rothman, K. (1976). Causes. American Journal of Epidemiology, 104, 587–592.

Sallis, J. F., Owen, N., & Fotheringham, M. J. (2000). Behavioral epidemiology: A systematic framework to classify phases of research on health promotion and disease prevention. Annals of Behavioral Medicine, 22(4), 294–298.

Semmelweis, I. (1988). The etiology, concept, and prophylaxis of childbed fever. In C. Buck, A. Llopis, E. Najera, & M. Terris (Eds.), The challenge of epidemiology: Issues and selected readings (pp. 46–59). Washington, D.C.: World Health Organization.

Sicilia, B., Miguel, C., Arribas, F., Zaborras, J., Sierra, E., & Gomollón, F. (2001). Environmental risk factors and Crohn's disease: A population-based, case-control study in Spain. Digestive and Liver Disease, 33, 762–767.

Simond, M., Godley, M. L., & Mouriquand, P. D. (1998). Paul-Louis Simond and his discovery of plague transmission by rat fleas: A centenary. Journal of the Royal Society of Medicine, 91(2), 101–104.

Singer, C. (1928). A short history of medicine. Oxford, UK: Clarendon Press.

Swinburn, B., & Egger, G. (2002). Preventive strategies against weight gain and obesity. Obesity Reviews, 3, 289–301.

U.S. Department of Health and Human Services. (1964). Smoking and health; report of the advisory committee to the surgeon general of the Public Health Service. Washington, DC: U.S. Government Printing Office.

U.S. Preventive Services Task Force. (2002). Aspirin for the primary prevention of cardiovascular events: Recommendation and rationale. Annals of Internal Medicine, 136, 157–160.

U.S. Preventive Services Task Force. (2009). Aspirin for the primary prevention of cardiovascular events: An update of the evidence. Retrieved from http://www .uspreventiveservicestaskforce.org/uspstf09/aspirincvd/aspcvdart.htm

Uzoigwe, J. C., Khaitsa, M. L., & Gibbs, P. S. (2007). Epidemiological evidence for Mycobacterium avium subspecies paratuberculosis as a cause of Crohn's disease. Epidemiology and Infection, 135(7), 1057–1068.

APPLICATION SECTION

Cigarette Smoking and Lung Cancer

Adapted from "Cigarette Smoking and Lung Cancer," Centers for Disease Control and Prevention Epidemiology Program Office Case Studies in Applied Epidemiology No. 731-703. This case study is based on the classic studies by Doll and Hill in which they showed an association between smoking and lung cancer. Two case studies were developed by Clark Heath, Godfrey Oakley, David Erickson, and Howard Ory in 1973. These two studies were later combined and were substantially revised and updated by Nancy Binkin and Richard Dicker in 1990. The current version was updated by Richard Dicker, with input from Julie Magri, in 2003.

Part I: Background

A causal relationship between cigarette smoking and lung cancer was first suspected in the 1920s on the basis of clinical observations. To test this apparent association, numerous epidemiologic studies were undertaken between 1930 and 1960. Two studies were conducted by Richard Doll and Austin Bradford Hill in Great Britain. The first was a case-control study begun in 1947 comparing the smoking habits of patients with lung cancer with the smoking habits of other patients. The second was a cohort study begun in 1951 recording causes of death among the British in relation to smoking habits. This case study deals first with the case-control study, then with the cohort study. Data for the case-control study were obtained from hospitalized patients in London and vicinity over a 4-year period (April 1948 to February 1952). Initially, 20 hospitals, and later more, were asked to notify the investigators of all patients admitted with a new diagnosis of lung cancer. These patients were then interviewed concerning their smoking habits, as were controls selected from patients with other disorders (primarily nonmalignant) who were hospitalized in the same facilities at the same time. Data for the cohort study were obtained from the population of all physicians listed in the British Medical Register who resided in England and Wales as of October 1951. Information about present and past smoking habits was obtained by questionnaire. Information about lung cancer came from death certificates and other mortality data that were recorded during the ensuing years.

CASE STUDY QUESTIONS

1. What makes the first study a case-control study?
2. What makes the second study a cohort study?
3. What are some possible reasons why hospitals were chosen for the case-control study?
4. For the case-control study, what are the advantages of selecting controls from the same hospitals as cases?
5. For the case-control study, what are the disadvantages of selecting controls from the same hospital as cases?
6. For the case-control study, how representative are hospitalized patients with lung cancer of all persons who have lung cancer?
7. For the case-control study, how representative are hospitalized patients without lung cancer of the general population who do not have lung cancer?
8. For the case-control study, what other sources of cases and controls could have been used?
9. For the case-control study, how might representative issues affect interpretation of the study's results?
10. For the case-control study, why might information obtained from a questionnaire about smoking produce biased results?
11. For the cohort study, what type of selection bias might be present?
12. For the cohort study, how might selection bias be minimized?

Part II: Case-Control Study

More than 1,700 patients with lung cancer, all younger than age 75 years, were eligible for the case-control study. About 15% of these persons were not interviewed because of death, discharge, severity of illness, or inability to speak English. An additional group of patients were interviewed but later excluded when the initial lung cancer diagnosis was proven to be mistaken. The final study group included 1,465 cases (1,357 males and 108 females). **Table I-1** shows the relationship between cigarette smoking and lung cancer among male cases and controls.

CASE STUDY QUESTIONS

1. Calculate the proportion of cases and controls who smoked.
2. What do you infer from these proportions?
3. Calculate the odds of smoking among the cases.
4. Calculate the odds of smoking among the controls.
5. Calculate the ratio of these odds.
6. What do you infer from the odds ratio about the relationship between smoking and lung cancer?

Table I-2 shows the frequency distribution of male cases and controls by average number of cigarettes smoked per day.

1. Compute the odds ratio by category of daily cigarette consumption, comparing each smoking category to nonsmokers.
2. Interpret these results.
3. What are other possible explanations for the apparent association?

Part III: Cohort Study

Data for the cohort study were obtained from the population of all physicians listed in the British Medical Register who resided in England and Wales as of October 1951. Questionnaires were mailed

Table I-1		
Smoking Status before Onset of the Present Illness, Lung Cancer Cases and Controls with Other Diseases, Great Britain, 1948–1952		
	Cases	**Controls**
Cigarette smoker	1,350	1,296
Nonsmoker	7	61
Total	1,357	1,357

Data from "Cigarette Smoking and Lung Cancer," Centers for Disease Control and Prevention Epidemiology Program Office Case Studies in Applied Epidemiology No. 731–703.

Table I-2			
Most Recent Amount of Cigarettes Smoked Daily before Onset of the Present Illness, Lung Cancer Cases and Controls with Other Diseases, Great Britain, 1948–1952			
Daily number of cigarettes	**Number of cases**	**Number of controls**	**Odds ratio**
0	7	61	Referent
1–14	565	706	
15–25	445	408	
25+	340	182	
All smokers	1,350	1,296	

Data from "Cigarette Smoking and Lung Cancer," Centers for Disease Control and Prevention Epidemiology Program Office Case Studies in Applied Epidemiology No. 731–704.

in October 1951 to 59,600 physicians. The questionnaire asked the physicians to classify themselves into one of three categories: (1) current smoker, (2) ex-smoker, or (3) nonsmoker. Smokers and ex-smokers were asked how much they smoked, their method of smoking, the age they started to smoke, and, if they had stopped smoking, how long it had been since they last smoked. Nonsmokers were defined as persons who had never consistently smoked as much as one cigarette per day for as long as 1 year. Usable responses to the questionnaire were received from 40,637 physicians (68%), of whom 34,445 were males and 6,192 were females.

CASE STUDY QUESTION

1. How might the response rate of 68% affect the study results?

Part IV: Analysis of Male Physician Respondents, 35 Years of Age or Older

The occurrence of lung cancer in physicians responding to the questionnaire was documented over a 10-year period (November 1951 through October 1961) from death certificates filed with the Registrar General of the United Kingdom and from lists of physician deaths provided by the British Medical Association. All certificates indicating that the decedent was a physician were abstracted. For each death attributed to lung cancer, medical records were reviewed to confirm the diagnosis. Diagnoses of lung cancer were based on the best evidence available; about 70% were from biopsy, autopsy, or sputum cytology (combined with bronchoscopy or X-ray evidence); 29% were from cytology, bronchoscopy, or X-ray alone; and only 1% were

Table I-3

Number and Rate (per 1,000 Person Years) of Lung Cancer Deaths by Number of Cigarettes Smoked per Day, Doll and Hill Physician Cohort Study, Great Britain, 1951–1961

Daily number of cigarettes	Deaths from lung cancer	Person years at risk	Mortality rate per 1,000 person years	Rate ratio	Rate difference per 1,000 person years
0	3	42,800		Referent	Referent
1–14	22	38,600			
15–25	54	38,900			
25+	57	25,100			
All smokers	133	102,600			

Data from "Cigarette Smoking and Lung Cancer," Centers for Disease Control and Prevention Epidemiology Program Office Case Studies in Applied Epidemiology No. 731–705.

from only case history, physical examination, or death certificate. Of 4,597 deaths in the cohort during the 10-year period, 157 were reported to have been caused by lung cancer; in 4 of the 157 cases this diagnosis could not be documented, leaving 153 confirmed deaths from lung cancer. **Table I-3** shows numbers of lung cancer deaths by daily number of cigarettes smoked at the time of the 1951 questionnaire (for male physicians who were nonsmokers and current smokers only). Person years of observation (person years at risk) are given for each smoking category. The number of cigarettes smoked was available for 136 of the persons who died from lung cancer.

CASE STUDY QUESTIONS

1. Compute lung cancer mortality rates, rate ratios, and rate differences for each smoking category. What do each of these measures mean?
2. What proportion of lung cancer deaths among all smokers can be attributed to smoking? What is the proportion called?
3. If no one had smoked, how many deaths from lung cancer would have been averted?

The cohort study also provided mortality rates for cardiovascular disease among smokers and nonsmokers. **Table I-4** presents lung cancer mortality data and comparable cardiovascular disease mortality data.

1. Which cause of death has a stronger association with smoking? Why?
2. Calculate the population attributable risk percentage for lung cancer mortality and for cardiovascular disease mortality.

Table I-4

Mortality Rates (per 1,000 Person Years), Rate Ratios, and Excess Deaths from Lung Cancer and Cardiovascular Disease by Smoking Status, Doll and Hill Physician Cohort Study, Great Britain, 1951–1961

	Smokers	Nonsmokers	All	Rate ratio	Excess deaths per 1,000 person years	Attributable risk percentage among smokers
Lung cancer	1.30	0.07	0.94	18.5	1.23	95%
Cardiovascular disease	9.51	7.32	8.87	1.30	2.19	23%

Data from "Cigarette Smoking and Lung Cancer," Centers for Disease Control and Prevention Epidemiology Program Office Case Studies in Applied Epidemiology No. 731–706.

How do they compare? How do they differ from the attributable risk percentage?

3. How many lung cancer deaths per 1,000 persons per year are attributable to smoking among the entire population? How many cardiovascular disease deaths?

4. For what cause of death burden of smoking greater? Why?

5. What do these data imply for the practice of public health and preventive medicine?

As noted at the beginning of this case study, Doll and Hill began their case-control study in 1947. They began their cohort study in 1951 (**Table I-5**).

Table I-5

Number and Rate (per 1,000 Person Years) of Lung Cancer Deaths for Current Smokers and Former Smokers by Years Since Quitting, Doll and Hill Physician Cohort Study, Great Britain, 1951–1961

Cigarette smoking status	Lung cancer deaths	Rate per 1,000 person years	Rate ratio
Current smokers	133	1.30	18.5
Former smokers, years since quitting:			
< 5 years	5	0.67	9.6
5–9 years	7	0.49	7.0
10–19 years	3	0.18	2.6
20+ years	2	0.19	2.7
Nonsmokers	3	0.07	1.0 (ref)

Data from "Cigarette Smoking and Lung Cancer," Centers for Disease Control and Prevention Epidemiology Program Office Case Studies in Applied Epidemiology No. 731-707.

Table I-6

Comparison of Measures of Association from Doll and Hill's 1948–1952 Case-Control Study and Doll and Hill's 1951–1961 Physician Cohort Study, by Number of Cigarettes Smoked Daily, Great Britain

Daily number of cigarettes smoked	Rate ratio from cohort study	Odds ratio from case-control study
0	1.0 (ref)	1.0 (ref)
1–14	8.1	7.0
15–24	19.8	9.5
25+	32.4	16.3
All smokers	18.5	9.1

Data from "Cigarette Smoking and Lung Cancer," Centers for Disease Control and Prevention Epidemiology Program Office Case Studies in Applied Epidemiology No. 731–708.

The rate ratios and odds ratios from the two studies by numbers of cigarettes smoked are given in **Table I-6**.

1. Compare the results of the two studies. Comment on the similarities and differences in the computed measures of association.
2. What are the advantages and disadvantages of case-control versus cohort studies?
3. Which type of study (case-control or cohort) would you have done first? Why? Why do a second study? Why conduct the other type of study?
4. Which of the following criteria for causality are met by the evidence presented from the two studies?

	Yes	No
Strong association		
Consistency among studies		
Exposure precedes disease		
Dose–response effect		
Biologic plausibility		

Case Study ▌▌

Oral Contraceptive Use and Ovarian Cancer

Adapted from "Oral Contraceptive Use and Ovarian Cancer," Centers for Disease Control and Prevention Epidemiology Program Office Case Studies in Applied Epidemiology No. 811-703. This case study was developed by Richard Dicker and Peter Layde in 1981. The current version was updated by Richard Dicker with input from the EIS Summer Course instructors.

Part I: Background

In 1980, ovarian cancer ranked as the fourth leading cause of cancer mortality among women in the United States. An estimated 18,000 new cases and more than 11,000 attributable deaths occurred among American women that year. Several studies had noted an increased risk of ovarian cancer among women of low parity, suggesting that pregnancy exerts a protective effect. By preventing pregnancy, oral contraceptives (OCs) might have been expected to increase the risk of ovarian cancer. On the other hand, by simulating pregnancy through suppression of pituitary gonadotropin release and inhibition of ovulation, OCs might have been expected to protect against the subsequent development of ovarian cancer. Because by 1980 OCs had been used by more than 40 million women in the United States, the public health impact of an association in either direction would have been substantial. To study the relationship between oral contraceptive use and ovarian cancer (as well as breast and endometrial cancers), the Centers for Disease Control and Prevention (CDC) initiated a case-control study, the Cancer and Steroid Hormone (CASH) Study, in 1980. Case patients were enrolled through eight regional cancer registries participating in the Surveillance, Epidemiology, and End Results (SEER) Program of the National Cancer Institute.

CASE STUDY QUESTIONS

1. Which investigations need to be reviewed by an institutional review board? Does this investigation need to be reviewed?
2. What types of bias are of particular concern in this case-control study? What steps might you take to minimize these potential biases?

As the investigators began to consider what data to collect with their questionnaire, they began to lay out the analyses they wanted to conduct. They did so by sketching out table shells—frequency distribution and two-way tables that contain appropriate titles, labels, measures, and statistics to be calculated, but no data. The tables followed a logical sequence from simple (descriptive epidemiology) to more complex (analytic epidemiology), which is often used when results are presented in a manuscript or oral presentation.

CASE STUDY QUESTION

1. List, in logical sequential order, the table shells you might use to analyze or present the CASH study data.

Part II Study Design

The study design included several features to minimize selection and information bias. Ascertainment bias of disease status (a type of selection bias) was minimized by attempting to enroll as cases all women aged 20–54 years with newly diagnosed, histologically confirmed, primary ovarian cancer who resided in one of the eight geographic areas covered by the cancer registries. Controls were women aged 20–54 years who were selected randomly using telephone numbers from the same geographic areas. Because 93% of U.S. households had telephones, virtually all women residing in the same areas as the cases were eligible to be controls. (Interestingly, all the enrolled women with ovarian cancer had telephones.)

To minimize interviewer bias, CDC investigators conducted group sessions to train interviewers in the administration of the pretested standard questionnaire. The same interviewers and questionnaires were used for both cases and controls. Neither cases nor controls were told of the specific a priori hypotheses to be tested in the study. Recall bias of OC exposure was minimized by showing participants a book with photographs of all OC preparations ever marketed in the United States and by using a calendar to relate contraceptive and reproductive histories to other life events.

The primary purpose of the CASH study was to measure and test the association between OC use and three types of reproductive cancer: breast cancer, endometrial cancer, and ovarian cancer. The enrollment of subjects into the study began in December 1980. During the first 10 months of the study, 179 women with ovarian cancer were enrolled, as were larger numbers of women with endometrial or breast cancer. During the same period, 1,872 controls were enrolled to equal the number of subjects with breast cancer. The same control group was used for the ovarian cancer analysis; however, the investigators excluded 226 women with no ovaries at the time of interview and four controls whose OC use was unknown, leaving 1,642 women to serve as controls. The distribution of exposure to OCs among ovarian cases and controls is shown in **Table II-1**.

CASE STUDY QUESTIONS

1. From these data, can you calculate the risk of ovarian cancer among OC users? Why or why not?
2. Describe the rationale behind using the odds ratio as an estimate of the risk ratio. When is the odds ratio not an appropriate estimate of the risk ratio?
3. What special information does the odds ratio give that you do not get from the chi-square statistic the and p-value? What additional information do you get from the p-value and the chi-square statistic? From a confidence interval?

Table II-1			
Ever-Use of OCs among Ovarian Cancer Cases and Controls, Cancer and Steroid Hormone Study, 1980–1981			
	Cases	Controls	
Ever user	93	959	1,052
Never user	86	683	769
Total	179	1,642	1,821

Data from "Oral Contraceptive Use and Ovarian Cancer," Centers for Disease Control and Prevention Epidemiology Program Office Case Studies in Applied Epidemiology No. 811–703.

4. How might you describe and interpret these results?
5. What is confounding? Under what circumstances would age be a confounder in this study?

Part III Confounding and Effect Modification

In the analysis of OC use and ovarian cancer, age was related both to OC use and to case-control status. (OC users were younger than never users; case patients were younger than controls.) Therefore, the investigators decided to stratify the data by age and calculate stratum-specific and, if appropriate, summary statistics of the stratified data. The Mantel-Haenszel (MH) procedure is a popular method for calculating a summary odds ratio and test of significance for stratified data.

CASE STUDY QUESTIONS

1. What is stratification? Why stratify data? How do you decide which variables to stratify?
2. What is effect modification? What is the process of finding it or recognive?
3. Using the data in **Table II-2**, calculate the odds ratio for the 40- to 49-year age stratum.
4. Using the data in Table II-2, calculate the expected value of cell A for the 40- to 49-year age stratum.
5. Using the data in Table II-2, calculate the MH chi-square for the 40- to 49-year age stratum.

The investigators had been taught to look for effect modification before looking for confounding.

CASE STUDY QUESTION

1. Do you think age is an effect modifier of the OC and ovarian cancer association?

The investigators concluded that age was not an effect modifier. They therefore decided to control for confounding by calculating an odds ratio adjusted for age, also called a summary odds ratio or MH odds ratio, as follows: They calculated an MH chi-square, from which they found a p-value. Finally, they calculated a 95% confidence interval of 0.45 to 0.92.

1. Using the stratified data in Table II-2, calculate the summary odds ratio adjusted for age.
2. Do you think age is a confounding variable in this analysis of the association between OC use and ovarian cancer?
3. What are other ways of eliminating confounding in a study?

Table II-2

Ever-Use of OCs and Risk of Ovarian Cancer, Stratified by Age, Cancer and Steroid Hormone Study, 1980–1981

Ages 20–39 years

	Cases	Controls	
Ever user	46	285	331
Never user	12	51	63
Total	58	336	394

Ages 40–49 years

	Cases	Controls	
Ever user	30	463	493
Never user	30	301	331
Total	60	764	824

Ages 50–54 years

	Cases	Controls	
Ever user	17	211	228
Never user	44	331	375
Total	61	542	603

Data from "Oral Contraceptive Use and Ovarian Cancer," Centers for Disease Control and Prevention Epidemiology Program Office Case Studies in Applied Epidemiology No. 811–704.

In the introduction to this case study, pregnancy was described as apparently protective against ovarian cancer. The investigators were interested in seeing whether the association between OC use and ovarian cancer differed for women of different parity. **Table II-3** shows parity-specific data.

Table II-3

Ever-Use of OCs and Risk of Ovarian Cancer, by Parity,* CASH Study, 1980–1981

Parity	Use of OCs	# Case patients	# Controls	Age-adjusted odds ratios (95% confidence intervals)
0	Ever user	20	67	0.3 (0.1–0.8)
	Never user	25	80	
1–2	Ever user	42	369	0.8 (0.4–1.5)
	Never user	26	199	
3+	Ever user	30	520	0.7 (0.4–1.2)
	Never user	35	400	

*Excludes seven controls (four never users and three ever users) and one case (ever user) with unknown parity.
Data from "Oral Contraceptive Use and Ovarian Cancer," Centers for Disease Control and Prevention Epidemiology Program Office Case Studies in Applied Epidemiology No. 811–705.

CASE STUDY QUESTION

1. Is there any evidence of effect modification in the data presented in Table II-3?

Part IV Implications

In their published report, the investigators wrote the following about the possible effect of modification by parity:

> Parity appeared to be an effect modifier of the association between oral contraceptive use and the risk of ovarian cancer ... [Table II-3]. Among nulliparous women, the age-standardized odds ratio was 0.3 (95% confidence interval: 0.1–0.8). Among parous women, however, the odds ratios were closer to, but still less than, 1.0. ... It is possible, therefore, that oral contraceptives are most protective for women not already protected by pregnancy.

Although this case study deals with the data collected over the first 10 months (phase 1) of the study, an additional 19 months of data (phase 2) were collected and analyzed subsequently. **Table II-4** summarizes the apparent role of parity as an effect modifier in the two phases of the study.

On the basis of the full study results, it appeared that the effect of OCs on ovarian cancer was not substantially different for nulliparous women and for parous women. Although there were no published studies of OCs and ovarian cancer when this study was launched, there were several by the time it was published. Almost all showed an apparently protective effect of OCs on ovarian cancer.

CASE STUDY QUESTION

1. What are the public health and/or policy implications of the apparently protective effect of OCs on ovarian cancer?

Table II-4			
Age-Adjusted Odds Ratios (aOR) and 95% Confidence Intervals for the Association of OC Use and Ovarian Cancer, by Parity and Phase of Study, CASH Study, 1980–1982			
Parity	Phase 1 (months 1–10)	Phase 2 (months 11–29)	Total (months 1–29)
	aOR (95% CI)	aOR (95% CI)	aOR (95% CI)
0	0.3 (0.1–0.8)	0.7 (0.5–1.2)	0.7 (0.4–1.0)
1–2	0.8 (0.4–1.5)	0.5 (0.3–0.7)	0.5 (0.4–0.8)
3+	0.7 (0.4–1.2)	0.5 (0.4–0.8)	0.6 (0.4–0.8)
Total	0.6 (0.4–0.9)	0.5 (0.4–0.7)	0.6 (0.5–0.7)

Data from "Oral Contraceptive Use and Ovarian Cancer," Centers for Disease Control and Prevention Epidemiology Program Office Case Studies in Applied Epidemiology No. 811–706.

Identifying Biomarkers That Predict Diabetes and Hypertension

We are interested in identifying whether selected biomarkers can predict diabetes and hypertension. Diabetes and hypertension were selected as outcome variables because they have been shown in previous research to be correlated and because of their large burden on society (Tidy, 2012; Townsend, 2007; WebMD, 2013). The treatment of hypertension insulin resistance is common among hypertensive patients, which puts each individual at risk for developing diabetes (Townsend, 2007). On the other hand, the causal direction has also been shown to go the other way as well (Tidy, 2012; WebMD, 2013).

A database of 1,225 individuals who were screened for certain health-related states or events was obtained in 2014. These individuals were reflective of the general population. The age range of individuals in the database was 18 to 88 years (M = 53.4, SD = 10.5). The data consisted of 707 males (57.7%) and 518 females (42.3%), with 1,164 Caucasian (95.0%) and 61 representing other racial groups (5%). The body mass index (BMI) ranged from 16.7 to 53.2 (M = 27.5, SD = 4.9), and the body fat percentage ranged from 13.9 to 73.2 (M = 48.3, SD = 9.3).

Table III-1			
Hypertension and Diabetes Status among Screening Participants, 2014			
	Diabetes	No diabetes	
Hypertension	38	184	222
No hypertension	50	953	1,003
Total	88	1,137	1,225

The body fat percentage was based on a measurement of just the abdominal region. Hypertension and diabetes status is presented in **Table III-1**.

Case Study Questions

1. What makes this a cross-sectional study?
2. What are the limitations with this study design for making causal inferences?
3. What is the conditional probability of diabetes among those with hypertension?
4. What is the conditional probability of diabetes among those without hypertension?
5. Is there a significant relationship between hypertension and diabetes? What is the chi-square value? What is the prevalence ratio and its 95% confidence interval?
6. Using logistic regression, the slope coefficient is 1.3702 (standard error = 0.2298). What are the odds ratio and the 95% confidence interval?
7. The correlation coefficient between BMI and body fat percentage is 0.608. Is this statistically significant based on a t test?
8. What assumptions do you make to represent the data using the correlation coefficient?
9. What assumptions do you make to use the t test?

Several regression models were run to determine whether BMI was significantly associated with selected variables, after adjusting for age, sex, and race (**Table III-2**). Models were also run with body fat percentage as the dependent variable.

Case Study Questions

1. Interpret the estimated regression slope coefficients. How does adjustment for age, sex, and race influence the interpretation?
2. What benefit, if any, is there to including age, sex, and race in the models, in terms of confounding?

Table III-2

Measures of Association among BMI, Body Fat Percentage, and Selected Variables, 2014

BMI	Slope estimate*	Standard error	% Body fat correlations	Slope estimate*	Standard error
Hypertension	2.14	0.36	Hypertension	3.06	0.64
Diabetes	3.73	0.53	Diabetes	4.09	0.95
Heart disease	0.21	0.81	Heart disease	0.32	1.43
High cholesterol	0.32	0.35	High cholesterol	0.61	0.63
Stroke	−1.81	1.97	Stroke	−0.3	3.51
Cancer	0.48	0.68	Cancer	0.2	1.2
Current smoker	−1.02	0.54	Current smoker	−1.36	0.96
Former smoker	0.8	0.36	Former smoker	1.47	0.64

*Adjusted for age, sex, and race.

3. What test statistics and assumptions are appropriate to assess the significance of the variables in each model?
4. Which variables are significant in the models involving BMI?
5. Which variables are significant in the models involving body fat percentage?
6. Is BMI associated with current or former smoking status? Explain.
7. Is body fat percentage associated with current or former smoking status? Explain.

A new age variable was created with three levels: 424 (< 50 years), 492 (50–59 years), and 309 (60+ years). The mean body fat percentages for the three age groups are presented in **Table III-3**.

An analysis of variance produced a model sum of squares of 7,936.82 and an error sum of squares of 98,519.97.

Case Study Questions

1. What assumptions are associated with analysis of variance?
2. Formulate the null and alternative hypotheses.
3. How many model degrees of freedom are there?

Table III-3

Mean Body Fat Percentage According to Age for 1,225 Adults, 2014

Age group	No.	Mean	Standard deviation
< 50	424	45.19	9.64
50–59	492	48.86	9.16
60+	309	51.76	9.31

Table III-4			
Diabetes by Obesity Status and Hypertension by Obesity Status in 1,225 Adults, 2014			
	Diabetes	**No diabetes**	
Obese (BMI ≥ 30)	88	226	314
Not obese (BMI < 30)	134	777	911
Total	222	1,003	1,225
	Hypertension	**No hypertension**	
Obese (BMI ≥ 30)	48	266	314
Not obese (BMI < 30)	40	871	911
Total	88	1,137	1,225

4. How many error degrees of freedom are there?
5. Evaluate the hypotheses using an F statistic.
6. What do you conclude about the difference among the means?
7. How many pair-wise mean comparisons can be made?
8. What is the Bonferroni correction?
9. Is there a significant difference between the means for the first two age groups?

Diabetes and hypertension status was categorized according to obesity status (**Table III-4**). Of interest is whether obesity is an indicator of diabetes and hypertension.

Case Study Questions

1. What is the probability of being obese among those who have diabetes (sensitivity)?
2. What is the probability of not being obese among those without diabetes (specificity)?
3. What is the probability of having diabetes among those who are obese (predictive value positive)?
4. What is the probability of not having diabetes among those who are not obese (predictive value negative)?
5. What is the overall ability of obesity to identify diabetes (overall accuracy)?
6. What is the probability of being obese among those who have hypertension (sensitivity)?
7. What is the probability of not being obese among those without hypertension (specificity)?
8. What is the probability of having hypertension among those who are obese (predictive value positive)?

9. What is the probability of not having hypertension among those who are not obese (predictive value negative)?
10. What is the overall ability of obesity to identify hypertension (overall accuracy)?
11. Does obesity do a better job of predicting diabetes or hypertension?

References

Tidy, C. (2012). Diabetes and high blood pressure. Retrieved from http://www.patient.co.uk/health/diabetes-and-high-blood-pressure

Townsend, R. R. (2007). Am I more likely to develop diabetes if I have high blood pressure? *The Journal of Clinical Hypertension, 5*(2), 175–176.

WebMD. (2013). Diabetes and high blood pressure. Retrieved from http://www.webmd.com/hypertension-high-blood-pressure/guide/high-blood-pressure

Physical and Mental Health Predictors of Exercise/Physical Activity

Sedentary behavior, cigarette smoking, high blood pressure, elevated blood glucose, being overweight, and obesity contribute to multiple chronic diseases (Cerami, Vlassara, & Brownlee, 1987; Healy et al., 2008; Katzmarzyk, Church, Craig, & Bouchard, 2009; U.S. Department of Health and Human Services [USDHHS], 1989; Vazquez, Duval, Jacobs, & Silventoinen, 2007; Yusuf, Giles, Croft, Anda, & Casper, 1998). In the United States, with the exception of smoking, each of these health risk factors has steadily increased in the past 2 decades (Centers for Disease Control and Prevention [CDC], 2013). The combination of these risk factors has been estimated to reduce life expectancy by 4.9 years in men and 4.1 years in women (Danaei et al., 2010). Along with a large burden of physical health problems, an estimated 25% of Americans aged 18 years and older have experienced a mental health illness in the previous year (Kessler, Chiu, Demler, & Walters, 2005). In 2009, the mean number of mentally unhealthy days (which includes stress, depression, and problems with emotions) in the past 30 days among adults was 3.5 (95% CI = 3.4–3.6), a result that was significantly greater for females than for males (4.0 [3.9–4.1] versus 2.9 [2.8–3.1]) (CDC, 2011).

Case Study Questions

1. Suppose you are interested in whether knowledge of risk for selected health problems will motivate increased physical activity/exercise among adults. Specifically, among those who have certain chronic conditions, you want to know whether learning about the condition motivated increased physical activity/exercise. To conduct your study, list the main elements of your study plan.
2. Formulate your main research question and hypothesis.
3. Why is it important to add a background and significance section to your study plan?
4. Suppose you can administer a questionnaire to individuals receiving health screenings at the Huntsman World Senior Games and adults attending the Good Life Expo. What study design would you use?
5. What are the limitations of using a convenience survey?
6. What variables would you include on your questionnaire?
7. What statistical issues should be considered?
8. Suppose you conducted a preliminary study and found that among those with hypertension/high blood pressure, 70% said their diagnosis motivated them to increase their exercise/physical activity each week. The mean time exercised or involved in physical activity was 60 minutes greater in this group. The overall standard deviation was 150 minutes. How many people with hypertension/high blood pressure do you need in your study if $\alpha = 0.05$ and $\beta = 0.20$?
9. Now suppose that 35% of the adult population experiences hypertension/high blood pressure. What overall sample size do you need to capture the number you obtained in the previous problem?
10. The actual number of individuals who completed the questionnaire was 674 from the Huntsman World Senior Games and 213 from the Good Life Expo. Data were collected in the fall of 2013. Is your sample size large enough to satisfy the requirement for evaluating your hypotheses with respect to hypertension/high blood pressure?

Data for selected demographic variables are presented by hypertension/high blood pressure status in **Table IV-1**.

Case Study Questions

1. Some participants did not complete every item in the questionnaire, resulting in a small number of missing data. Do you expect this to bias the results?

Table IV-1				
Hypertension/High Blood Pressure Status According to Selected Variables				
	Hypertension/high blood pressure*		Aerobic exercise at least 150 minutes per week	
	Yes	No	Yes	No
Sex				
Male	157	260	235	204
Female	137	291	198	249
Age				
18–49	11	49	10	52
50–59	40	135	86	94
60–69	99	200	172	139
70–79	111	145	145	129
80+	33	23	20	40
Smoking status				
Never	200	407	308	315
Used to smoke	78	114	106	91
Still smoke	9	24	13	21
Missing	7	7	6	27
Alcohol drinking in past 3 days				
Yes	125	303	209	162
No	467	242	220	265
Missing	12	7	4	27

*Based on the question, have you ever been told by a doctor or other health professional that you have hypertension/high blood pressure?

2. What potential bias may exist in the data because of self-reporting?
3. What steps could be taken to improve accuracy and completion of questionnaire responses?
4. How might you modify Table IV-1 to make it more informative?
5. Is hypertension/high blood pressure significantly associated with sex, age, smoking, or alcohol drinking?
6. Is participation in 150 minutes or more per week of aerobic exercise significantly associated with sex, age, smoking, or alcohol drinking?
7. Since participants at the Huntsman World Senior Games are aged 50 years and older, and those at the Good Life Expo are aged 18 years and older, could the location variable confound your results in the previous question?
8. The mean minutes of exercise/physical activity each week was calculated among those who were previously diagnosed

with hypertension/high blood pressure and by whether they said it motivated them to participate more in exercise/physical activity. Did the diagnosis motivate those with hypertension/high blood pressure to participate in more exercise/physical activity?

More exercise/physical activity	No.	Mean	Standard deviation
Yes	195	212.45	284.64
No	69	152.10	143.10

The final section of the survey asked participants which factors motivated them to be physically active. The results for these questions are given in **Table IV-2**. The reported motivators were analyzed according to the amount (< 150 minutes/week versus ≥ 150 minutes/week) and type of exercise (aerobic and anaerobic).

Table IV-2

Motivation Factors for Exercise/Physical Activity

	No.	%	Aerobic exercise 1–149 minutes versus none		Aerobic exercise ≥150 minutes versus none	
			OR*	95% CI†	OR*	95% CI†
To help manage stress						
Yes	473	64.6	1.90	1.09–3.30	2.37	1.33–4.20
No	259	35.4	1.00		1.00	
For social opportunities						
Yes	476	66.2	2.28	1.29–4.02	2.89	1.58–5.28
No	243	33.8	1.00		1.00	
To prevent or slow physical decline						
Yes	727	90.3	2.96	1.57–5.61	5.99	2.86–12.55
No	78	9.7	1.00		1.00	
To prevent or slow cognitive decline						
Yes	689	88.9	2.02	1.04–3.96	2.58	1.24–5.39
No	86	11.1	1.00		1.00	
To feel physically better now						
Yes	780	95.5	5.49	2.36–12.76	13.80	5.01–38.03
No	37	4.5	1.00		1.00	
To feel mentally better now						
Yes	744	93.2	7.20	3.38–15.30	10.98	4.78–25.23
No	54	6.8	1.00		1.00	

*OR = odds ratio.
†Adjusted for age, sex, and location.

Case Study Questions

1. What type of regression model was used to analyze these data?
2. Interpret the meaning of the odds ratios.
3. Is there sufficient information in Table IV-2 to know whether the odds ratios are statistically significant?
4. Why are the odds ratios greater for 150+ versus none compared with 1–149 versus none? What does this suggest about the relationship between the factors in Table IV-2 as motivators for aerobic exercise?
5. If you were developing an intervention, what factors might you focus on?
6. Why might it be useful to test for interaction effects among the factors in Table IV-2 and age, sex, and location?

Almost two-thirds of the participants responded that they are motivated to exercise or be physically active to help manage stress. A previous diagnosis of a health-related state or event may contribute to exercising or being physically active to help manage stress. Whether exercise/physical activity was pursued to help manage stress according to selected chronic diseases is presented in **Table IV-3**.

Table IV-3		
Exercise/Physical Activity to Help Manage Stress by Chronic Disease History		
	Exercise/physically active to help manage stress	
Told by a doctor or health professional that they have:	Yes	No
Prediabetes		
Yes	61	48
No	410	206
Diabetes		
Yes	26	28
No	441	226
Hypertension/high blood pressure		
Yes	162	169
No	305	84
Depression		
Yes	80	18
No	389	240
Anxiety		
Yes	85	19
No	386	239

Case Study Questions

1. Based on the data in Table IV-3, calculate the prevalence of exercise/physical activity motivated by each of the chronic conditions.
2. Calculate the prevalence ratios for each chronic condition.
3. Calculate a 95% confidence interval for each prevalence ratio.
4. What do you conclude from your results?

In the United States, research has shown that women in general tend to be more health conscious, in the sense that they are less likely to use illicit drugs, binge drink, or smoke cigarettes (USDHHS, 2009). They are also more likely than men to have health insurance and to have access to regular and consistent medical care and better nutrition (Imamura et al., 2015; USDHHS, 2009). They also may be more likely than men to be motivated to exercise or be physically active based on the following reasons: help manage stress; provide social opportunities; prevent or slow down physical health problems in the future; prevent or slow down cognitive decline in the future; feel physically better now; and feel mentally better now (**Table IV-4**).

Case Study Questions

1. Calculate the odds ratio for each model.
2. Calculate the 95% confidence interval for each odds ratio.
3. What do you conclude?

Table IV-4						
Logistic Regression Analysis						
	Help manage stress	Provide social opportunities	Prevent or slow down physical health problems in the future	Prevent or slow down cognitive decline in the future	Feel physically better now	Feel mentally better now
Slope estimate* female vs male	0.6370	0.5006	0.6638	0.7948	0.3826	0.5595
Standard error*	0.1626	0.1705	0.2543	0.2488	0.3505	0.2977

*Adjusted for age and location.

References

Centers for Disease Control and Prevention. (2011). Mental illness surveillance among adults in the United States. Retrieved from http://www.cdc.gov.erl.lib.byu.edu/mmwr/preview/mmwrhtml/su6003a1.htm

Centers for Disease Control and Prevention. (2013). Prevalence and trends data. Retrieved from http://apps.nccd.cdc.gov/brfss/

Cerami, A., Vlassara, H., & Brownlee, M. (1987). Glucose and aging. *Scientific American*, 256(5), 90–96.

Danaei, G., Rimm, E., Oza, S., Kulkarni, S., Murray, C., & Ezzati, M. (2010). The promise of prevention: The effects of four preventable risk factors on national life expectancy and life expectancy disparities by race and county in the United States. *PLoS Medicine*, 7. doi:10.1371/journal.pmed.1000248

Healy, G., Wijndaele, K., Dunstan, D., Shaw, J. E., Salmon, J., Zimmet, P. Z., & Owen, N. (2008). Objectively measured sedentary time, physical activity, and metabolic risk. *Diabetes Care*, 31, 369–371.

Imamura, F., Micha, R., Khatibzadeh, S., Fahimi, S., Shi, P., Powles, J., ... Global Burden of Diseases Nutrition and Chronic Diseases Expert Group (NutriCoDE). (2015). Dietary quality among men and women in 187 countries in 1990 and 2010: a systematic assessment. *The Lancet Global Health*, 3(3):e132–42.

Katzmarzyk, P., Church, T., Craig, C., & Bouchard, C. (2009). Sitting time and mortality from all causes, cardiovascular disease, and cancer. *Medicine and Science in Sports and Exercise*, 41(5), 998–1005.

Kessler, R., Chiu, W., Demler, O., & Walters, E. (2005). Prevalence, severity, and comorbidity of twelve-month DSM-IV disorders in the national comorbidity survey replication (NCS-R). *Archives of General Psychiatry*, 62(6), 617–627.

U.S. Department of Health and Human Services. (1989). *Reducing the health consequences of smoking: 25 years of progress* (DHHS Publication No. CDC 89-8411). Rockville, MD: Centers for Disease Control, Office on Smoking and Health.

U.S. Department of Health and Human Services. (2009). *Healthy People 2010 women's and men's health: A comparison of select indicators*. Washington, DC: U.S. Government Printing Office.

Vazquez, G., Duval, S., Jacobs, D. J., & Silventoinen, K. (2007). Comparison of body mass index, waist circumference and waist/hip ratio in predicting incident diabetes: A meta-analysis. *Epidemiologic Reviews*, 29, 115–128.

Yusuf, H., Giles, W., Croft, J., Anda, R., & Casper, M. (1998). Impact of multiple risk factor profiles on determining cardiovascular disease risk. *Preventive Medicine*, 27, 1–9.

Index

Note: Page numbers followed by f, or t indicate figures, or tables respectively.